Livestock Immunity to Ticks

'Dis die smeulende vuur wat swaarkry
En tog nie die kos kan gaarkry.
Maar die vrolike vlam, wat klap en kraak,
Dis hy wat sy taak tot vermaaklikheid maak,
En die swaarkry met lekkerkry klaarkry.'

From my mother. An alliterative limerick attributed to C. J. Langenhoven (1873–1932), lawyer, politician, author and champion of the Afrikaans language. Rough translation:

It's the smouldering fire that struggles
And yet can't cook the meal.
But the happy flame, that snaps and crackles
Turns its task into entertainment,
And finishes the struggle with pleasure.

Livestock Immunity to Ticks

Johann Schröder

CABI

CABI is a trading name of CAB International

CABI
Nosworthy Way
Wallingford
Oxfordshire OX10 8DE
UK

Tel: +44 (0)1491 832111
E-mail: info@cabi.org
Website: www.cabi.org

CABI
200 Portland Street
Boston
MA 02114
USA

T: +1 (617)682-9015
E-mail: cabi-nao@cabi.org

A catalogue record for this book is available from the British Library, London, UK.

ISBN-13: 9781800625747 (hardback)
9781800625754 (ePDF)
9781800625761 (ePub)

DOI: 10.1079/9781800625761.0000

Commissioning Editor: Alexandra Lainsbury
Editorial Assistant: Emma McCann
Production Editor: Rosie Hayden

Typeset by Exeter Premedia Services Pvt Ltd, Chennai, India
Printed and bound in the UK by CPI Group (UK) Ltd, Croydon, CR0 4YY

Contents

Acknowledgements

Inspired by Ivan Horak, I started collecting and counting ticks on cattle with fascination in 1976. In 1983 Peter Willadsen and David Kemp told me about the idea of using a hidden tick gut antigen as a vaccine. In 2019 Mario Pablo Estrada and Alina Rodriguez-Mallon, who had turned the Bm86 antigen into a commercial success, showed me the refinements they were adding to that pioneering discovery. This literature review pays inadequate tribute to the legacy of dedicated scientists and researchers.

Ron Glanville graciously provided a copy of his 1985 promotional thesis, with its invaluably comprehensive bibliography.

Renowned scientific photographer, Lynne de Vos, helped with reproduction of the illustrations.

CABI's editorial team provided the prompt, encouragement and assistance.

Nomenclature

Tick taxonomy has undergone changes during the period covered by this review (Keirans, 1992; Apanaskevich and Horak, 2008; Guglielmone *et al.*, 2009; Horak, 2009). This evolution has benefitted from developments in molecular biology and the use of genome sequencing to solve phylogenetic conundrums.

An example is the genus *Boophilus*, which was incorporated into the genus *Rhipicephalus*. Sequencing of the mitochondrial 16S rRNA and cytochrome oxidase subunit I (COI) genes revealed that what was previously called *Boophilus* (syn. *Rhipicephalus*) *microplus* consists of five clades. In addition to *R. microplus* clades A (South America, Africa and Asia), B (southern China, northern India) and C (India and Malaysia), there are *R. australis* (Australia) and *R. annulatus* (Burger *et al.*, 2014; Low *et al.*, 2015). In this volume, other than in the references, which are listed as published, citations of older publications use the latest agreed version of a tick's species designation in the text, thus *Boophilus annulatus* is given as [*B.*] *R. annulatus*, *Boophilus decoloratus* as [*B.*] *R. decoloratus*, *Boophilus microplus* as either [*B.*] *R. microplus* or as [*B. microplus*] *R. australis*, depending on the context.

The reviewed literature contains numerous references to ticks by their vernacular or lay designations, for example 'bottle tick', 'bont [= variegated, invariably *Amblyomma* spp.] tick', 'bush tick', 'castor bean tick', 'cattle tick', 'scrub tick', 'wattle tick' and 'zebra tick'. These are often inconsistent, non-specific and confusing, and are avoided in this review, in which I consistently use the zoological names.

Although widely used in the literature, the Latin names *Bos indicus* and *Bos taurus* are avoided in this volume, because they are not strictly speaking two separate species of cattle (Norval et al., 1992). To acknowledge phenotypic breed differences in tick susceptibility, the breed names, or the terms European/Zebu, or taurine/indicine are used as far as possible.

References

Apanaskevich, D.A. and Horak, I.G. (2008) The genus *Hyalomma*. VI. Systematics of *H.* (*Euhyalomma*) *truncatum* and the closely related species, *H.* (*E.*) *albiparmatum* and *H.* (*E.*) *nitidum* (Acari: Ixodidae). *Experimental & Applied Acarology* 44,115–136.

Burger, T.D., Shao, R. and Barker, S.C. (2014) Phylogenetic analysis of mitochondrial genome sequences indicates that the cattle tick, *Rhipicephalus* (*Boophilus*) *microplus*, contains a cryptic species. *Molecular Phylogenetics and Evolution* 76, 241–253. http://dx.doi.org/10.1016/j.ympev.2014.03.017

Guglielmone, A.A., Robbins, R.G., Apanaskevich, D.A., Petney, T.N., Estrada-Peña, A. and Horak, I.G. (2009) Comments on controversial tick (Acari: Ixodida) species names and species described or resurrected from 2003 to 2008. *Experimental & Applied Acarology* 48, 311–327.

Horak, I.G. (2009) A century of tick taxonomy in South Africa. *Onderstepoort Journal of Veterinary Research* 76, 69–74.

Keirans, J.E (1992) Systematics of the Ixodida (Argasidae, Ixodidae, Nuttaliellidae): an overview and some problems. In: Fivaz, B., Petney, T. and Horak, I. (eds) *Tick Vector Biology. Medical and Veterinary Aspects*. Springer, Heidelberg, pp. 1–21.

Low, V.L., Tay, S.T., Kho, K.L. *et al*. (2015) Molecular characterisation of the tick *Rhipicephalus microplus* in Malaysia: new insights into the cryptic diversity and distinct genetic assemblages throughout the world. *Parasites & Vectors* 8, 341. https://doi.org/10.1186/s13071-015-0956-5

Norval, R.A.I., Berry, B.D. and Young, A.S. (1992) *The Epidemiology of Theileriosis in Africa*. Academic Press, London.

Abbreviations and Acronyms

Abbreviation	Description	Context[a]
ACh	acetylcholine	1.3.2.1
AChE	acetylcholinesterase	1.3.2.1
ADP/AMP/ATP	Adenosine di-/mono-/triphosphate	Ch. 4
AKR	Akarin(s)	5.2.5
APC	Antigen-presenting cell	3.5
ASF(V)	African swine fever (virus)	1.3.3
AZA	azadirachtin	2.2.2
Beef CRC3	Cooperative Research Centre for Beef Genetic Technologies	5.2.2, 5.2.4
BoLA	Bovine leucocyte antigen	4.1.1
Bt	*Bacillus thuringiensis*	2.1.6
Cas-9	CRISPR-associated protein 9	5.2.2
CCHF(V)	Crimean-Congo haemorrhagic fever (virus)	1.3.3, 5.2.5
cDNA	Complementary DNA	1.3.2, 5.1
cfu	Colony-forming unit	2.1.6
CMI	Cell-mediated immunity	Ch. 4
COI[b]	Cytochrome c oxidase subunit 1	1.1.3
CRISPR	Clustered regularly interspaced short palindromic repeats	5.2.2
CRT	Calreticulin	3.4, 4.5.2, 5.2.4
CTL	C-type lectin	Ch. 3
Cry	Crystalline Bt protein	2.1.6
DAMP	Danger associated molecular pattern	3.1.3
DEG	Differentially expressed genes	2.2.1, 3.3.2

Continued

Abbreviation	Description	Context[a]
DNA	Deoxyribonucleic acid	Numerous
dsRNA	Double-stranded RNA	5.2.2, 5.5
EAFIM	Engorged adult female immersion method	2.2
ECG	Electrocardiogram	1.3.2.1
EFFPE	Engorged female filter paper envelope	2.2
EGF	Epidermal growth factor	5.1.3
ELI	Expression library immunization	5.2
ELISA	Enzyme-linked immunosorbent assay	5.4.3
ER	Endoplasmic reticulum	3.4
FPN	Fipronil	4.6
GABA	(Gamma) γ-aminobutyric acid	4.4
GC/MS	Gas chromatography/mass spectrometry	2.2.2
GM	Genetically modified	2.1.7
GM-CSF	Granulocyte macrophage-colony stimulating factor	5.4.2
HSP	Heat shock protein	5.2.4
IFN-γ	Interferon-gamma, gamma interferon	3.1.2
Ig-A, -E, -G, -M	Immunoglobulin-A, -E, -G, -M; antibodies	1.3.4, 4.1.3
IgSF	Immunoglobulin superfamily	4.1
IL 1, IL 6, IL 10	Interleukin 1, 6, 10	Ch. 3
IMD	'Immune deficiency' antibacterial defence response signalling pathway	Ch. 3
indel	Insertion/deletion (of amino acids in genome sequences)	5.2.5
IP	Intellectual Property	6.2
IP-10	Interferon-γ-induced/inducible protein 10	3.4
Iris	*Ixodes ricinus* immunosuppressor	3.4, 4.5
ISH	*In situ* hybridization	5.2.3
ITM	Infect-and-treat method	5.1
iTreg	Induced CD4+ regulatory T-cells	4.1.2
ITS	Internal transcribed spacer	1.1.3
KLH	Keyhole limpet hemocyanin	4.5.4, 5.2.5, 5.5.1
LPT	Larval packet test	2.2
LSD(V)	Lumpy skin disease (virus)	1.3.3
LTT	Larval tarsal test	2.2
MBL	Mannose-binding lectin	3.1.3
miRNA	Micro RNA	3.4, 4.4
mRNA	Messenger RNA	5.2
MP	Metalloprotease	3.4, 5.2.3
MSF	Mediterranean spotted fever	1.3.3

Continued

Abbreviation	Description	Context[a]
ncRNA	Non-coding RNA	3.4, 4.4
NF-κB	Nuclear factor of κ light polypeptide gene enhancer in B-cells	Ch. 3
NK	Natural killer	Ch. 3
NLR	(Nucleotide oligomerization and binding domain) NOD-like receptor	Ch. 3
nTreg	Natural (thymically derived) CD4+ regulatory T-cells	4.1.2
PAMP	Pathogen-associated molecular pattern	Ch. 3
PBMC	Peripheral blood mononuclear cell(s)	3.3.2, 4.4
PRM	Pattern recognition molecule	3.1
PRR	Pathogen recognition receptor	Ch. 3
qRT-PCR	Quantitative reverse transcription polymerase chain reaction	5.2.2
QTL	Quantitative trait loci	2.3
RACE	Rapid amplification of cDNA ends	5.2.5 serpins
RLH	(Retinoic acid inducible gene-I) RIG-I-like helicases	Ch. 3
RNA	Ribonucleic acid	Numerous
RNAi	RNA interference (gene silencing)	5.2.2, 5.5
rRNA	Ribosomal RNA	2.1.7
RV	Reverse vaccinology	5.2.1
SEM	Scanning electron microscope/micrograph	2.1.8
serpin	Serine protease inhibitor	1.3.1, 3.4, 4.5
SGE	Salivary gland extract	4.6.6
SIP	Secreted insecticidal Bt proteins	2.1.6
SLP	Surface layer Bt proteins	2.1.6
SNP	Single nucleotide polymorphism	2.2.1, 2.3
STAT	Signal transducer and activator of transcription	4.1.2
SUB	Subolesin	5.2.5
TBEV	Tick-borne encephalitis virus	1.3.3
TBM	Tingible body macrophage	4.1.2, 4.4.1
TBV	Tick-borne virus	1.3.3; Table 1.2
TCR	T-cell receptor	Ch. 4
T_{FH}	Follicular helper T-cell	4.1.2
TGF-β	Transforming growth factor β	Ch. 3
TLR	Toll-like receptor	Ch. 3
TNF	Tumour necrosis factor	Ch. 3
TOT	Transovarial transfer	1.3.3
Treg	Regulatory T-cells	4.1.2
TROSPA	Tick receptor for outer surface protein A	5.2.5

Continued

Abbreviation	Description	Context[a]
TRP64	Tick recombinant protein 64	5.2.4
TSGP	Tick salivary gland protein	1.3.2
TST	Trans-stadial transfer	1.3.3
VIP	Vegetative insecticidal Bt toxins	2.1.6
VLP	Virus-like particle	5.4.3
VPTA	Vapour phase toxicity assay	2.2.2
WGS	Whole-genome sequencing	

[a]In this volume.

[b]In some publications, this gene is referred to as 'cox 1' which is potentially confusing, as 'cox' is the acronym usually assigned to cyclooxygenase in the inflammation cytokine cascade.

1 Introduction: The Significance of Ticks

Abstract

Being eight-legged in their adult stage, ticks are related to mites, spiders and scorpions. They are parasitic and occur worldwide in abundant numbers. Their occurrence depends on meteorological factors, habitat suitability and the availability of the wide range of hosts they infest in search of a blood meal. Ticks are directly and indirectly harmful to their hosts in a variety of ways, ranging from mechanical damage and intoxication, to eliciting allergic reactions, and acting as vectors for a number of bacterial, protozoal and viral pathogens. They find their hosts by various means, in which semiochemicals play a large part. Climate change is one of the factors influencing the geographic distribution of ticks, but migratory birds are probably the most overlooked long-distance transport medium for ticks and the pathogens they carry.

1.1 Background

1.1.1 Scope

In 2009, the world list of valid tick names comprised 692 ixodid ('hard') and 186 argasid ('soft') tick species (Horak, 2009). There have been differences of opinion among acarologists as to the taxonomic validity of some of the names (Guglielmone *et al.*, 2009). The two families of these eight-legged arthropod (Acarines) ectoparasites have distinctly different life histories. Both are obligate parasites, requiring regular blood meals for sustenance, maturation of ovaries and successful reproduction. They intermittently infest mammals, birds, reptiles and amphibians to complete their life cycles, but spend greater proportions of their lives in the environment than on the host.

It is beyond the scope of this volume to elaborate on the global economic impact of ticks. Numerous publications have reported estimates of the extent of this loss, which is made up of the cost of lost production, the cost of prevention of tick infestation and the cost of the impact, prevention and treatment of tick-borne disease (Peter *et al.*, 2005; Grisi *et al.*, 2014; Mapholi *et al.*, 2014; Rodriguez *et al.*, 2020; Strydom *et al.*, 2023). Ticks are harmful, with few redeeming features, although the case is made that, in a natural ecosystem in equilibrium, parasites exert a fitness selection pressure. Domestication disturbs this balance through the introduction of susceptible hosts, increased stocking density and stress (Uilenberg, 1992; Malan *et al.*, 1997).

Ticks exert their pathogenic effects on their hosts in a variety of ways, commencing with the discomfort and pain caused by their presence and bite wounds and proceeding to blood loss, which can be considerable. Tick bites involve the secretion of saliva which can cause toxicity in varying degrees and types. Ticks can serve as mechanical and biological vectors of a variety of viral, microbial and protozoal pathogens. Tick bites can give rise to allergic reactions. Once ticks detach, they leave wounds as potential portals of entry for other pathogens, and downgrading the quality of the leather subsequently produced from those skins or hides.

The tick infestation challenge can be overwhelming, leading to death of the host, but several factors have an impact on the number of parasitic ticks at any one time. These factors range from grooming and preening to habitat alteration, pasture composition and innate and adaptive host resistance (Chapters 2, 3 and 4, this volume). Early conviction that eradication was a viable option for tick control (Laws and Manning, 1910), gave way to the realization that in only a small number of instances has human intervention with chemicals achieved this aim (George *et al.*, 2002; Walker, 2011).

Both free-living and parasitic ticks have been enumerated by various means to provide context to their importance and to elucidate their geographic and seasonal prevalence.

DOI: 10.1079/9781800625761.0001

Parasitic ticks have been counted both on live animals (Baker and Ducasse, 1967; MacLeod *et al.*, 1977; Londt *et al.*, 1979; Horak *et al.*, 2009) and on cadavers (Schröder, 1980; Horak, 1999). Because the former requires appropriate immobilization of the animal, counts might be restricted to predilection sites to provide an estimate of total tick burden (MacLeod *et al.*, 1977; Matthee *et al.*, 1997; Magesa *et al.*, 2023) or just one side of the animal's body (Schröder 1981–1984, unpublished observations) and extrapolated for an estimation of total tick burden. Much more reliable results are obtained with the so-called destructive sampling method, where the carcass is flayed and the hide or skin minutely examined, with or without the use of tick-detaching chemicals (MacIvor *et al.*, 1987). More information on the collection of free-living ticks is provided below ('Hunting and questing').

1.1.2 Occurrence

Free-living ticks can be nidicolous, spending their entire lives in the nests, burrows or caves used as dwellings by their hosts, as is the case for most argasid ticks, such as *A. persicus* (Monti *et al.*, 2023), but also *Ixodes angustus* (Durden *et al.*, 2018). They tend to be more host specific. Non-nidicolous ticks spend long periods away from their hosts in the environment which is more typical for the ixodids (Ostfeld *et al.*, 2006).

Models of tick populations can be useful in understanding population dynamics (Stokowski and Allen, 2024). The computerized CLIMEX system was devised to map and predict the geographic distribution of poikilothermic organisms (such as insects and ticks) based on meteorological data in situations where too little biological information is available for building a population model. The ticks included for validation were [*B. microplus*] *R. australis* (in Australia), *Rhipicephalus appendiculatus* and *Amblyomma variegatum* (in Africa) (Sutherst, 1985; Sutherst and Maywald, 1985). The phenology of a three-host tick, *Haemaphysalis longicornis*, was subsequently studied in Australia at two sites under different environmental conditions (Sutherst and Bourne, 1991).

CLIMEX has also been used to predict the possible spread of *Ixodes holocyclus* in Australia in response to different climate change scenarios. Other models have followed, analysing the distribution of *Ixodes ricinus* in Australia (Teo *et al.*, 2021), and *I. ricinus* and *Dermacentor reticulatus* in Europe (Noll *et al.*, 2023), the climate suitability of the New World for *A. variegatum* (Estrada-Peña *et al.*, 2007) and the suitability of ecological niches for *Ornithodoros* spp. in Iran (Moradi-Asl and Jafari, 2020). Habitat preferences of ticks infected with spotted fever group *Rickettsia* spp. have been evaluated based on collections of questing and feeding ticks (Gual-Gonzalez *et al.*, 2024). A recently published model enables researchers to analyse tick population and infection dynamics models (Stokowski and Allen, 2024).

Even after different models were used for the same data, it was clear that, in addition to climate variables and habitat features, host availability and anthropogenic impacts such as global travel and international animal trade constitute additional determinants of local and regional occurrence of ticks (Hassan and Salih, 2013; Noll *et al.*, 2023), for example the introduction of [*B. microplus*] *R. australis* into New Caledonia (Hüe *et al.*, 2013) and *H. longicornis* into the United States (Lilak *et al.*, 2024). Intensive acaricide application to cattle resulted in the displacement of *A. hebraeum* to ecologically less favourable habitats in Zimbabwe, because they could be sustained on wild hosts (Norval *et al.*, 1994).

Microclimate also has to be considered, as illustrated by *Amblyomma variegatum*, whose presence in the highlands of Madagascar was questioned (Uilenberg *et al.*, 1979, cited by Walker and Olwage, 1987) and attributed to regular reintroduction. Survival of unfed and fed nymphs and moulted adults over the June–September colder period in the Malagasy highland at altitudes above 1600m proved the importance of the microenvironment for free-living tick survival (Rahajarison *et al.*, 2014).

Climate change may be responsible for the appearance of ticks in new locations (Mapholi *et al.*, 2014; Martello *et al.*, 2014; Garcia-Vozmediano *et al.*, 2020; Rudolf *et al.*, 2021; Teo *et al.*, 2021) and for extended periods (Probst *et al.*, 2024). *Haemaphysalis concinna* has been found in 34 Eurasian countries, potentially carrying at least 40 bacterial and viral human pathogens, and can parasitize 119 host species, a large number of which are birds, which means that they play a crucial role in the aerial transmission of tick-borne microbes (Liu *et al.*, 2024), as has been shown for passerine migratory birds (Budachetri *et al.*, 2017b). Predictive modelling suggests that *H. concinna* could survive in regions where it has never previously been recorded, such as central and south America, south-east Oceania and southern Africa (Liu *et al.*, 2024).

Some tick species initially introduced by stock movement can displace or overwhelm species that were there before. *R. microplus* is an example of this invasive behaviour, having displaced the native *R. decoloratus* in parts of Africa (Horak *et al.*, 2009; Etiang *et al.*, 2024). It is suspected that *R. microplus* males reach sexual maturity a day or two before *R. decoloratus* males do. Matings between the precocious males of the former and receptive females of the latter species are presumably sterile, causing *R decoloratus* numbers to dwindle. This is difficult to understand, considering that multiple copulations do occur in *R. microplus* and assuming that it also happens in *R. decoloratus*. As sperm from the most recently placed spermatophore dominates the female's offspring, one could assume that a *R. decoloratus* female impregnated first by a male *R microplus* and then by *R. decoloratus* would predominantly produce eggs of the latter species (Kaufman, 2004).

1.1.3 Molecular biology

Advances in molecular biology have made profound impacts on the study of ticks and tick-borne diseases (Jongejan *et al.*, 2007). Gene evolution occurs in various ways including vertical descent (speciation), gene duplication, gene loss, horizontal gene transfer and gene rearrangement by fission or fusion. Genes that are related by common descent are called homologues. Orthologues are homologues derived from a single ancestral gene via speciation (vertical descent) from the last common ancestor of the compared genomes, and typically performing equivalent functions. Homologues related by duplication are called paralogues and might perform different functions in different genomes (Koonin, 2005). The ancestral Tree of Life and the gradation of lineage-specific conservation divided into Core of Life, Lineages of Life and Edges of Life (Mans *et al.*, 2016) give insight into the phylogenetic relationship of Ixodida, or 'ticks', with other Eukaryotes.

Taxonomy has benefitted from reinterpretation of phylogenetic relationships, previously based on macro- and microscopic appraisal of anatomical features. Sequencing the transcriptomes of different life cycle stages, and unfed and partially engorged ticks, has provided insights into stage-specific processes and energy metabolism (Bellgard *et al.*, 2012; Vechtova *et al.*, 2020; Wang *et al.*, 2024). Given the gene sequence divergence between *I. scapularis* (as a representative prostriate tick) and *R. microplus* (representing the Metastriata), having access to the *R. microplus* genome eliminated a serious limit to molecular research efforts (Bellgard *et al.*, 2012). The *Ix*1000G project was mooted as a framework for the assemblage of genomic data from thousands of *Ixodes* ticks to better understand genetic diversity and the transmission of disease (Murgia *et al.*, 2019).

Tick microbiome sequences have revealed their importance to tick physiology and their vulnerability to vectored pathogens and host immune reactions. But short-term field studies and procedural errors have also led to misleading conclusions on the nature of some tick–host relationships (Estrada-Peña *et al.*, 2013, 2021). Although *Bartonella* spp. DNA has been detected in more than one tick species, the host–vector–pathogen relationship was still to be elucidated (Billeter *et al.*, 2008). Recent inability to distinguish *I. ricinus* from *I. inopinatus* utilizing the entire mitochondrial genome highlights the need for careful evaluation of molecular data in answering questions of tick taxonomy and geographic distribution (Rollins *et al.*, 2023). Using partial sequences of the TROSPA and COI genes, instead of 16s rDNA and morphology, *I. inopinatus* was found to be a dominant tick in Algeria, and to occur in Italy coincidentally with *I. ricinus* and hybrids of the two species (Daněk *et al.*, 2024).

1.2 Life Histories

Despite their differences in appearance and life history, hard and soft ticks share conserved gene regions. Sialomic (salivary gland proteomic) analysis revealed that they both secrete major salivary proteins (Mans *et al.*, 2003b, 2008), with divergent functions.

Although first described more than a century ago, and in more than one species, parthenogenesis in hard and soft ticks is considered a rare, sporadic and uncharacteristic phenomenon (Nuttall, 1915; Oliver, 1971; Oliver *et al.*, 1993; Qui *et al.*, 2020). The parthenogenic population of *Haemaphysalis longicornis* has a triploid karyotype, can complete engorgement without copulation and produce viable female-only offspring. Three enzymes are differentially expressed during the embryonic development of the parthenogenetic ticks (Qui *et al.*, 2020). Based on the sequence similarity (differences below 2%) of the examined genes, it was decided to consider the parthenogenic ticks as a meta-population rather than a cryptic species (Chen *et al.*, 2014).

Described for *Ornithodoros moubata* as early as 1948, multiple copulations are known to occur for both argasid and ixodid ticks, based on the presence of multiple sperm capsules in the female seminal receptacle (Kaufman, 2004). In the case of *R microplus*, multiple paternity has been demonstrated by microsatellite analysis of the progeny of individual females (Cutullé *et al.*, 2010).

There is a considerable body of published information on the role of pheromones in tick behaviour. Assembly pheromones occur mostly in argasid ticks and concentrate free-living ticks in optimal microenvironments. Aggregation/attachment pheromones are produced by parasitic male ixodid ticks that have fed and completed their spermatogenesis and appear to be species specific. Preattachment or prefeeding pheromones induce attachment of sex partners near each other. Attractant sex pheromones are emitted by attached feeding female ticks of many species. One chemical, 2,6-dichlorophenol, has been identified (Gothe, 1987), but there are bound to be species differences and other molecules. Hexane extracts of *Amblyomma cajennense* yielded 2,6-dichlorophenol that failed to act as an attractant and mounting sex pheromone for *R. sanguineus* (Louly *et al.*, 2008).

1.2.1 Argasids ('soft' ticks)

These ticks, also known as 'tampans', are represented by the three genera *Argas*, *Otobius* and *Ornithodoros*. Their soft and wrinkled integument in the unfed state allows for rapid engorgement when a bloodmeal is taken (Mans and Neitz, 2004). The life history roughly follows the pattern of egg → larva → nymph → adult. In the case of *Otobius megnini* the number of nymphal stages can vary from one to three in different geographic regions (Nava *et al.*, 2009; Diyes and Rajakaruna, 2017), and the adult is not parasitic, with mating occurring off the host. Living, as they do, deep in the external auditory meatus of their host, the biosecurity risk of inadvertent transboundary translocation of larvae and nymphs is easily foreseen (Keirans and Pound, 2003).

The fowl tampan, *Argas persicus*, is a so-called 'ornithophilic nidicolous' tick (Monti *et al.*, 2023), found in close association with domestic fowl. Doubt about its existence in southern Africa, after all preserved specimens had upon examination proven to be *Argas walkerae*, was dispelled when a specimen from a museum collection in Windhoek proved to be *A. persicus* (Eastwood, 1972).

Argasids vary in the extent of their host ranges, partly explained by evolutionary differences in the number of copies of genes encoding for salivary proteins between *Ornithodoros savignyi* and *Ornithodoros moubata*, with the latter having the narrower host range, and the evolution influenced by host and environmental factors (Mans *et al.*, 2003a). The wider host range of *O. savignyi* might be accounted for by, and provides justification for, the fact that up to four subspecies have since been recognized, based on morphology and molecular analysis (Charles and Basu, 2021). *Ornithodoros coriaceus* parasitize deer and cattle (Hokama and Howarth, 1977).

1.2.2 Ixodids ('hard' ticks)

These ticks have a sturdy shield or scutum that covers the entire dorsal surface of adult males but only a small anterior portion of that of female ticks, allowing them to ingest larger blood meals. As can be seen in Fig. 1.1, the mouthparts consist of a hypostome which penetrates the host's skin by way of its two cutting chelicerae and two palps that lie flat on the skin once the hypostome is fully inserted.

Larvae hatch from eggs in the environment and infest the first host. The nymphal and adult stages of these ticks are also parasitic. Upon engorgement, the larvae and nymphs detach from the host to moult to the next stage. Copulation occurs on the host. Engorged females drop off the host to lay their eggs. Engorged detached larvae and nymphs of single host ('oligoxenic') ticks remain on the host to reattach after moulting.

The time taken for each of the life cycle stages is subject to environmental conditions, of which temperature was found to be more important than relative humidity for [*B. microplus*] *R. australis* in southern Queensland (Snowball, 1957). Under ideal conditions, single-host ticks can complete their life cycle from egg to egg within 9 weeks. In the case of multihost ('polyxenic') ticks, the nymphs drop off to moult to adulthood before finding the next host ('two-host'), or all replete stages drop off, with new nymphs and adults having to find the next host after moulting ('three-host' ticks). Under ideal environmental conditions, three-host ticks probably need at least 1 year to complete their life cycle, but it can take up to 6 years (Vechtova *et al.*, 2020), with extended survival probably enabled by a process of autophagy (Umemiya-Shirafuji *et al.*, 2014). *H. longicornis* has been shown to enhance its overwintering survival by responding to cold stress with a decrease in its water content and increases in its glycerol and protein content in nymphs and adults (Yu *et al.*, 2014).

1.2.3 Hunting and questing

Host-seeking behaviour varies between ticks and tick life cycle stages, which influences the method of collection of field specimens (Kensinger and Allan, 2011; Dantas-Torres *et al.*, 2013). Some species and stages rely on 'questing' (Wilkinson, 1953; Sutherst *et al.*, 1978; Fourie *et al.*, 1996; Estrada-Peña *et al.*, 2013), sitting in waiting on vegetation. Collection by flagging and blanket dragging is better suited to these (Spickett *et al.*, 1992; Schroder *et al.*, 2006; Horak *et al.*, 2006, 2011; Dantas-Torres *et al.*, 2013; Uys *et al.*, 2015; Wojan *et al.*, 2022). Analysing the numbers of questing ticks collected over 164 consecutive months at the same two sites in the Kruger National Park gave valuable insights into the complex interaction between ticks, hosts and their environment (Horak *et al.*, 2011).

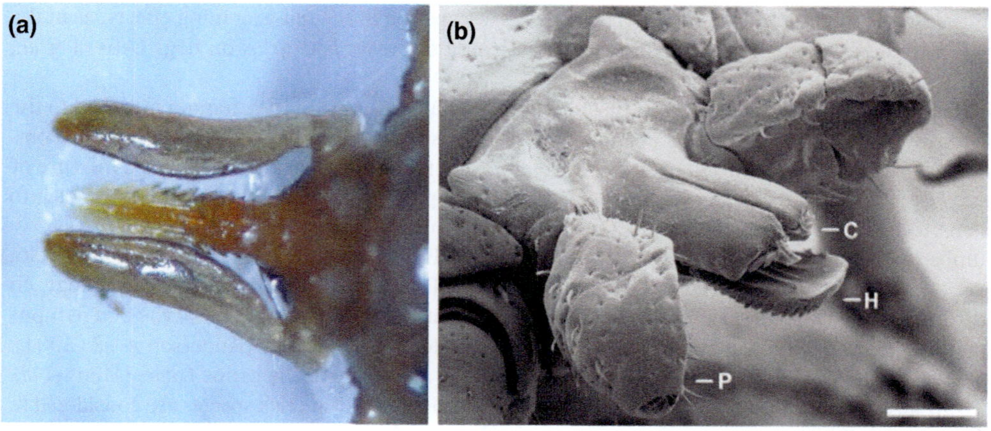

Fig. 1.1. Ixodid tick mouthparts showing the hypostome with the rear-facing anchoring barbs, the chelicerae and the two palps. (a) Light microscope image (50 × magnification) of *Ixodes holocyclus*, ventral view. From Steen *et al.* (2006) with permission from Elsevier, conveyed through Copyright Clearance Center, Inc. (b) SEM image (scale bar 200 µ) of *Dermacentor marginatus*, semi-frontal view. From Suppan *et al.* (2018) under the terms of the Creative Commons Attribution License.

Other species and stages are hunters and actively pursue their quarry with the aid of semiochemicals, such as carbon dioxide (Nevill, 1964) and kairomones in the case of *A. walkerae* infesting chickens (Beelitz and Gothe, 1991). Hunting ticks can easily be collected, for example in dry ice tick traps (Nevill, 1964; Hokama and Howarth, 1977; Mount and Dunn, 1983; Mans and Neitz, 2004; Labruna *et al.*, 2007; Kensinger and Allan, 2011) but adding a synthetic aggregation-attachment pheromone such as *o*-nitrophenol will enhance the capture of adult female *Amblyomma hebraeum* (Norval *et al.*, 1989) and *A. variegatum* (Barré *et al.*, 1997). There appears to be no difference in attractant potency between natural and synthetic pheromones, nor between natural extracts of *A. variegatum* from different geographic locations (Sonenshine *et al.*, 2000).

Multihost ticks are evidently better equipped to detect hosts and mates than oligoxenics, judging by the duplication of the olfactory receptor gene in *H. anatolicum* (Wang *et al.*, 2024).

1.2.4 Host selection and attachment

The long-held view that ticks are relatively host specific (Hoogstraal and Aeschlimann, 1982, cited by Tatchell, 1987; Durden and Keirans, 1996) is challenged by the fact that distribution and seasonal dynamics of some tick species can be predicted based on climatic factors (Sutherst and Maywald, 1985; Cumming, 1998), and by the lack of tick–host coevolution in most cases (Estrada-Peña *et al.*, 2023). The perception of host specificity may be an artefact of incomplete sampling, because the number of different hosts seems to increase in linear relationship to the number of collections (Cumming, 1998). Body size and habitat also determine geographic distribution and host selection, with small mammals preferentially hosting immature ixodid ticks (Horak *et al.*, 2005; Nava *et al.*, 2008), larger ungulates being more important hosts for adult ticks, and grazers supporting fewer adult ticks than browsers and intermediate feeders (Gallivan and Horak, 1997; De Matos *et al.*, 2009). The preferred questing height of larvae, nymphs and adults of *R. appendiculatus* was found to increase in that order in Zimbabwe, which could also account for adults being more prevalent on larger hosts (Short *et al.*, 1989). Goats in particular, possibly due to their preference for browsing, are capable of successfully hosting ticks often regarded as specific to cattle, as shown in various locations in southern Africa and New Zealand (Baker and Ducasse, 1968; Heath *et al.*, 1987; Bryson *et al.*, 2002; Nyangiwe and Horak, 2007; De Matos *et al.*, 2009).

Many ticks are characterized by their preferred site of attachment to the host (Baker and Ducasse, 1967; Tatchell, 1987; Papadopoulos *et al.*, 1996; Izdebska and Cydzik, 2010; Tadesse *et al.*, 2012), influencing the common names assigned to some tick species, such as brown ear tick for *R. appendiculatus* and spinose ear tick for *O. megnini*. This preference, also referred to as ‘topical specificity’, is ascribed to a number of factors, of which the relationship of host skin thickness and tick mouthpart (gnathosoma) length (Izdebska and Cydzik, 2010) is probably most relevant. Two *Hyalomma* spp. were found to prefer the thin-skinned perineum and inguinal areas on two breeds of sheep and also the relative wool-less feet of Merinos (Fourie and Kok, 1995). The site of attachment is also influenced by semiochemicals, with attractant aggregation-attachment pheromones usually secreted by the adult male (Gothe, 1987; Norval *et al.*, 1989; Barré *et al.*, 1997; Sonenshine *et al.*, 2000; Stachurski, 2000). Some tick attachment sites might also be influenced by attempts to escape the host’s self-grooming efforts, as in the case of *Ixodes holocyclus* on dogs (Atwell *et al.*, 2000).

To ensure that they remain attached to the host’s dermis for the several days needed to complete their bloodmeal, ticks secrete a mixture of glycoproteins and lipoproteins that hardens into a cement (Lynn *et al.*, 2022b).

Hard ticks are divided into the Metastriata and Prostriata based on their morphology. In the latter, the anal groove of larvae and nymphs is anterior of the anus (Anderson *et al.*, 2004). They all belong to the genus *Ixodes* (Mans *et al.*, 2016). Metastriate tick species are considered to have a short hypostome, e.g. *Dermacentor* and *Rhipicephalus* spp. Prostriate species have longer, barbed mouthparts, e.g. *Ixodes holocyclus*, with hypostomes up to 980 μ long, and are regarded as not needing a cement for attachment (Francischetti *et al.*, 2009; Hall-Mendelin *et al.*,

2011). This distinction might not be that simple, because although morphologically classed as metastriates (Anderson *et al.*, 2004), the mouthparts of *Amblyomma* and *Hyalomma* spp, are otherwise regarded as quite long (Schröder, 1980). And although classed as prostriates with long mouthparts and less need for attachment cement, the cement of *Ixodes* spp. has been studied as a potential source of immunogenic proteins (Lynn *et al.*, 2022b).

Rather than use the position of the anal groove to classify ticks on the length of their mouthparts, a non-taxonomical classification into Brevi- (short) and Longirostrata is easier to interpret. It is also genomically explicable with Brevirostrata having greater need for the attachment cement, having been demonstrated by cDNA library analysis to have more glycine-rich proteins, noteworthy for their adhesive and tensile characteristics, in their salivary glands (Maruyama *et al.*, 2010; de Castro *et al.*, 2016), and monoxenous ticks having a greater variety of these proteins than ticks that feed on several hosts (heteroxenous) (Maruyama *et al.*, 2010).

In addition to its anchoring function, tick cement also seals the bite wound to prevent loss of fluids and ingress of bacteria from the host skin surface to the feeding pool, and to improve the blood suction efficiency of the muscular pharynx (Suppan *et al.*, 2018).

1.2.5 Refugia

Game and nature reserves, with sustainable populations of suitable hosts, serve as reservoirs for tick populations (Horak, 1980; Horak *et al.*, 1983, 1987, 1989, Horak *et al.*, 2017, 2021, 2022; Duncan and Monks, 1992; Gallivan and Horak, 1997; Horak and Boomker, 1998; MacIvor and Horak, 2003; Schroder *et al.*, 2006; Golezardy and Horak, 2007; Michel and Bengis, 2012; Kariuki *et al.*, 2012, Kariuki *et al.*, 2019; Uys *et al.*, 2015). Given ticks' wide and mostly non-specific host preference, sympatric wild hosts can offer a refuge from human intervention for ticks found on livestock.

Examples of this sylvatic component of the livestock tick life history abound, such as the futile attempts to eliminate ticks from cattle in a paddock shared by native hare and antelope (Laws and Manning, 1910), ticks on cattle co-grazing with impala (Horak, 1982) or African buffalo (Walker *et al.*, 2014), *O. coriaceus* on deer and cattle in California and Mexico (Hokama and Howarth, 1977), and the occurrence of *A. persicus* in chicken nest boxes frequented by wild birds in Italy (Monti *et al.*, 2023).

1.3 Pathogenic Effects

The harmful effects of ticks (Schröder, 1980; Uilenberg, 1992; Ndhlovu *et al.*, 2009; Hurtado and Giraldo-Ríos, 2018) can be direct through mechanical damage, blood loss and/or intoxication, for example. Signs of these effects can be clinically inapparent, such as reduced live weight gain, which was shown to be logarithmically related to burdens of *Amblyomma americanum* on beef calves in the US (Barnard, 1985), but cattle in visibly poor condition have been seen to carry more ticks (Tadesse *et al.*, 2012).

Ticks also damage their hosts indirectly, by transmitting other pathogens or creating portals of entry for subsequent infection or infestation. Painful bites in the interdigital space can cause lameness in cattle and sheep, for example by *Hyalomma* spp. and *Amblyomma* spp., known for their long mouthparts, (Thomas, 1950; Uilenberg, 1992; Kok and Fourie, 1995) and species of *Rhipicephalus* (Walker, 1990). Ticks and tick-borne diseases are estimated to affect 80% of the world's cattle, causing significant production losses (Bellgard *et al.*, 2012; Strydom *et al.*, 2023).

Indiscriminate host selection (see section 1.2.4) means that there are many accounts of argasid and ixodid tick species, whose 'natural' hosts are domestic and wild animals, infesting humans, usually when they intrude on the tick's habitat (Swanepoel, 1959; Naudé *et al.*, 2001; Horak *et al.*, 2002; Labruna *et al.*, 2007; van Nunen *et al.*, 2009; Grady *et al.*, 2011; Hook *et al.*, 2015; Kwak, 2018; Rodriguez-Vivas *et al.*, 2020). *H. longicornis* is a recently arrived invasive species in the north-eastern USA and its discovery on a variety of synanthropic mammals introduces another dimension to consideration of the epidemiology of tick-borne disease in humans (Ferreira *et al.*, 2023). Alternatively, human patients can present with symptoms of tick-borne disease without a precise recollection of a tick bite (Senanayake *et al.*, 2012). A long list of tick species infesting humans in the USA, and the diseases they cause or transmit, has recently been published (Eisen, 2022).

1.3.1 Bite wounds

Ixodid ticks need several days to complete their bloodmeal. Tick bites damage the skin mechanically, and the penetrating wound is made worse by tick saliva with its main components of hyaluronidase, cement and anticoagulant (Gaspar, 1995; Gaspar *et al.*, 1996; Gashaw and Mersha, 2013). Their saliva enables them to counter the host's haemostatic, inflammatory and immune mechanisms (Hall-Mendelin *et al.*, 2011; Boeuf *et al.*, 2019). Tick saliva components include enzymes, enzyme inhibitors, immunoglobulin-binding proteins and cytokine expression modulators (Steen *et al.*, 2006).

Protease inhibitors are important components of tick saliva and include serine protease (serpins) and Kunitz inhibitors (Chmelař *et al.*, 2017). Saliva from *I. ricinus* has been shown to cause dissociation of fibroblasts, interpreted as the means by which a feeding pool is formed in the dermis around the mouthparts of a feeding tick (Boeuf *et al.*, 2019). Histologically, the bovine skin reaction to *I. holocyclus* was shown to consist first of mast cell degranulation and infiltration of eosinophils, also seen around attachment sites of [*B.*] *R. microplus*, followed by basophils (Allen *et al.*, 1977) and neutrophils (Saleem *et al.*, 2019). In rabbits infested with larvae and nymphs of *Hyalomma rufipes*, macrophage activity increases the size of the lesion (Arthur, 1973). Fig. 1.2 provides a graphic presentation of a variety of tick saliva components that participate in maintaining a feeding pool for the attached tick.

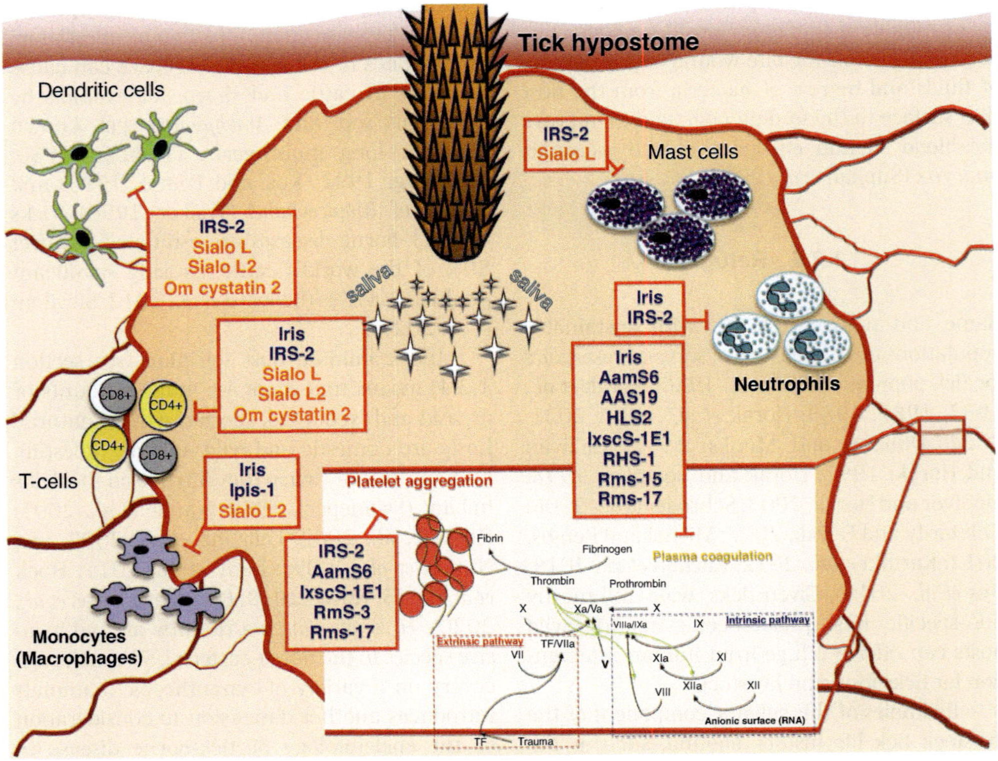

Fig. 1.2. Tick saliva serpins and cystatins active at the site of tick attachment. From Chmelař *et al.* (2017) under the terms of the Creative Commons Attribution License (CC BY).

Secondary bacterial infection and myiasis potentially worsen the extent of this damage. Ticks with long mouthparts (*Amblyomma* spp., *Hyalomma* spp.) leave open wounds when they detach after engorgement. Tick bite wounds readily become infested by Old World screw-worm (*Chrysomya bezziana*) fly larvae (Perkins, 1987; Spickett *et al.*, 1989a).

The local inflammatory skin reaction at tick bite sites leaves scars that affect subsequent leather quality (Allen *et al.*, 1977; Saleem *et al.*, 2019). In Ethiopia, only a small percentage of harvested hides and skins qualify for processing to top-grade leather due to blemishes, some of which are caused by ticks (Gashaw and Mersha, 2013; Kahsay *et al.*, 2015; Amde, 2017; Saleem *et al.*, 2019). Manual visual inspection, searching for defects in the leather grading process, is time-consuming, inconsistent, inefficient and costly, and can be automated (Liong *et al.*, 2019; Gan *et al.*, 2022).

1.3.2 Intoxication

Based on the homology of proteins in tick saliva with those of scorpion, spider, snake, platypus and bee venoms, the contention was that ticks should be regarded as venomous ectoparasites (Cabezas-Cruz and Valdés, 2014). Both tick venom and tick toxins (toxic components of tick secretions) are recognized (Mans *et al.*, 2004a). Whereas ca. 99–100% of other arachnid (scorpions and spiders) species are venomous, fewer than 8% of known tick species are capable of causing paralysis, the most important form of tick toxicosis (Mans *et al.*, 2004a; Pienaar *et al.*, 2018). A graphic illustration of tick toxicoses is provided in Fig. 1.3 (Apari and Földvári, 2021). The phylogenetic relationship of the various toxic tick species is shown in Fig. 1.4 (Cabezas-Cruz and Valdés, 2014).

There is a variety of tick salivary gland proteins (TSGPs), initially attributed to morphologically distinct granular cell types (Hall-Mendelin *et al.*, 2011). The discovery that cell types with similar morphologies do not necessarily express the same proteins, whereas the same proteins can be expressed by cell types with different morphologies, indicated that an alternative classification method of the salivary gland proteome might be more reliable (Mans *et al.*, 2004b).

The benefit ticks derive from their toxins is enigmatic (Mans *et al.*, 2002, 2004a), and it has been suggested that the toxins are a vestigial remnant of ticks' evolution from a predatory to a parasitic lifestyle (Mans *et al.*, 2003b). Several evolutionary roles have been hypothesized; paralysing the host to prevent grooming, causing tachycardia to enhance blood supply, and preventing necroptosis (regulated cell death) to prevent rejection of ticks all seem plausible. Less credible is the hypothesis that tick toxins cause the demise of tick-transmitted pathogens systemically inside the host (Apari and Földvári, 2021), but recent evidence does point to vector dysbiosis (microbiome disturbance) caused by transmitted pathogens (Bonnet *et al.*, 2017; Adegoke *et al.*, 2020).

Paralysis

It took a number of unrelated individual case reports on different continents during the 19th and early 20th centuries, with records dating back to 1824, for 'tick paralysis' to be recognized as a syndrome. It was the first described form of tick toxicosis and although more species are implicated, definite confirmation of paralysis due to ticks has been described for 27–43 species of 8–10 genera (Todd, 1914; Gothe *et al.*, 1979; Mans *et al.*, 2004a). In their comprehensive review of clinical cases, Stanbury and Huyck (1945) list tick paralysis in domestic animals in Australia (*I. holocyclus*), South Africa (*Ixodes pilosus*, *Ixodes rubicundus*), North America (*Dermacentor andersoni*) and Crete (*I. ricinus*, *Haemaphysalis punctata*). The first record of tick paralysis in Australia is attributed to Bancroft in 1884 (Dodd, 1921). Subsequent to this, mention of tick paralysis in Australian veterinary literature appears desultory until the report of a workshop held in 1974, with presentations on epidemiology, host–parasite relationships and pathophysiology. It was concluded that more information was needed (Bagnall and Doube, 1975). The highlights of 100 years' research on tick paralysis in Australia were considered to be the production of tick antivenene, advances in veterinary critical care medicine and the

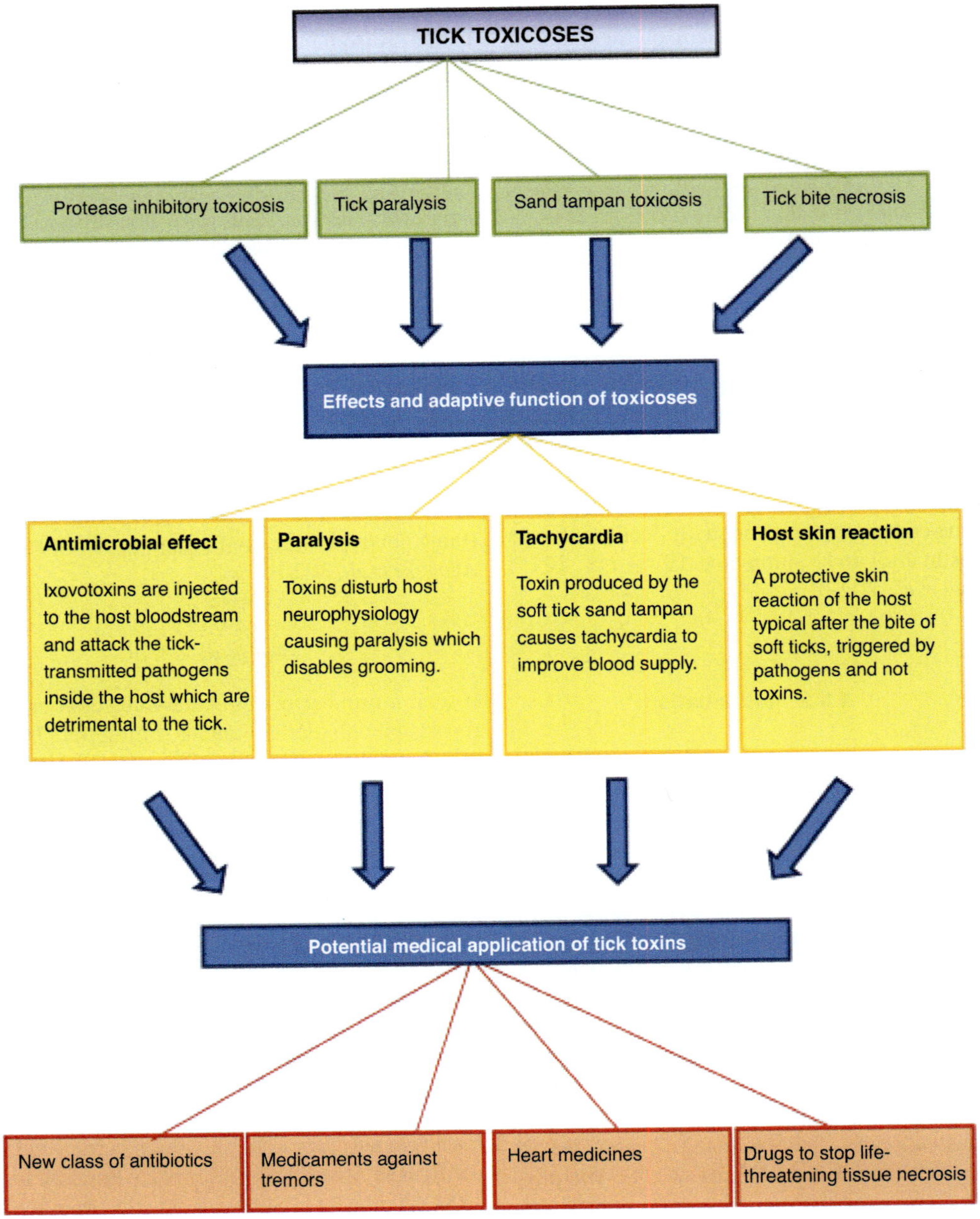

Fig. 1.3. Schematic representation of the different tick toxicoses. From Apari and Földvári (2021) under the terms of the Creative Commons Attribution License.

development of isooxazoline acaricides (Padula *et al.*, 2020).

A paralysis toxin was isolated from *A. (Persicargas) walkerae* to address the enigma of paralysis induction by postlarval stages, that spend less feeding time on the host. Only replete larvae were found to induce paralysis in day-old chickens (Viljoen *et al.*, 1990).

Dermacentor and *Argas* paralyses are characterized by reduction in motor nerve conduction velocity, decreased compound action potentials of nerves and their corresponding

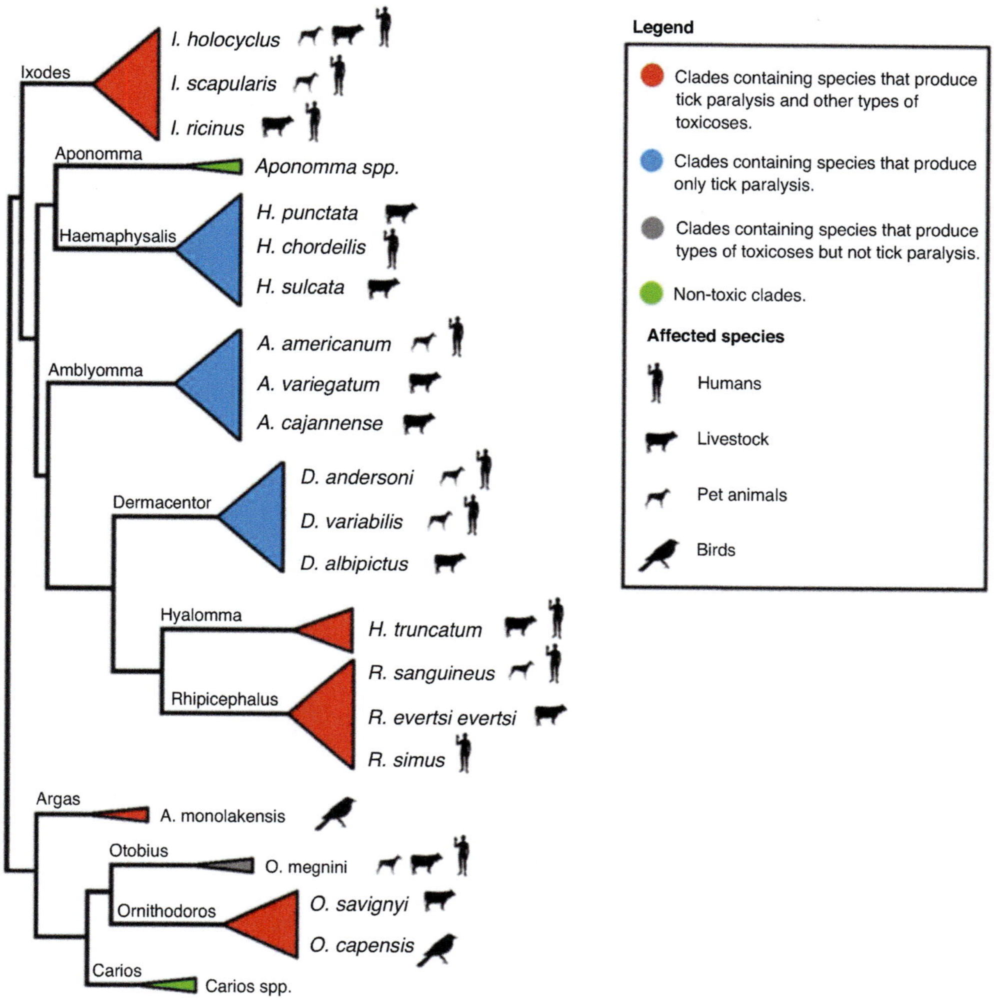

Fig. 1.4. Phylogenetic relationships of toxic tick genera. From Cabezas-Cruz and Valdés (2014) under the terms of the Creative Commons Attribution License.

muscles, and impaired afferent fibre impulse propagation. The myocardium and stimulus-conducting system of the heart are not directly affected, and the effects can be influenced by blocking acetylcholinesterase (AChE). Later work, using homogenates of *A.* (*P.*) *walkerae in vitro* on rat brain synaptosomes, demonstrated inhibition of [^{3}H]-glycine release, which is reconcilable with decreased synthesis or release of acetylcholine at the neuromuscular junction (Maritz *et al.*, 2000, 2001).

The paralysis syndrome of *I holocyclus* differs from those caused by *Dermacentor andersoni, D. variabilis* and *A.* (*P.*) *walkerae* in respect of the functional integrity of the peripheral nerves, but the pathogenic mechanism could not be explained at that stage (Gothe *et al.*, 1979). It has since been shown to be due to inhibition of acetylcholine (ACh) at the motor nerve neuromuscular junction (Webster *et al.*, 2013a). In humans, *I. holocyclus* is characterized by an ascending, symmetrical, flaccid paralysis, worsening in the 24–48 hour following removal of the tick. Fatal respiratory failure can be the outcome without timely intervention (Grattan-Smith *et al.*, 1997).

In addition to humans, tick paralysis in Australia affects cattle, horses, sheep, cats and dogs. It is attributed to *I. holocyclus* and, to a lesser extent, to *Ixodes cornuatus* (Dodd, 1921; Padula, 2016; Barker and Barker, 2020), which is more restricted in its habitat (Hall-Mendelin *et al.*, 2011).

Using salivary glands and viscera dissected from engorged female *I. holocyclus* collected from cats and dogs displaying signs of paralysis, complementary DNA (cDNA, coding DNA) was sequenced and aligned with the previously reported HT1 protein sequence. Eighteen different and non-redundant sequences were designated HT2–HT19. HT1, HT2, HT3 and HT4 sequences were synthesized and tested for specific binding to rat synaptosomes, and their neurotoxic capacity determined in a neonatal mouse assay. HT4 in particular produced rapid pronounced respiratory distress in all animals (Rodriguez-Valle *et al.*, 2018). The cDNA sequence of the HT1 neurotoxin had previously been determined by RACE-PCR and the toxin expressed as a fusion protein in *E. coli*. Vaccination raised antibodies and partial protection against the native toxin in mouse assays but not in vaccinated dogs challenged with live ticks (Masina, 1999).

The manifestation of *I. holocyclus* intoxication in dogs progresses in five stages of an ascending paralysis, from inappetence and lethargy, hindlimb ataxia, through quadriplegia and recumbency, to death from respiratory failure. Clinical examination revealed dysfunction of the efferent motor system, some disturbance of afferent pathways (reduced reflexes) and involvement of the autonomic nervous system. Recumbent dogs suffer a progressive fall in respiratory rate, accompanied by hypoxaemia, with increased alveolar–arterial oxygen tension difference (Ilkiw, 1987; Ilkiw and Turner, 1987a, b; Ilkiw *et al.*, 1988; Padula, 2016). Repeat ECGs from dogs during intoxication revealed a prolonged QT interval and altered T-wave morphology, reflecting delayed cardiac repolarization. Resolution of these changes took longer than clinical recovery (Campbell and Atwell, 2002). Pulmonary oedema was seen in some histological sections from dogs that succumbed. The respiratory failure of paralysed cats and dogs is deemed to be a combination of respiratory muscle paralysis, leading to hypoventilation, and pulmonary parenchyma pathology, causing hypoxaemia (Webster *et al.*, 2013a, b). It was considered that the pulmonary congestion and oedema could be the result of either cardiac failure or increased permeability of the blood–air barrier (Webster *et al.*, 2013a).

Karoo paralysis in South Africa was reported in 1892, is of particular importance in sheep and is caused by *I. rubicundus*. It mainly occurs in autumn (March to May) when adult tick activity is highest, and resembles the paralysis caused by *I. holocyclus* in that it is ascending and flaccid (Stampa and Du Toit, 1958; Stampa, 1959; Spickett and Heyne, 1988). A survey lasting 3 years found 12 of 15 examined species of native mammals in the Karoo to be infested with *I. rubicundus* (Horak *et al.*, 1987). Paralysis of rabbits by *I. rubicundus* nymphs was related to tick numbers and its onset hastened by cold conditions, attributed to a synchronous toxin release (Spickett *et al.*, 1989b).

The geographical distribution in South Africa of *I. pilosus*, which favours a higher rainfall environment, differs markedly from that of *I. rubicundus*, found in more arid regions. In addition to cattle (Theiler, 1950), it was found also to infest grey rhebok (*Pelea capreolus*) (Horak *et al.*, 1986). The male feeds by parasitizing the female on or off the host (Norval, 1974). It is considered of minor economic importance (Rechav, 1991) and is not implicated in paralysis, despite its inclusion in an earlier review (Stanbury and Huyck, 1945).

The spring lamb paralysis syndrome in South Africa is caused by *Rhipicephalus evertsi evertsi* (Clark, 1938; Horak *et al.*, 1991), and is a graded response related to infestation level and inversely related to host age and weight. Geographically patchy distribution of paralysis due to *R. e. evertsi* led to the initial belief that strains differed in their toxicity, as had been postulated for *Dermacentor* spp. and *Ixodes* spp. (Hamel and Gothe, 1978). Experimental comparison of 16 isolates from different locations failed to demonstrate differences but showed that *R. e. evertsi* had to attain an engorged mass of 15–21 mg to become toxic to sheep. The degree of paralysis could be graded by the quotient of engorging tick mass to sheep live mass in mg/kg, from 2.1 to 3.4 mg/kg for slight leg weakness to 21–60 mg/kg for total paralysis (Gothe and Bezuidenhout, 1986). The subspecies *R. e.*

mimeticus was shown to be similarly toxic (Gothe *et al.*, 1986). A neurotoxin, characterized to a molecular weight of 68 kDa, was isolated from the salivary glands of female *R. e. evertsi* meeting the previous mass parameters (Viljoen *et al.*, 1986).

Western blot assays demonstrated that a monoclonal antibody against the *R. e. evertsi* spring lamb paralysis-inducing toxin recognized protein bands of similar molecular mass and amino acid composition to the *I. rubicundus* Karoo paralysis toxin. The same antibody also rendered some degree of protection against *A. (P.) walkerae* toxin in day-old chickens (Crause *et al.*, 1994).

Regional loss of sensory and motor nerve function was described in a man who lost the use of his arm following a bite in the axilla from one male *Hyalomma transiens*. Full motor function returned within a few days after removal of the tick, but a small area of cutaneous anaesthesia remained several months after the incident (Erasmus, 1952). In a similar case, paralysis of the forearm flexor muscles remained after the *Hyalomma truncatum* was removed from the patient's axilla, leading to muscle wasting in the ensuing months (Swanepoel, 1959).

Other tick toxicoses

In addition to paralysis, 'sweating sickness' in cattle, characterized by moist eczema related to hyperaemia of epithelial surfaces such as the skin and mucosae and initially attributed to *Hyalomma transiens* (Neitz, 1954), is caused by strains of *H. truncatum*. Clinical signs such as salivation, lachrymation and diarrhoea have also been described (Mans *et al.*, 2004a). Crude salivary gland extracts were analysed immunologically by Western blot and shown to differ between strains that induce sweating sickness and those that do not (Burger *et al.*, 1991).

Thomas (1950) describes localized skin necrosis surrounding the attachment sites of individual *Hyalomma* spp. in dogs and cattle.

Mass overnight mortalities in sheep and cattle confined to pens where *O. savignyi* were known to occur were at first attributed to rapid exsanguination (Howell *et al.*, 1975; Mans and Neitz, 2004) but were suspected to be caused by a highly potent toxin (Howell, 1966). Saliva collected from field-trapped adult female ticks was analysed chromatographically and shown to consist of a complex mixture of components (Neitz *et al.*, 1969). The toxic fraction had an LD_{50} in mice of 206–220 μg/kg (Howell *et al.*, 1975). Other components of the saliva of *O. savignyi* were found to inhibit enzymes in the coagulation cascade, such as an inhibitor of activated coagulation factor X (Gaspar, 1995; Gaspar *et al.*, 1996) and the platelet aggregation inhibitors apyrase and savignygrin (Mans *et al.*, 2003a; Mans and Neitz, 2004; Stutzer *et al.*, 2009). Using an isolated rat heart perfusion system, other toxins identified in *O. savignyi* saliva were shown to have myocardial effects such as ventricular block and ventricular tachycardia, which could be demonstrated electrocardiographically. The authors concluded that sand tampan toxicosis and tick paralysis were unrelated phenomena (Mans *et al.*, 2002).

There are toxic effects of tick bites that do not necessarily cause clinical signs, such as various methods of interfering with or modulating the host's immune response. These are dealt with in Chapters 3 and 4.

1.3.3 Pathogen transmission – bacteria, viruses and protozoa

A multitude of infectious pathogens is transmitted by ticks (de la Fuente *et al.*, 2017) and it is considered to be their main importance (Wu-Chuang *et al.*, 2021). By way of example, incomplete summaries are given in Table 1.1. Bacteria, Table 1.2. Viruses and Table 1.3. Protozoa. Mixed infections of tick-borne bacteria and protozoa occur (Lejal *et al.*, 2019) and were found to be more likely than single infections in a molecular survey of a variety of cattle breeds in Cameroon (Abanda *et al.*, 2019). In the WHO European region, 23 species of Rickettsiales were detected in wild and domestic animal samples and in 55 species of ticks (Guccione *et al.*, 2023). A recently published list provides exhaustive information on zoonotic bacterial, viral and parasitic tick-borne pathogens transmitted by 32 tick species in the western Balkan states of Albania, Bosnia and Herzegovina, Croatia, Montenegro, North Macedonia and Serbia (Kapo *et al.*, 2024).

Ticks with a wide host range (see section 1.2.4) are exposed to a wider range of pathogens,

Table 1.1. Some bacteria/bacterial diseases transmitted by ticks.

Pathogen/disease	Vector	Host	Authors
Anaplasma marginale	*[B.] R. decoloratus, [B.] R. annulatus, [B.] R. microplus*	Cattle	Urquhart *et al.*, 1996
Anaplasma capra	*Ixodes kashmiricus*	Goat	Numan *et al.*, 2023
Anaplasma phagocytophilum [*Ehrlichia phagocytophila*] / Human granulocytic anaplasmosis (/ehrlichiosis)	*Ixodes ricinus, Ixodes scapularis, H lusitanicum*	Human	Bakken and Dumler, 2000; Allan and Sonenshine, 2002; Grady *et al.*, 2011; Lejal *et al.*, 2019; Vechtova *et al.*, 2020; Díaz-Sánchez *et al.*, 2021; Sloupenska *et al.*, 2021; Lesiczka, 2023
Ehrlichia ruminantium / Heartwater	*Amblyomma hebraeum*	Cattle, sheep, goats	Liebenberg *et al.*, 2020
	Amblyomma tholloni		Kariuki *et al.*, 2019
Bartonella spp.	*I. scapularis*	Human	Billeter *et al.*, 2008; Sloupenska *et al.*, 2021
Bartonella henselae / Cat scratch disease	*I. scapularis, I. ricinus, R. sanguineus*	Human	Schutze, 2000; Sanogo *et al.*, 2003; Wechtaisong *et al.*, 2020
Borrelia afzelli / Lyme borreliosis (Europe)	*.I ricinus*	Human	Hamilton *et al.*, 2021
Borrelia burgdorferi / Lyme disease	*I. scapularis*	Human	Allan and Sonenshine, 2002; Pal *et al.*, 2004; Grady *et al.*, 2011
	I. ricinus		Lejal *et al.*, 2019; Vechtova *et al.*, 2020
Borrelia miyamotoi / relapsing fever	*I. ricinus, I. scapularis*		Lejal *et al.*, 2019; Lynn *et al.*, 2022a
Borrelia persica	*Ornithodoros tholozani*	Human	Rafinejad *et al.*, 2011
Borrelia spp. / relapsing fever	*O. tholozani, Ornithodoros lahorensis*	Human	Moradi-Asl and Jafari, 2020
Coxiella burnetii / Q fever	*H. lusitanicum*	Human	Díaz-Sánchez *et al.*, 2021
Francisella tularensis / Tularaemia	*H. lusitanicum*	Human	Grady *et al.*, 2011; Borde *et al.*, 2017; Díaz-Sánchez *et al.*, 2021
Rickettsia africae / African tick bite fever	*A. hebraeum*	Human	Baker *et al.*, 1977; Horak *et al.*, 2002
Rickettsia australis/ Australian scrub typhus	*Ixodes holocyclus*	Human	Teo *et al.*, 2021
Rickettsia conorii / Mediterranean spotted fever (MSF), tick bite fever, tick typhus, Israeli spotted fever	*Rhipicephalus simus, R. sanguineus, Hyalomma* spp.	Human, dog	Baker *et al.*, 1977; Horak *et al.*, 2002; Levin *et al.*, 2011; Spernovasilis *et al.*, 2021
Rickettsia felis	*I. ricinus*		Lejal *et al.*, 2019

Continued

Table 1.1. Continued

Pathogen/disease	Vector	Host	Authors
Rickettsia helvetica	*I. ricinus*		Lejal *et al*., 2019
Rickettsia rickettsii / Rocky Mountain spotted fever	*I. ricinus*	Human	Grady *et al*., 2011; Vechtova *et al*., 2020
Rickettsia parkeri / (spotted fever group)	*Amblyomma maculatum*	Human	Wright *et al*., 2015
Rickettsia sibirica mongolitimonae/ MSF-	*Haemaphysalis concinna*	Human	Rudakov *et al*., 2019; Jakimovski *et al*., 2022
like, Siberian tick typhus	*Rhipicephalus turanicus*	Human	Fouche *et al*., 2017, 2021

Table 1.2. Some viral diseases transmitted by ticks.

Disease	Vector	Host	Authors
Hepatitis B	*Hyalomma marginatum rufipes*	Human	Horak *et al*., 2002
	Ornithodoros moubata		Jupp *et al*., 1987
Crimean-Congo haemorrhagic fever	*Hyalomma marginatum rufipes, Hyalomma* spp.	Human	Horak *et al*., 2002; Jakimovski *et al*., 2023
	H marginatum, H. dromedarii, H. excavatum, H. anatolicum, H. scupense	Cattle, sheep, goat	Kasi *et al*., 2020
	H. lusitanicum	Deer	Díaz-Sánchez *et al*., 2021
African swine fever	*O. moubata*	Pig	Haresnape *et al*., 1988; Wilkinson *et al*., 1988
	Ornithodoros zumpti		Craig *et al*., 2021
Lumpy skin disease	*Amblyomma hebraeum, Rhipicephalus appendiculatus, R. decoloratus*	Cattle	Lubinga *et al*., 2013, 2014a, b, 2015, ; Tuppurainen *et al*., 2011, Tuppurainen *et al*., 2013a, bTuppurainen *et al*. (2013a)
	Rhipicephalus annulatus		Rouby *et al*., 2017
Nairobi sheep disease	*Rhipicephalus pulchellus*	Sheep, goat	Pegram, 1976; Marczinke and Nichol, 2002; Gong *et al*., 2015; Krasteva *et al*., 2020
	Haemaphysalis intermedia, H. wellingtoni, Rhipicephalus haemaphysaloides	Sheep	Gong *et al*., 2015
Louping ill	*I. ricinus*	Sheep	Stockman, 1916; Reid and Chianini, 2007; Hubálek and Rudolf, 2012
Tick-borne encephalitis	*I. ricinus*	Cattle, goat	Mathews-Martin *et al*., 2024
	I. persulcatus	Wild hosts	Muto *et al*., 2015

Table 1.3. Some protozoa transmitted by ticks.

Pathogen	Vector	Host	Authors
B. bigemina	*Rhipicephalus annulatus, R. australis, R. bovis, R. decoloratus*	Cattle	Urquhart *et al.*, 1996; Freeman *et al.*, 2010
[*B. argentina*] *B. bovis*			
B. caballi	*Dermacentor nuttalli,* [*B.*] *R. microplus*	Equids	Battsetseg *et al.*, 2001, 2002
B. divergens	*I. ricinus*	Cattle, humans	Kjemtrup and Conrad, 2000; Zintl *et al.*, 2003; Hornok *et al.*, 2014
B. equi	*Dermacentor nuttalli,* [*B.*] *R. microplus*	Equids	Battsetseg *et al.*, 2001, 2002
B. major	*Haemaphysalis punctata*	Cattle	Hornok *et al.*, 2014
B. microti[a]	*I. dammini*	Human	Senanayake *et al.*, 2012; Goethert, 2021
B. motasi	*H. punctata*	Sheep	Lewis *et al.*, 1981
	H. longicornis, H. qinghaiensis		Tian *et al.*, 2013
B. ovata	*Haemaphysalis* spp.	Cattle	Sivakumar *et al.*, 2022
B. venatorum	*I. ricinus*	Deer, sheep	Gray *et al.*, 2019; Lejal *et al.*, 2019
Theileria annulata / Tropical theileriosis	*Hyalomma scupense, R. microplus*	Cattle	Ben Said *et al.*, 2012; Cui *et al.*, 2018
T. hippotragi	*R. e. evertsi*	Cattle	Benade, 2010
T. lestoquardi (syn. *T. hirci*)	*Hyalomma marginatum, H. anatolicum, H. excavatum, H. impeltatum, Rhipicephalus turanicus, R. sanguineus, Dermacentor marginatus*	Sheep, goats	Tian *et al.*, 2013; El Imam and Taha, 2015
T. luwenshuni	*H. longicornis, H. qinghaiensis, H. punctata*	Sheep, goats	Tian *et al.*, 2013; Phipps *et al.*, 2016
T. mutans	*Amblyomma* spp.	Cattle	de Vos and Roos, 1981; Sugimoto and Fujisaki, 2001
T. orientalis[b] / Oriental theileriosis	*Dermacentor nuttalli*	Cattle	Altangerel *et al.*, 2011
	Haemaphysalis longicornis		Marendy *et al.*, 2019
T. ovis	(*Rhipicephalus bursa?*)	Sheep, goats	Schnittger *et al.*, 2003
T. parva[c] / East Coast fever	*Rhipicephalus appendiculatus, R. zambeziensis*	Cattle, buffalo	Uilenberg, 1999; Chaisi *et al.*, 2011
	Rhipicephalus pulchellus	Cattle	Nana *et al.*, 2010
T. recondita	*H. punctata*	Sheep, goats	Alani and Herbert, 1988
T. separata	*R. e. evertsi*	Sheep	El Imam *et al.*, 2016

Continued

Table 1.3. Continued

Pathogen	Vector	Host	Authors
T. sinensis	*H. qinghaiensis, I. kashmiricus*	Cattle, sheep, goat, yak	Yin *et al*., 2004; Numan *et al*., 2023
T. taurotragi	*R. appendiculatus*	Cattle	de Vos and Roos, 1981; Benade, 2010
T. uilenbergi	*H. qinghaiensis*	Sheep	Yin *et al*., 2007
T. velifera	*Amblyomma* spp., *R. e. evertsi*	Cattle	Berger, 1979; Lawrence, 1979; de Vos and Roos, 1981

[a]The taxonomic status is controversial and it is considered to belong in neither the *Babesia* or *Theileria* genus (Goethert, 2021).
[b]Incl. *T. sergenti, T. buffeli.*
[c]*Sensu lato – incl. T. p. parva, T. p. bovis* and *T. p. lawrencei* (Schröder, 2023).

while the number of hosts a tick feeds on during its lifespan will enhance or expand its transmission potential. Single-host ticks partially overcome this limitation by transovarial transfer to their offspring (de la Fuente *et al.*, 2017).

Transmission of pathogens by ticks can be purely mechanical, as a 'contaminant' on the tick's mouthparts, but there is often a biological interaction between vector and pathogen. The pathogen has to overcome the tick host's innate immune system and the midgut infection barrier, to gain access to the salivary glands and ovaries. A disturbance in the tick's microbiome (see section 1.3.2) might result in changes in the integrity of the peritrophic membrane, which can affect pathogen infection (de la Fuente *et al.*, 2017). Tick-borne pathogens manipulate the gene expression of their vector hosts to ensure their survival, replication and transmission (Budachetri *et al.*, 2017a; Hamilton *et al.*, 2021). The acquisition, development and transmission of pathogens comprise multistage processes. The release of pathogens coincides with the excretion of excess water during the bloodmeal and infectivity may be enhanced by tick saliva components which modulate host responses (see sections 3.4 and 4.5, this volume) (Nene *et al.*, 2004). There is accumulating evidence that tick-transmitted pathogens can manipulate the composition of tick saliva to improve their survival, transmission and evasion of host responses (Boeuf *et al.*, 2019; Pham *et al.*, 2021).

An example of biological transmission of a bacterium is *Borrelia burgdorferi*, in which a major surface lipoprotein is upregulated to enable invasion of the salivary glands of *I. scapularis* (Pal *et al.*, 2004). Successful transmission of the spirochaete to the next host involves the tick's salivary pharmacopoeia of anti-inflammatory, antihaemostatic and anti-immune molecules (Nuttall *et al.*, 2000). Transmission is preceded by the establishment of the acellular peritrophic membrane, formed by secretion from the midgut epithelium in some ixodid species, appearing 18 hours after the beginning of the bloodmeal, surrounding the bloodmeal and protecting the midgut epithelium. Integrity of the peritrophic membrane is necessary for colonization of the tick gut by *B. burgdorferi* (Boulanger and Wikel, 2021).

Using a transcriptomic approach, differentially expressed genes in the midgut of unfed, 24 h-fed and replete *I. ricinus* nymphs during the transmission of *Borrelia afzelii*, the predominant cause of Lyme borreliosis in Europe, were demonstrated. Silencing five of the validated genes was shown to delay the infection process and decrease infection prevalence, offering the possibility of a novel preventive strategy for this disease (Mahmood *et al.*, 2021).

Further light is cast on the role of tick saliva in the transmission of *B. burgdorferi* with the description of the effects of sialostatins from *I. scapularis* inhibiting the role of cathepsins (Pham *et al.*, 2021).

Borrelia miyamotoi is potentially transmitted by multiple routes, also by *I. scapularis*, with bacteria disseminated throughout the tissues of all three stages of unfed ticks, including the salivary glands and female ovarian tissue, but with transovarial transmission probably the primary one (Lynn *et al.*, 2022a). *Rickettsia parkeri* is transmitted transovarially and transstadially by *Amblyomma maculatum*, as another example of biological transmission (Wright *et al.*, 2015).

Because the principal vector of *Anaplasma marginale* is the single-host *Rhipicephalus* spp., transovarial transfer was long assumed as this Rickettsia's mode of transmission. This has been proven not to be the case (Panizza *et al.*, 2022), with male ticks transferring from host to host considered to be the principal transmission method (Carter P., personal communication, Lismore, 2023).

Babesia spp. and *Theileria* spp. are the only important protozoal genera transmitted by ticks, and both belong to the phylum Apicomplexa. Continuity of transmission of protozoa by ticks is mostly achieved by transovarial (TOT; single-host ticks) or trans-stadial (TST; multihost ticks) transfer to the next stage (Schröder, 2023).

Worldwide, ticks are second only to mosquitoes as vectors of arboviruses of veterinary and public health importance (Lutomiah *et al.*, 2014). The 27 tick-borne viruses (TBVs) detected in Europe by 2012 were grouped by clinical syndrome into those that (i) cause febrile reactions (with/without weakness, myalgia, arthralgia, polyarthritis and skin rash), (ii) affect the central nervous system (meningitis, encephalomyelitis, paresis/paralysis) and (iii) cause haemorrhagic disease. Virus transmission in ticks can be vertical (TOT or TST) or horizontal, during copulation. Under conditions of TOT, ticks play the role of long-term virus reservoir (Hubálek and Rudolf, 2012).

The most important TBVs belong to six families, the most important of which are the Flaviviridae and Bunyaviridae, that include numerous viruses that cause encephalitis or haemorrhagic fever in humans (Brackney and Armstrong, 2016). By 2017, more than 350 bunyaviruses had been identified and classified into five genera, many of them transmitted by arthropods, some by ticks (Pereira *et al.*, 2017). TBVs that cause disease in humans and animals appear to represent a small fraction of the tick virome (Brackney and Armstrong, 2016). The dendogram in Fig. 1.5 displays the phylogenetic relationships of a number of tick-borne encephalitis viruses (TBEVs) (Böhm *et al.*, 2017).

There is ample evidence of the role played by ticks in the biological transmission of the capripoxvirus causing lumpy skin disease (LSD) in cattle. They are not mere mechanical vectors. Instances of vertical (TST and TOT) transmission in more than one species of oligoxenic and polyxenic ticks have been described (Tuppurainen *et al.*, 2011, Tuppurainen *et al.*, 2013a; Lubinga *et al.*, 2013, 2014a, b, 2015). Ticks of various species are the main transmitters of the Nairovirus genus in Africa and Asia. Nairoviruses are zoonotic and Nairobi sheep disease virus causes acute haemorrhagic gastroenteritis in sheep and goats (Pegram, 1976; Marczinke and Nichol, 2002; Gong *et al.*, 2015; Krasteva *et al.*, 2020). *O. moubata* inhabits human dwellings and animal burrows and is considered an important vector of African swine fever (ASF) (Haresnape *et al.*, 1988; Wilkinson *et al.*, 1988) but has also proven itself to be capable of mechanical transmission of hepatitis B virus (Jupp *et al.*, 1987).

Ascribing vector status to ticks based on the detection of bacterial (16S rRNA) or protozoal (18S rRNA) DNA alone (Sanogo *et al.*, 2003; Dietrich *et al.*, 2010) is fraught and controversial (Telford and Wormser, 2010; Uilenberg *et al.*, 2018; Wechtaisong *et al.*, 2020).

1.3.4 Meat allergy

Between 2003 and 2007, 25 human patients living in the Northern Beaches region of Sydney, Australia, reported an allergic reaction several hours after ingesting more than one type of red meat (beef, lamb, pork or venison). They all had a history of a painful tick bite during 1–6 months prior to the allergic reaction (van Nunen *et al.*, 2009). The allergen was identified to be galactose-α−1,3-galactose (alpha-gal), a cross-reactive carbohydrate determinant present in most mammals but absent in humans, Old World monkeys and other great apes. The allergy is elicited by IgE antibodies specific for alpha-gal (Commins *et al.*, 2009; Commins and Platts-Mills, 2009; Langley *et al.*, 2022). Humans lost the ability to synthesize alpha-gal through evolutionary inactivation of the α−1,3-galactosyltransferase gene and gained the ability to produce high antibody titres to the antigen (Pacheco *et al.*, 2021; Langley *et al.*, 2022).

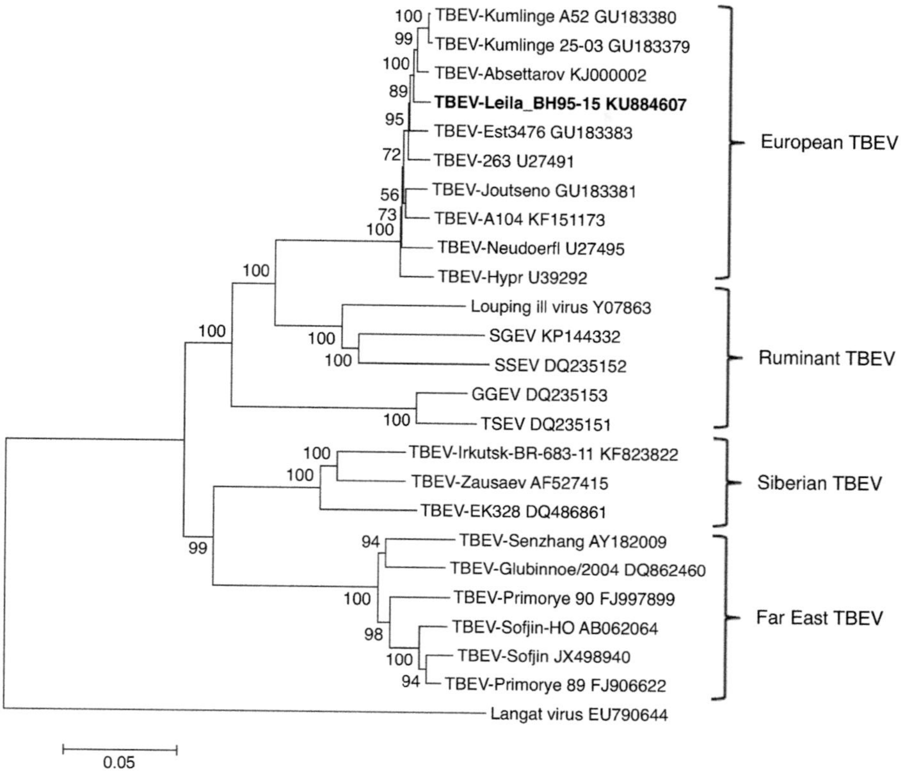

Fig. 1.5. Phylogenetic relationships of Eurasian TBEVs. From Böhm *et al*. (2017) under the terms of the Creative Commons Attribution License.

Tick-induced mammalian meat allergy related to immunoglobulin-E (IgE) antibodies against alpha-gal has now been reported in 17 countries, on all six continents, and alpha-gal has been demonstrated on the mouthparts or in the salivary glands or guts of tick species such as *Amblyomma americanum*, *Amblyomma sculptum*, *Amblyomma variegatum*, *Dermacentor variabilis*, *Haemaphysalis longicornis*, *Ixodes (Endopalpiger) australiensis*, *Ixodes cajennense*, *Ixodes holocyclus*, *Ixodes nipponensis*, *Ixodes ricinus* and *Ixodes scapularis* (Commins *et al*., 2011; Commins and Platts-Mills, 2013; van Nunen, 2014; Araujo *et al*., 2016; Kwak *et al*., 2018; Crispell *et al*., 2019).

Although non-primate mammals can synthesize alpha-gal and are therefore not expected to mount an immune response to this self-antigen, bites of *I. ricinus* have been shown to induce immunity to alpha-gal in dogs, raising the question of possible meat allergy in these animals, similar to that in humans (Hodžić *et al*., 2019).

There seem to be three possible origins of alpha-gal found in ticks:

- residual glycoprotein from a blood meal on a non-primate mammal,
- endogenous alpha-gal synthesized by the tick, or
- alpha-gal produced by the tick's microbiota (Mateos-Hernández *et al*., 2020).

1.3.5 Tick bite allergy

Tick anaphylaxis is rare in countries other than Australia (van Nunen, 2015). Salivary antigens from ticks such as *Rhipicephalus bursa* and *Hyalomma marginatum* can lead directly to an IgE response and anaphylaxis, without the involvement of alpha-gal (Mateos-Hernández *et al*., 2017).

References

Abanda, B., Paguem, A., Abdoulmoumini, M., Kingsley, M.T., Renz, A. *et al.* (2019) Molecular identification and prevalence of tick-borne pathogens in Zebu and Taurine cattle in North Cameroon. *Parasites & Vectors* 12, 448. DOI: 10.1186/s13071-019-3699-x.

Adegoke, A., Kumar, D., Bobo, C., Rashid, M.I., Durrani, A.Z. *et al.* (2020) Tick-borne pathogens shape the native microbiome within tick vectors. *Microorganisms* 8/9, 1299. DOI: 10.3390/microorganisms8091299.

Alani, A.J. and Herbert, I.V. (1988) Morphology and transmission of *Theileria recondita* (Theileriidae: Sporozoa) isolated from *Haemaphysalis punctata* from North Wales. *Veterinary Parasitology* 28, 283–291.

Allan, S.A. and Sonenshine, D.E. (2002) Evidence of an assembly pheromone in the black-legged deer tick, *Ixodes scapularis*. *Journal of Chemical Ecology* 28/1, 15–27.

Allen, J.R., Doube, B.M. and Kemp, D.H. (1977) Histology of bovine skin reactions to *Ixodes holocyclus* Neumann. *Canadian Journal of Comparative Medicine* 41/1, 26–35.

Altangerel, K., Battsetseg, B., Battur, B., Sivakumar, T., Batmagnai, E. *et al.* (2011) The first survey of *Theileria orientalis* infection in mongolian cattle. *Veterinary Parasitology* 182/1-2, 343–348. DOI: 10.1016/j.vetpar.2011.05.040.

Amde, B. (2017) Major factors affecting hide and skin production, quality and the tanning industry in Ethiopia. *Advances in Biological Research* 11/3, 116–125. DOI: 10.5829/idosi.abr.2017.116.125.

Anderson, J.M., Ammerman, N.C. and Norris, D.E. (2004) Molecular differentiation of metastriate tick immatures. *Vector Borne Zoonotic Diseases* 4/4, 334–342.

Apari, P. and Földvári, G. (2021) Harm or protection? The adaptive function of tick toxins. *Evolutionary Applications* 14/2, 271–277. DOI: 10.1111/eva.13123.

Araujo, R.N., Franco, P.F., Rodrigues, H., Santos, L.C. and McKay, C.S. (2016) *Amblyomma sculptum* tick saliva: α-Gal identification, antibody response and possible association with red meat allergy in Brazil. *International Journal for Parasitology* 46/3, 213–220. DOI: 10.1016/j.ijpara.2015.12.005.

Arthur, D.R. (1973) The histopathology of skin following bites by *Hyalomma rufipes* (Koch 1844), and a theory on feeding by this tick. *Journal of the Entomological Society of Southern Africa* 36/1, 117–124.

Atwell, R.B., Campbell, F.E. and Court, E. (2000) The attachment sites of the paralysis tick (*Ixodes holocyclus*) on dogs. *Australian Veterinary Practitioner* 30/2, 68–71.

Bagnall, B.G. and Doube, B.M. (1975) The Australian paralysis tick *Ixodes holocyclus*. *Australian Veterinary Journal* 51/3, 159–160.

Baker, J.A.F., Thompson, G.E. and Miles, J.O. (1977) Resistance to toxaphene by the bont tick, *Amblyomma hebraeum* (Koch). *Journal of the South African Veterinary Association* 48/1, 59–65.

Baker, M.K. and Ducasse, F.B.W. (1967) Tick infestation of livestock in Natal. I. The predilection sites and seasonal variations of cattle ticks. *Journal of the South African Veterinary Medical Association* 38/4, 447–453.

Baker, M.K. and Ducasse, F.B.W. (1968) Tick infestation of livestock in Natal. The rôle played by goats as reservoirs of the economically important cattle ticks. *Journal of the South African Veterinary Medical Association* 39/3, 55–59.

Bakken, J.S. and Dumler, J.S. (2000) Human *Granulocytic ehrlichiosis*. *Clinical Infectious Diseases* 31, 554–560.

Barker, D. and Barker, S.C. (2020) Survey of cases of tick-paralysis and the presence of the eastern paralysis tick, *Ixodes holocyclus*, and the southern paralysis tick, *Ixodes cornuatus*, in the Greater Melbourne Area. *Australian Veterinary Journal* 98/1-2, 2–10. DOI: 10.1111/avj.12883.

Barnard, D.R. (1985) Injury thresholds and production loss functions for the Lone Star Tick, *Amblyomma americanum* (Acari: Ixodidae), on pastured, preweaner beef cattle, *Bos taurus*. *Journal of Economic Entomology* 78/4, 852–855.

Barré, N., Garris, G.I. and Lorvelec, O. (1997) Field sampling of the tick *Amblyomma variegatum* (Acari: Ixodidae) on pastures in Guadeloupe; attraction of CO_2 and/or tick pheromones and conditions of use. *Experimental & Applied Acarology* 21, 95–108.

Battsetseg, B., Xuan, X., Ikadai, H., Bautista, J.L., Byambaa, B. *et al.* (2001) Detection of *Babesia caballi* and *Babesia equi* in *Dermacentor nuttalli* adult ticks. *International Journal for Parasitology* 31/4, 384–386.

Battsetseg, B., Lucero, S., Xuan, X., Claveria, F.C., Inoue, N. *et al.* (2002) Detection of natural infection of *Boophilus microplus* with *Babesia equi* and *Babesia caballi* in Brazilian horses using nested polymerase chain reaction. *Veterinary Parasitology* 107/4, 351–357.

Beelitz, P. and Gothe, R. (1991) Investigations on the host seeking and finding of *Argas* (*Persicargas*) *walkerae* (Ixodoidea: Argasidae). *Parasitology Research* 77, 622–628.

Bellgard, M.I., Moolhuijzen, P.M., Guerrero, F.D., Schibeci, D., Rodriguez-Valle, M. *et al.* (2012) CattleTickBase: An integrated internet-based bioinformatics resource for *Rhipicephalus* (*Boophilus*) *microplus*. *International Journal for Parasitology* 42/2, 161–169. DOI: 10.1016/j.ijpara.2011.11.006.

Benade, J.A. (2010) Immunization of roan antelope (*Hippotragus equinus*) using *in vitro* cultured *Theileria* species (sable) schizonts. M. Med. Vet. (Wildlife Diseases) thesis, University of Pretoria, South Africa.

Ben Said, M., Galai, Y., Canales, M., Nijhof, A.M., Mhadhbi, M. *et al.* (2012) Hd86, the Bm86 tick protein ortholog in *Hyalomma scupense* (syn. *H. detritum*): Expression in *Pichia pastoris* and analysis of nucleotides and amino acids sequences variations prior to vaccination trials. *Veterinary Parasitology* 183/3-4, 215–223. DOI: 10.1016/j.vetpar.2011.07.049.

Berger, J. (1979) *Theileria velifera* demonstrated in cattle in the Eastern cape Province of the Republic of South Africa. *Journal of the South African Veterinary Association* 50/1, 45–46.

Billeter, S.A., Levy, M.G., Chomel, B.B. and Breitschwerdt, E.B. (2008) Vector transmission of *Bartonella* species with emphasis on the potential for tick transmission. *Medical and Veterinary Entomology* 22, 1–15.

Boeuf, A., Schnell, G., Bernard, Q., Kern, A., Westermann, B. *et al.* (2019) Dissociating effect of salivary gland extract from *Ixodes ricinus* on human fibroblasts: Potential impact on *Borrelia* transmission. *Ticks and Tick-Borne Diseases* 10/2, 433–441. DOI: 10.1016/j.ttbdis.2018.12.005.

Böhm, B., Schade, B., Bauer, B., Hoffmann, B., Hoffmann, D. *et al.* (2017) Tick-borne encephalitis in a naturally infected sheep. *BMC Veterinary Research* 13/1, 267. DOI: 10.1186/s12917-017-1192-3.

Bonnet, S.I., Binetruy, F., Hernández-Jarguín, A.M. and Duron, O. (2017) The tick microbiome: Why non-pathogenic microorganisms matter in tick biology and pathogen transmission. *Frontiers in Cellular and Infection Microbiology* 7, 236. DOI: 10.3389/fcimb.2017.00236.

Borde, J.P., Zange, S., Antwerpen, M.H., Georgi, E., Buttlar, H. *et al.* (2017) Five cases of vector-borne *Francisella tularensis holarctica* infections in southwestern Germany and genetic diversity. *Ticks and Tick-Borne Diseases* 8/5, 808–812. DOI: 10.1016/j.ttbdis.2017.06.009.

Boulanger, N. and Wikel, S. (2021) Induced transient immune tolerance in ticks and vertebrate host: A keystone of tick-borne diseases. *Frontiers in Immunology* 12, 625993. DOI: 10.3389/fimmu.2021.625993.

Brackney, D.E. and Armstrong, P.M. (2016) Transmission and evolution of tick-borne viruses. *Current Opinion in Virology* 21, 67–74. DOI: 10.1016/j.coviro.2016.08.005.

Bryson, N.R., Tice, G.A., Horak, I.G., Stewart, C.G. and Plessis, B.J.A. (2002) Ixodid ticks on indigenous goats owned by small-scale farmers in four communal grazing areas in South Africa. *Journal of the South African Veterinary Association* 73/1, 26–30.

Budachetri, K., Crispell, G. and Karim, S. (2017a) Amblyomma maculatum SECIS binding protein 2 and putative selenoprotein P are indispensable for pathogen replication and tick fecundity. *Insect Biochemistry and Molecular Biology* 88, 37–47. DOI: 10.1016/j.ibmb.2017.07.006.

Budachetri, K., Williams, J., Mukherjee, N., Sellers, M., Moore, F. *et al.* (2017b) The microbiome of neotropical ticks parasitizing on passerine migratory birds. *Ticks and Tick-Borne Diseases* 8/1, 170–173. DOI: 10.1016/j.ttbdis.2016.10.014.

Burger, D.B., Crause, J.C., Spickett, A.M. and Neitz, A.W.H. (1991) A comparative study of proteins present in sweating-sickness-inducing and non-inducing strains of *Hyalomma truncatum* ticks. *Experimental and Applied Acarology* 13, 59–63.

Cabezas-Cruz, A. and Valdés, J.J. (2014) Are ticks venomous animals? *Frontiers in Zoology* 11, 47. Available at: http://www.frontiersinzoology.com/content/11/1/47 (accessed 18 December 2024).

Campbell, F.E. and Atwell, R.B. (2002) Long QT syndrome in dogs with tick toxicity (*Ixodes holocyclus*). *Australian Veterinary Journal* 80/10, 611–616.

Chaisi, M.E., Sibeko, K.P., Collins, N.E., Potgieter, F.T. and Oosthuizen, M.C. (2011) Identification of *Theileria parva* and *Theileria* sp. (buffalo) 18S rRNA gene sequence variants in the African Buffalo

(*Syncerus caffer*) in southern Africa. *Veterinary Parasitology* 182/2–4, 150–162. DOI: 10.1016/j.vetpar.2011.05.041.

Charles, R.A. and Basu, A.K. (2021) A review of the afrotropical sand tampan, *Ornithodoros savignyi*: A complex species. *CABI Reviews* 16, 036. DOI: 10.1079/PAVSNNR202116036.

Chen, X., Xu, S., Yu, Z., Guo, L., Yang, S. *et al.* (2014) Multiple lines of evidence on the genetic relatedness of the parthenogenetic and bisexual *Haemaphysalis longicornis* (Acari: Ixodidae). *Infection, Genetics and Evolution* 21, 308–314. DOI: 10.1016/j.meegid.2013.12.002.

Chmelař, J., Kotál, J., Langhansová, H. and Kotsyfakis, M. (2017) Protease inhibitors in tick saliva: The role of serpins and cystatins in tick-host-pathogen interaction. *Frontiers in Cellular Infection and Microbiology* 7, 216. DOI: 10.3389/fcimb.2017.00216.

Clark, R. (1938) A note on paralysis in lambs caused apparently by *Rhipicephalus evertsi*. *Journal of the South African Veterinary Medical Association* 9/3, 143–145.

Commins, S.P. and Platts-Mills, T.A.E. (2009) Anaphylaxis syndromes related to a new mammalian cross-reactive carbohydrate determinant. *Journal of Allergy and Clinical Immunology* 124/4, 652–657. DOI: 10.1016/j.jaci.2009.08.026.

Commins, S.P. and Platts-Mills, T.A.E. (2013) Tick bites and red meat allergy. *Current Opinions on Allergy and Clinical Immunology* 13/4, 354–359. DOI: 10.1097/ACI.0b013e3283624560.

Commins, S.P., Satinover, S.M., Hosen, J., Mozena, J., Borish, L. *et al.* (2009) Delayed anaphylaxis, angioedema, or urticaria after consumption of red meat in patients with IgE antibodies specific for galactose-α-1,3-galactose. *Journal of Allergy and Clinical Immunology* 123/2, 426–433. DOI: 10.1016/j.jaci.2008.10.052.

Commins, S.P., James, H.R., Kelly, E.A., Pochan, S.L., Workman, L.J. *et al.* (2011) The relevance of tick bites to the production of IgE antibodies to the mammalian oligosaccharide galactose-α-1,3-galactose. *Journal of Allergy and Clinical Immunology* 127(5), 1286–1293. DOI: 10.1016/j.jaci.2011.02.019.

Craig, A.F., Heath, L., Crafford, J.E., Richt, J.A. and Swanepoel, R. (2021) Updated distribution and host records for the argasid tick *Ornithodoros* (*Pavlovskyella*) *zumpti*: A potential vector of african swine fever virus in South Africa. *Onderstepoort Journal of Veterinary Research* 88/1, a1960. DOI: 10.4102/ojvr.v88i1.1960.

Crause, J.C., Wyngaardt, S., Gothe, R. and Neitz, A.W.H. (1994) A shared epitope found in the major paralysis inducing tick species of Africa. *Experimental & Applied Acarology* 18, 51–59.

Crispell, G., Commins, S.P., Archer-Hartman, S.A., Choudhary, S., Dharmarajan, G. *et al.* (2019) Discovery of alpha-gal-containing antigens in North American tick species believed to induce red meat allergy. *Frontiers in Immunology* 10, 1056. DOI: 10.3389/fimmu.2019.01056.

Cui, Y., Wang, X., Zhang, Y., Yan, Y., Dong, H. *et al.* (2018) First confirmed report of outbreak of Theileriosis/Anaplasmosis in a cattle farm in Henan, China. *Acta Tropica* 177, 207–210. DOI: 10.1016/j.actatropica.2017.08.029.

Cumming, G.S. (1998) Host preference in African ticks (Acari: Ixodida): A quantitative data set. *Bulletin of Entomological Research* 88, 379–406.

Cutullé, C., Jonsson, N.N. and Seddon, J.M. (2010) Multiple paternity in *Rhipicephalus microplus* confirmed by microsatellite analysis. *Experimental and Applied Acarology* 50/1, 51–58. DOI: 10.1007/s10493-009-9298-3.

Daněk, O., Hrbatová, A., Volfová, K., Ševčíková, S., Lesiczka, P. *et al.* (2024) Italian peninsula as a hybridization zone of *Ixodes inopinatus* and *I. ricinus* and the prevalence of tick-borne pathogens in *I. inopinatus*, *I. ricinus*, and their hybrids. *Parasites & Vectors* 17/1, 196. DOI: 10.1186/s13071-024-06271-z.

Dantas-Torres, F., Lia, R.P., Capelli, G. and Otranto, D. (2013) Efficiency of flagging and dragging for tick collection. *Experimental and Applied Acarology* 61, 119–127.

de Castro, M.H., Klerk, D., Pienaar, R., Latif, A.A., Rees, D.J. *et al.* (2016) *De novo* assembly and annotation of the salivary gland transcriptome of *Rhipicephalus appendiculatus* male and female ticks during blood feeding. *Ticks and Tick-Borne Diseases* 7/4, 536–548. DOI: 10.1016/j.ttbdis.2016.01.014.

de la Fuente, J., Antunes, S., Bonnet, S., Cabezas-Cruz, A., Domingos, A.G. *et al.* (2017) Tick–pathogen interactions and vector competence: Identification of molecular drivers for tick-borne diseases. *Frontiers in Cellular and Infection Microbiology* 7, 114. DOI: 10.3389/fcimb.2017.00114.

De Matos, C., Sitoe, C., Neves, L., Nöthling, J.O. and Horak, I.G. (2009) The comparative prevalence of five ixodid tick species infesting cattle and goats in Maputo Province, Mozambique. *Onderstepoort Journal of Veterinary Research* 76, 201–208.

de Vos, A.J. and Roos, J.A. (1981) The isolation of *Theileria*? *Taurotragi* in South Africa. *Onderstepoort Journal of Veterinary Research* 48/3, 149–153.

Díaz-Sánchez, S., Fernández, A.M., Habela, M.A., Calero-Bernal, R., Mera, I.G.F. *et al.* (2021) Microbial community of *Hyalomma lusitanicum* is dominated by *Francisella*-like endosymbiont. *Ticks and Tick-Borne Diseases* 12/2, 101624. DOI: 10.1016/j.ttbdis.2020.101624.

Dietrich, F., Schmidgen, T., Richter, D., Matuschka, F., Vonthein, R. *et al.* (2010) Prevalence of *Bartonella henselae* and *Borrelia burgdorferi* sensu lato DNA in *Ixodes ricinus* ticks in Europe. *Applied and Environmental Microbiology* 76/5, 1395–1398. DOI: 10.1128/AEM.02788-09.

Diyes, G.C.P. and Rajakaruna, R.S. (2017) Life cycle of spinose ear tick, *Otobius megnini* (Acari: Argasidae) infesting the racehorses in Nuwara Eliya, Sri Lanka. *Acta Tropica* 166, 164–176.

Dodd, S. (1921) Tick paralysis. *Journal of Comparative Pathology and Therapeutics* 34, 309–323.

Duncan, I.M. and Monks, N. (1992) Tick control on eland (*Taurotragus oryx*) and buffalo (*Syncerus caffer*) with flumethrin 1% pour-on through a Duncan applicator. *Journal of the South African Veterinary Association* 63/1, 7–10.

Durden, L.A. and Keirans, J.E. (1996) Host–parasite co-extinction and the plight of tick conservation. *American Entomologist* 42/2, 87–91.

Durden, L.A., Gerlach, R.F., Beckmen, K.B. and Greiman, S.E. (2018) Hyperparasitism and non-nidicolous mating by male *Ixodes angustus* ticks (Acari: Ixodidae). *Journal of Medical Entomology* 55/3, 766–768. DOI: 10.1093/jme/tjy012.

Eastwood, E.B. (1972) First record of *Argas persicus* from Southern Africa. *Journal of Parasitology* 58/2, 251.

Eisen, L. (2022) Tick species infesting humans in the United States. *Ticks and Tick-Borne Diseases* 13, 102025. DOI: 10.1016/j.ttbdis.2022.102025.

El Imam, A.H. and Taha, K.M. (2015) Malignant ovine theileriosis (*Theileria lestoquardi*): A review. *Jordan Journal of Biological Sciences* 8/3, 165–174. DOI: 10.12816/0026953.

El Imam, A.H., Hassan, S.M., Gameel, A.A., El Hussein, A.M., Taha, K.M. *et al.* (2016) Molecular identification of different *Theileria* and *Babesia* species infecting sheep in Sudan. *Annals of Parasitology* 62/1, 47–54. DOI: 10.17420/ap6201.31.

Erasmus, L.D. (1952) Regional tick paralysis. Sensory and motor changes caused by a male tick, genus *Hyalomma*. *South African Medical Journal* 26/50, 985–987.

Estrada-Peña, A., Pegram, R.G., Barré, N. and Venzal, J.M. (2007) Using invaded range data to model the climate suitability for *Amblyomma variegatum* (Acari: Ixodidae) in the new world. *Experimental and Applied Acarology* 41/3, 203–214. DOI: 10.1007/s10493-007-9050-9.

Estrada-Peña, A., Gray, J.S., Kahl, O., Lane, R.S. and Nijhof, A.M. (2013) Research on the ecology of ticks and tick-borne pathogens – methodological principles and caveats. *Frontiers in Cellular and Infection Microbiology* 3/29, 1–12. DOI: 10.3389/fcimb.2013.00029.

Estrada-Peña, A., Cevidanes, A., Sprong, H. and Millan, J. (2021) Pitfalls in tick and tick-borne pathogens research, some recommendations and a call for data sharing. *Pathogens* 10/6, 712. DOI: 10.3390/pathogens10060712.

Estrada-Peña, A., Guglielmone, A.A. and Nava, S. (2023) World-wide host associations of the tick genus *Ixodes* suggest relationships based on environmental sharing rather than on co-phylogenetic events. *Parasites & Vectors* 16/1, 75. DOI: 10.1186/s13071-022-05641-9.

Etiang, P., Atim, S.A., Nkamwesiga, J., Nalumenya, D., Byaruhanga, C. *et al.* (2024) Identification and distribution of *Rhipicephalus microplus* in selected high-cattle density districts in Uganda: Signaling future demand for novel tick control approaches. *BMC Veterinary Research* 20, 119. DOI: 10.1186/s12917-024-03979-z.

Ferreira, F.C., González, J., Milholland, M.T., Tung, G.A. and Fonseca, D.M. (2023) Ticks (Acari: Ixodida) on synanthropic small and medium-sized mammals in areas of the northeastern United States infested with the asian longhorned tick, *Haemaphysalis longicornis*. *International Journal for Parasitology* 53/14, 809–819. DOI: 10.1016/j.ijpara.2023.06.003.

Fouche, G., Sakong, B.M., Adenubi, O.T., Dzoyem, J.P., Naidoo, V. *et al.* (2017) Investigation of the acaricidal activity of the acetone and ethanol extracts of 12 South African plants against the adult ticks of *Rhipicephalus turanicus*. *Onderstepoort Journal of Veterinary Research* 84/1, a1523. DOI: 10.4102/ojvr.v84i1.1523.

Fouche, G., Sakong, B.M., Adenubi, O.T., Dzoyem, J.P., Naidoo, V. *et al.* (2021) Corrigendum: Investigation of the acaricidal activity of the acetone and ethanol extracts of 12 South African plants against the adult ticks of *Rhipicephalus turanicus*. *Onderstepoort Journal of Veterinary Research* 88(1), a1950. DOI: 10.4102/ojvr.v88i1.1950.

Fourie, L.J. and Kok, D.J. (1995) Attachment preferences of *Hyalomma truncatum* and *Hyalomma marginatum* rufipes ticks (Acari: Ixodidae) on two sheep breeds. *Onderstepoort Journal of Veterinary Research* 62, 211–213.

Fourie, L.J., Kok, D.J., Krugel, L., Snyman, A. and Van der Lingen, F. (1996) Control of Karoo paralysis ticks through vegetation management. *Medical and Veterinary Entomology* 10, 39–43.

Francischetti, I.M., Sá-Nunes, A., Mans, B.J., Santos, I.M. and Ribeiro, J.M.C. (2009) The role of saliva in tick feeding. *Frontiers in Bioscience* 14, 2051–2088.

Freeman, J.M., Kappmeyer, L.S., Ueti, M.W., McElwain, T.F., Baszler, T.V. *et al.* (2010) A *Babesia bovis* gene syntenic to *Theileria parva p67* is expressed in blood and tick stage parasites. *Veterinary Parasitology* 173/3–4, 217–218. DOI: 10.1016/j.vetpar.2010.06.024.

Gallivan, G.J. and Horak, I.G. (1997) Body size and habitat as determinants of tick infestations of wild ungulates in South Africa. *South African Journal of Wildlife Research* 27/2, 63–70.

Gan, Y.S., Yau, W.-C., Liong, S.-T. and Chen, C.-C. (2022) Automated classification system for tick-bite defect on leather. *Mathematical Problems in Engineering* Article ID 5549879. DOI: 10.1155/2022/5549879.

Garcia-Vozmediano, A., Krawczyk, A.I., Sprong, H., Rossi, L., Ramassa, E. *et al.* (2020) Ticks climb the mountains: ixodid tick infestation and infection by tick-borne pathogens in the western alps. *Ticks and Tick-Borne Diseases* 11/5, 101489. DOI: 10.1016/j.ttbdis.2020.101489.

Gashaw, B.A. and Mersha, C.K. (2013) Pathology of tick bite lesions in naturally infested skin and hides of ruminants: A review. *Acta Parasitologica Globalis* 4/2, 59–63. DOI: 10.5829/idosi.apg.2013.4.2.74215.

Gaspar, A.R.M. (1995) Biochemical investigations into anticoagulants in salivary glands of the tick *Ornithodoros savignyi* Audouin (1827). PhD thesis, University of Pretoria, South Africa.

Gaspar, A.R.M., Joubert, A.M., Crause, J.C. and Neitz, A.W.H. (1996) Isolation and characterization of an anticoagulant from the salivary glands of the tick, *Ornithodoros savignyi*. *Experimental & Applied Acarology* 20, 583–598.

George, J.E., Davey, R.B. and Pound, J.M. (2002) Introduced ticks and tick-borne diseases: The threat and approaches to eradication. *Veterinary Clinics Food Animal Practice* 18, 401–416.

Goethert, H.K. (2021) What *Babesia microti* is now. *Pathogens* 10, 1168. DOI: 10.3390/pathogens10091168.

Golezardy, H. and Horak, I.G. (2007) Ticks (Acari: Ixodidae) collected from animals in three western, semi-arid nature reserves in South Africa. *Onderstepoort Journal of Veterinary Research* 74, 81–85.

Gong, S., He, B., Wang, Z., Shang, L., Wei, F. *et al.* (2015) Nairobi sheep disease virus RNA in ixodid ticks, China, 2013. *Emerging Infectious Diseases* 21/4, 718–720. DOI: 10.3201/eid2104.141602.

Gothe, R. (1987) Tick pheromones. *Onderstepoort Journal of Veterinary Research* 54, 439–441.

Gothe, R. and Bezuidenhout, J.D. (1986) Studies on the ability of different strains or populations of female *Rhipicephalus evertsi evertsi* (Acarina: Ixodidae) to produce paralysis in sheep. *Onderstepoort Journal of Veterinary Research* 53, 19–24.

Gothe, R., Kunze, K., and Hoogstraal, H. (1979) Review article: The mechanisms of pathogenicity in the tick paralyses. *Journal of Medical Entomology* 16/5: 357 – 369. DOI: 10.1093/jmedent/16.5.357.

Gothe, R., Gold, Y. and Bezuidenhout, J.D. (1986) Investigations into the paralysis-inducing ability of *Rhipicephalus evertsi* mimeticus and that of hybrids between this subspecies and *Rhipicephalus evertsi evertsi*. *Onderstepoort Journal of Veterinary Research* 53, 25–29.

Grady, C.A., McDonald, D.R., Poppen, C.F. and Pritt, B.S. (2011) *Dermacentor* tick attached to tympanic membrane. *Lancet* 378, 347. DOI: 10.1016/S0140-6736(11)60981-1.

Grattan-Smith, P.J., Morris, J.G., Johnston, H.M., Yiannikas, C., Malik, R. *et al.* (1997) Clinical and neurophysiological features of tick paralysis. *Brain* 120, 1975–1987.

Gray, A., Capewell, P., Loney, C., Katzer, F., Shiels, B.R. *et al.* (2019) Sheep as host species for zoonotic *Babesia venatorum*, United Kingdom. *Emerging Infectious Diseases* 25/12, 2257–2260. DOI: 10.3201/eid2512.190459.

Grisi, L., Leite, R.C., Martins, J.R., de Barros, T.M., Andreotti, R. *et al.* (2014) Reassessment of the potential economic impact of cattle parasites in Brazil. *Brazilian Journal of Veterinary Parasitology* 23/2, 150–156. DOI: 10.1590/s1984-29612014042.

Gual-Gonzalez, L., Self, S.C.W., Zellars, K., Meyer, M., Dye-Braumuller, K.C. *et al.* (2024) Eco-epidemiology of *Rickettsia amblyommatis* and *Rickettsia parkeri* in naturally infected ticks (Acari: Ixodida) from South Carolina. *Parasites & Vectors* 17, 33. DOI: 10.1186/s13071-023-06099-z.

Guccione, C., Colomba, C., Iaria, C. and Cascio, A. (2023) Rickettsiales in the WHO European region: An update from a one health perspective. *Parasites & Vectors* 16/1, 41. DOI: 10.1186/s13071-022-05646-4.

Guglielmone, A.A., Robbins, R.G., Apanaskevich, D.A., Petney, T.N., Estrada-Peña, A. *et al.* (2009) Comments on controversial tick (Acari: Ixodida) species names and species described or resurrected from 2003 to 2008. *Experimental & Applied Acarology* 48, 311–327.

Hall-Mendelin, S., Craig, S.B., Hall, R.A., O'Donoghue, P., Atwell, R.B. *et al.* (2011) Tick paralysis in Australia caused by *Ixodes holocyclus* Neumann. *Annals of Tropical Medicine & Parasitology* 105/2, 95–106. DOI: 10.1179/136485911X12899838413628.

Hamel, H.D. and Gothe, R. (1978) Influence of infestation rate on tick-paralysis in sheep induced by *Rhipicephalus evertsi evertsi* Neumann, 1897. *Veterinary Parasitology* 4, 183–191.

Hamilton, P.T., Maluenda, E., Sarr, A., Belli, A., Hurry, G. *et al.* (2021) *Borrelia afzelii* infection in the rodent host has dramatic effects on the bacterial microbiome of *Ixodes ricinus* ticks. *Applied and Environmental Microbiology* 87, e00641-21. DOI: 10.1128/AEM.00641-21.

Haresnape, J.M., Wilkinson, P.J. and Mellor, P.S. (1988) Isolation of African swine fever virus from ticks of the *Ornithodoros moubata* complex (Ixodoidea: Argasidae) collected within the African swine fever enzootic area of Malawi. *Epidemiology and Infection* 101, 173–185. DOI: 10.1017/S0950268800029332.

Hassan, S.M. and Salih, D.A. (2013) An overview of factors responsible for geographic distribution pattern of Ixodid ticks in the Sudan. *Sokoto Journal of Veterinary Sciences* 11/2, 1–9. DOI: 10.4314/sokjvs.v11i2.1.

Heath, A.C.G., Tenquist, J.D. and Bishop, D.M. (1987) Goats, hares, and rabbits as hosts for the New Zealand cattle tick, *Haemaphysalis longicornis*. *New Zealand Journal of Zoology* 14/4, 549–555. DOI: 10.1080/03014223.1987.10423028.

Hodžić, A., Mateos-Hernández, L., Leschnik, M., Alberdi, P., Rego, R.O.M. *et al.* (2019) Tick bites induce anti-α-gal antibodies in dogs. *Vaccines* 7, 114. DOI: 10.3390/vaccines7030114.

Hokama, Y. and Howarth, J.A. (1977) Dry-ice (CO_2) trap for efficient field collection of *Ornithodoros coriaceus* (Acarina: Argasidae). *Journal of Medical Entomology* 13/4-5, 627–628. DOI: 10.1093/jmedent/13.4-5.627.

Hoogstraal, H. and Aeschlimann, A. (1982) Tick–host specificity. *Bulletin de La Societe Entomologique Suisse* 55, 5–32.

Hook, S.A., Nelson, C.A. and Mead, P.S. (2015) U.S. public's experience with ticks and tick-borne diseases: Results from national healthstyles surveys. *Ticks and Tick-Borne Diseases* 6, 483–488. DOI: 10.1016/j.ttbdis.2015.03.017.

Horak, I.G. (1980) The control of parasites in antelope in small game reserves. *Journal of the South African Veterinary Association* 51/1, 17–19.

Horak, I.G. (1982) Parasites of domestic and wild animals in South Africa. XV. The seasonal prevalence of ectoparasites on impala and cattle in the northern Transvaal. *Onderstepoort Journal of Veterinary Research* 49, 85–93.

Horak, I.G. (1999) Parasites of domestic and wild animals in South Africa. XXXVII. Ixodid ticks on cattle on Kikuyu grass pastures and in valley Bushveld in the Eastern Cape Province. *Onderstepoort Journal of Veterinary Research* 66, 175–184.

Horak, I.G. (2009) A century of tick taxonomy in South Africa. *Onderstepoort Journal of Veterinary Research* 76, 69–74.

Horak, I.G. and Boomker, J. (1998) Parasites of domestic and wild animals in South Africa. XXXV. Ixodid ticks and bot fly larvae in the Bontebok National Park. *Onderstepoort Journal of Veterinary Research* 65, 205–211.

Horak, I.G., Sheppey, K., Knight, M.M. and Beuthin, C.L. (1986) Parasites of domestic and wild animals in South Africa XXI. Arthropod parasites of vaal ribbok, bontebok and scrub hares in the western Cape Province. *Onderstepoort Journal of Veterinary Research* 53, 187–197.

Horak, I.G., Moolman, L.C. and Fourie, L.J. (1987) Some wild hosts of the Karoo paralysis tick, *Ixodes rubicundus* Neumann, 1904 (Acari: Ixodidae). *Onderstepoort Journal of Veterinary Research* 54, 49–51.

Horak, I.G., Keep, M.E., Spickett, A.M. and Boomker, J. (1989) Parasites of domestic and wild animals in South Africa. XXIV. Arthropod parasites of bushbuck and common duiker in the Weza State Forest, Natal. *Onderstepoort Journal of Veterinary Research* 56, 63–66.

Horak, I.G., Williams, E.J. and Schalkwyk, P.C. (1991) Parasites of domestic and wild animals in South Africa. XXV. Ixodid ticks on sheep in the North-Eastern Orange Free State and in the Eastern Cape Province. *Onderstepoort Journal of Veterinary Research* 58, 115–123.

Horak, I.G., Potgieter, F.T., Walker, J.B., de Vos, V. and Boomker, J. (1983) The Ixodid tick burdens of various large ruminant species in South African nature reserves. *Onderstepoort Journal of Veterinary Research* 50, 221–228.

Horak, I.G., Boshoff, C.R., Cooper, D.V., Foggin, C.M., Govender, D. *et al.* (2017) Parasites of domestic and wild animals in South Africa. XLIX. Ticks (Acari: Ixodidae) infesting white and black Rhinoceroses in Southern Africa. *Onderstepoort Journal of Veterinary Research* 84(1), a1301. DOI: 10.4102/ojvr.v84i1.1301.

Horak, I.G., Fourie, L.J., Heyne, H., Walker, J.B. and Needham, G.R. (2002) Ixodid ticks feeding on humans in South Africa: With notes on preferred hosts, geographic distribution, seasonal occurrence and transmission of pathogens. *Experimental and Applied Acarology* 27, 113–136.

Horak, I.G., Fourie, L.J. and Braack, L.E.O. (2005) Small mammals as hosts of immature ixodid ticks. *Onderstepoort Journal of Veterinary Research* 72/3, 255–261.

Horak, I.G., Gallivan, G.J., Spickett, A.M. and Potgieter, A.L.F. (2006) Effect of burning on the numbers of questing ticks collected by dragging. *Onderstepoort Journal of Veterinary Research* 73/3, 163–174.

Horak, I.G., Nyangiwe, N., Matos, C. and Neves, L. (2009) Species composition and geographic distribution of ticks infesting cattle, goats and dogs in a temperate and in a subtropical region of South-East Africa. *Onderstepoort Journal of Veterinary Research* 76, 263–276.

Horak, I.G., Gallivan, G.J. and Spickett, A.M. (2011) The dynamics of questing ticks collected for 164 consecutive months off the vegetation of two landscape zones in the Kruger National Park (1988-2002). I. Total ticks, *Amblyomma hebraeum* and *Rhipicephalus decoloratus*. *Onderstepoort Journal of Veterinary Research* 78/1, 32. DOI: 10.4102/ojvr.v78i1.32.

Horak, I.G., Boomker, J., Junker, K. and Gallivan, G.J. (2021) Some gastrointestinal nematodes and ixodid ticks shared by several wildlife species in the Kruger National Park, South Africa. *Parasitology* 148/6, 740–746. DOI: 10.1017/S0031182021000135.

Horak, I.G., Junker, K. and Krasnov, B.R. (2022) Similarity in ixodid tick communities harboured by wildlife and livestock in the Albany Thicket biome of South Africa. *Parasitology* 149, 667–674. DOI: 10.1017/S0031182022000129.

Hornok, S., Mester, A., Takács, N., Mera, I.G.F., Fuente, J. *et al.* (2014) Re-emergence of bovine piroplasmosis in Hungary: Has the etiological role of Babesia divergens been taken over by *B.* major and Theileria buffeli? *Parasites & Vectors* 7/1, 434. DOI: 10.1186/1756-3305-7-434.

Howell, C.J. (1966) Collection of salivary gland secretion from the argasid *Ornithodoros savignyi* Adouin (1827) by the use of a pharmacological stimulant. *Journal of the South African Veterinary Medical Association* 37/2, 236–239.

Howell, C.J., Neitz, A.W.H. and Potgieter, D.J.J. (1975) Some toxic, physical and chemical properties of the oral secretion of the sand tampan, *Ornithodoros savignyi* Audouin (1827). *Onderstepoort Journal of Veterinary Research* 42/3, 99–102.

Hubálek, Z. and Rudolf, I. (2012) Tick-borne viruses in Europe. *Parasitology Research* 111/1, 9–36. DOI: 10.1007/s00436-012-2910-1.

Hüe, T., Graille, M., Mortelecque, A., Desoutter, D., Delathière, J.M. *et al.* (2013) Diagnostic methods used to monitor an outbreak of babesiosis (*Babesia bovis*) in a herd of feral cattle in New Caledonia. *Australian Veterinary Journal* 91/ 6, 254–258. DOI: 10.1111/avj.12059.

Hurtado, O.J.B. and Giraldo-Ríos, C. (2018) Economic and health impact of the ticks in production animals. In: Abubakar, M. and Perera, P.K. (eds) *Ticks and Tick-Borne Pathogens*. InTechOpen, London.

Ilkiw, J.E. (1987) Infestation in the dog by the paralysis tick *Ixodes holocyclus*. 1. Clinical and histological findings. *Australian Veterinary Journal* 64/5, 137–139.

Ilkiw, J.E. and Turner, D.M. (1987a) Infestation in the dog by the paralysis tick *Ixodes holocyclus*. 2. Blood-gas and pH, haematological and biochemical findings. *Australian Veterinary Journal* 64/5, 139–142.

Ilkiw, J.E. and Turner, D.M. (1987b) Infestation in the dog by the paralysis tick *Ixodes holocyclus*. 3. Respiratory effects. *Australian Veterinary Journal* 64/5, 142–144.

Ilkiw, J.E., Turner, D.M. and Goodman, A.H. (1988) Infestation in the dog by the paralysis tick, *Ixodes holocyclus*. 4. Cardiovascular effects. *Australian Veterinary Journal* 65/8, 232–235.

Izdebska, J.N. and Cydzik, K. (2010) Analysis of the reasons for differences in topical specificity among various species of tick (Acari, Ixodidae) infesting *European Bison*. *European Bison Conservation Newsletter* 3, 75–84.

Jakimovski, D., Mateska, S., Simin, V., Bogdan, I., Mijatović, D. *et al.* (2022) Mediterranean spotted fever-like illness caused by *Rickettsia sibirica mongolitimonae* North Macedonia, June 2022. *Euro Surveillance* 27/42, 2200735. DOI: 10.2807/1560-7917.ES.2022.27.42.2200735.

Jakimovski, D., Grozdanovski, K., Rangelov, G., Pavleva, V., Banović, P. *et al.* (2023) Cases of Crimean-Congo haemorrhagic fever in North Macedonia, July to August 2023. *Euro Surveillance* 28/34, 2300409. DOI: 10.2807/1560-7917.ES.2023.28.34.2300409.

Jongejan, F., Nene, V., Fuente, J., Pain, A. and Willadsen, P. (2007) Advances in the genomics of ticks and tick-borne pathogens. *Trends in Parasitology* 23/9, 391–396. DOI: 10.1016/j.pt.2007.07.004.

Jupp, P.G., Joubert, I.J., Cornell, A.J., Swanefelder, C. and Prozesky, O.W. (1987) An experimental assessment of the tampan tick Ornithodoros moubata as vector of hepatitis B virus. *Medical and Veterinary Entomology* 1/4, 361–368.

Kahsay, T., Negash, G., Hagos, Y. and Hadush, B. (2015) Pre-slaughter, slaughter and post-slaughter defects of skins and hides at the Sheba Tannery and Leather Industry, Tigray region, northern Ethiopia. *Onderstepoort Journal of Veterinary Research* 82/1, 931. DOI: 10.4102/ojvr.%20v82i1.931.

Kapo, N., Zuber Bogdanović, I., Gagović, E., Žekić, M., Veinović, G. *et al.* (2024) Ixodid ticks and zoonotic tick-borne pathogens of the Western Balkans. *Parasites & Vectors* 17, 45. DOI: 10.1186/s13071-023-06116-1.

Kariuki, E.K., Penzhorn, B.L. and Horak, I.G. (2012) Ticks (Acari: Ixodidae) infesting cattle and African buffaloes in the Tsavo conservation area, Kenya. *Onderstepoort Journal of Veterinary Research* 79/1, 437. DOI: 10.4102/ojvr.%20v79i1.437.

Kariuki, E.K., Kutima, H., Kock, M., Horak, I.G., Jooste, R. *et al.* (2019) Ixodid ticks (Acari: Ixodidae) collected from African savanna elephants (*Loxodonta africana*) and African forest elephants (*Loxodonta cyclotis*). *Onderstepoort Journal of Veterinary Research* 86/1, e1–e5. DOI: 10.4102/ojvr.v86i1.1781.

Kasi, K.K., von Arnim, F., Schulz, A., Rehman, A., Chudhary, A. *et al.* (2020) Crimean-Congo haemorrhagic fever virus in ticks collected from livestock in Balochistan, Pakistan. *Transboundary and Emerging Diseases* 67, 1543–1552. DOI: 10.1111/tbed.13488.

Kaufman, W.R. (2004) Assuring paternity in a promiscuous world: Are there lessons for ticks among the insects? *Parasitology* 129, S145–S160. DOI: 10.1017/S0031182004004846.

Keirans, J.E. and Pound, J.M. (2003) An annotated bibliography of the spinose ear tick, *Otobius megnini* (Dugès, 1883). *Systematic & Applied Acarology Special Publications* 13, 1–68.

Kensinger, B.J. and Allan, B.F. (2011) Efficacy of dry ice-baited traps for sampling *Amblyomma americanum* (Acari: Ixodidae) varies with life stage but not habitat. *Journal of Medical Entomology* 48/3, 708–711.

Kjemtrup, A.M. and Conrad, P.A. (2000) Human babesiosis: An emerging tick-borne disease. *International Journal for Parasitology* 30/12–13, 1323–1337. DOI: 10.1016/S0020-7519(00)00137-5.

Kok, D.J. and Fourie, L.J. (1995) The role of *Hyalomma* ticks in foot infestations and temporary lameness of sheep in a semi-arid region of South Africa. *Onderstepoort Journal of Veterinary Research* 62, 201–206.

Koonin, E.V. (2005) Orthologs, paralogs, and evolutionary genomics. *Annual Review of Genetics* 39, 309–338. DOI: 10.1146/annurev.genet.39.073003.114725.

Krasteva, S., Jara, M., Frias-De-Diego, A. and Machado, G. (2020) Nairobi sheep disease virus: a historical and epidemiological perspective. *Frontiers in Veterinary Science* 7, 419. DOI: 10.3389/fvets.2020.00419.

Kwak, M. (2018) The first records of human infestation by the hard tick *Ixodes* (*Endopalpiger*) *australiensis* (Acari: Ixodidae), with a review of human infestation by ticks in Australia. *Experimental and Applied Acarology* 74, 185–190. DOI: 10.1007/s10493-018-0217-3.

Kwak, M., Somerville, C. and Van Nunen, S. (2018) A novel Australian tick *Ixodes* (*Endopalpiger*) *australiensis* inducing mammalian meat allergy after tick bite. *Asia Pacific Allergy* 8/3, e31. DOI: 10.5415/apallergy.2018.8.e31.

Labruna, M.B., Pacheco, R.C., Ataliba, A.C. and Szabó, M.P.J. (2007) Human parasitism by the capybara tick, *Amblyomma dubitatum* (Acari: Ixodidae). *Entomological News* 118/1, 77–80.

Langley, D.B., Schofield, P., Nevoltris, D., Jackson, J., Jackson, J.J.L. *et al.* (2022) Genetic and structural basis of the human anti-α-galactosyl antibody response. *Proceedings of the National Academy of Sciences of the USA* 119/28, e2123212119. DOI: 10.1073/pnas.2123212119.

Lawrence, J.A. (1979) The differential diagnosis of the bovine theilerias of Southern Africa. *Journal of the South African Veterinary Association* 50/4, 311–313.

Laws, H.E. and Manning, B. (1910) Eradication of ticks by the starvation method. *Agricultural Journal of the Cape of Good Hope* 37/1, 9–17.

Lejal, E., Marsot, M., Chalvet-Monfray, K., Cosson, J., Moutailler, S. *et al.* (2019) A three-years assessment of *Ixodes ricinus*-borne pathogens in a French peri-urban forest. *Parasites & Vectors* 12/1, 551. DOI: 10.1186/s13071-019-3799-7.

Lesiczka, P.M. (2023) Distant genetic variants of *Anaplasma phagocytophilum* from *Ixodes ricinus* attached to people. *Parasites & Vectors* 16/1, 80. DOI: 10.1186/s13071-023-05654-y.

Levin, M.L., Killmaster, L.F. and Zemtsova, G.E. (2011) Domestic dogs (*Canis familiaris*) as reservoir hosts for *Rickettsia conorii*. *Vector-Borne and Zoonotic Diseases* 12/1, 28–33. DOI: 10.1089/vbz.2011.0684.

Lewis, D., Holman, M.R., Purnell, R.E., Young, E.R., Herbert, I.V. *et al.* (1981) Investigations on *Babesia motasi* isolated from Wales. *Research in Veterinary Science* 31/2, 239–243. DOI: 10.1016/S0034-5288(18)32501-3.

Liebenberg, J., Steyn, H.C., Josemans, A.I., Faber, I. and Zweygarth, E. (2020) *In vitro* propagation and genome sequencing of three 'atypical' *Ehrlichia ruminantium* isolates. *Onderstepoort Journal of Veterinary Research* 87/1, a1769. DOI: 10.4102/ojvr.v87i1.1769.

Lilak, A.A., Pecor, D.B., Matulis, G., Potter, A.M., Wofford, R.N. *et al.* (2024) Data release: Targeted systematic literature search for tick and tick-borne pathogen distributions in six countries in sub-Saharan Africa from 1901 to 2020. *Parasites & Vectors* 17/1, 84. DOI: 10.1186/s13071-023-06086-4.

Liong, S.-T., Gan, Y.S., Huang, Y.-C., Yuan, C.-A. and Chang, H.-C. (2019) Automatic defect segmentation on leather with deep learning. *arXiv* 1903, 12139. DOI: 10.48550/arXiv.1903.12139.

Liu, J., Han, X.Y., Ye, R.Z., Xu, Q., Wang, X.Y. *et al.* (2024) An integrated data analysis reveals distribution, hosts, and pathogen diversity of *Haemaphysalis concinna*. *Parasites & Vectors* 17, 92. DOI: 10.1186/s13071-024-06152-5.

Londt, J.G.H., Horak, I.G. and De Villers, I.L. (1979) Parasites of domestic and wild animals in south africa. XIII. The seasonal incidence of adult ticks (Acarina: Ixodidae) on cattle in the northern Transvaal. *Onderstepoort Journal of Veterinary Research* 46, 31–39.

Louly, B.C.C., Silveira, D.N., Soares, S.F., Ferri, P.H., Melo, A.C.C. *et al.* (2008) More about the role of 2,6-dichlorophenol in tick courtship: identification and olfactometer bioassay in *Amblyomma cajennense* and *Rhipicephalus sanguineus*. *Memórias Do Instituto Oswaldo Cruz* 103/1, 60–65.

Lubinga, J.C., Tuppurainen, E.S.M., Stoltsz, W.H., Ebersohn, K., Coetzer, J.A.W. *et al.* (2013) Detection of lumpy skin disease virus in saliva of ticks fed on lumpy skin disease virus-infected cattle. *Experimental and Applied Acarology* 61/1, 129–138. DOI: 10.1007/s10493-013-9679-5.

Lubinga, J.C., Clift, S.J., Tuppurainen, E.S., Stoltsz, W.H., Babiuk, S. *et al.* (2014a) Demonstration of lumpy skin disease virus infection in *Amblyomma hebraeum* and *Rhipicephalus appendiculatus* ticks using immunohistochemistry. *Ticks and Tick-Borne Diseases* 5, 113–120. DOI: 10.1016/j.ttbdis.2013.09.010.

Lubinga, J.C., Tuppurainen, E.S.M., Coetzer, J.A.W., Stoltsz, W.H. and Venter, E.H. (2014b) Transovarial passage and transmission of LSDV by *Amblyomma hebraeum*, *Rhipicephalus appendiculatus* and *Rhipicephalus decoloratus*. *Experimental and Applied Acarology* 62, 67–75. DOI: 10.1007/s10493-013-9722-6.

Lubinga, J.C., Tuppurainen, E.S.M., Mahlare, R., Coetzer, J.A.W., Stoltsz, W.H. *et al.* (2015) Evidence of transstadial and mechanical transmission of lumpy skin disease virus by *Amblyomma hebraeum* ticks. *Transboundary and Emerging Diseases* 62/2, 147–182. DOI: 10.1111/tbed.12102.

Lutomiah, J., Musila, L., Makio, A., Ochieng, C., Koka, H. *et al.* (2014) Ticks and tick-borne viruses from livestock hosts in arid and semiarid regions of the eastern and northeastern parts of Kenya. *Journal of Medical Entomology* 51/1, 269–277. DOI: 10.1603/me13039.

Lynn, G.E., Breuner, N.E., Hojgaard, A., Oliver, J., Eisen, L. *et al.* (2022a) A comparison of horizontal and transovarial transmission efficiency of *Borrelia miyamotoi* by *Ixodes scapularis*. *Ticks and Tick-Borne Diseases* 13/5, 102003. DOI: 10.1016/j.ttbdis.2022.102003.

Lynn, G.E., Černý, J., Kurokawa, C., Diktaș, H., Matias, J. *et al.* (2022b) Immunization of guinea pigs with cement extract induces resistance against *Ixodes scapularis* ticks. *Ticks and Tick-Borne Diseases* 13/6, 102017. DOI: 10.1016/j.ttbdis.2022.102017.

MacIvor, K.M.D. and Horak, I.G. (2003) Ixodid ticks of Angora and Boer goats, grysbok, common duikers, kudus and scrub hares in Valley Bushveld in the Eastern Cape Province, South Africa. *Onderstepoort Journal of Veterinary Research* 70, 113–120.

MacIvor, K.M.D., Horak, I.G., Holton, K.C. and Petney, T.N. (1987) A comparison of live and destructive sampling methods of determining the size of parasitic tick populations. *Experimental & Applied Acarology* 3, 131–143.

MacLeod, J., Colbo, M.H., Madbouly, M.H. and Mwanaumo, B. (1977) Ecological studies of ixodid ticks (Acari: Ixodidae) in Zambia. III. Seasonal activity and attachment sites on cattle, with notes on other hosts. *Bulletin of Entomological Research* 67/1, 161–173. DOI: 10.1017/S0007485300010981.

Magesa, W.S., Haji, I., Kinimi, E., Nzalawahe, J.S. and Kazwala, R. (2023) Distribution and molecular identification of ixodid ticks infesting cattle in Kilombero and Iringa districts, Tanzania. *BMC Veterinary Research* 19, 121. DOI: 10.1186/s12917-023-03652-x.

Mahmood, S., Sima, R., Urbanova, V., Trentelman, J.J., Krezdorn, N. *et al.* (2021) Identification of tick *Ixodes ricinus* midgut genes differentially expressed during the transmission of *Borrelia afzelii* spirochetes using a transcriptomic approach. *Frontiers in Immunology* 11, 612412. DOI: 10.3389/fimmu.2020.612412.

Malan, F.S., Horak, I.G., de Vos, V. and Van Wyk, J.A. (1997) Wildlife parasites: Lessons for parasite control in livestock. *Veterinary Parasitology* 71, 137–153.

Mans, B.J. and Neitz, A.W.H. (2004) The sand tampan, *Ornithodoros savignyi*, as a model for tick–host interactions. *South African Journal of Science* 100, 283–288.

Mans, B.J., Steinmann, C.M.L., Venter, J.D., Louw, A.I. and Neitz, A.W.H. (2002) Pathogenic mechanisms of sand tampan toxicoses induced by the tick, *Ornithodoros savignyi*. *Toxicon* 40/7, 1007–1016. DOI: 10.1016/50041-0101(02)00098-3.

Mans, B.J., Louw, A.I. and Neitz, A.W. (2003a) The influence of tick behavior, biotope and host specificity on concerted evolution of the platelet aggregation inhibitor savignygrin, from the soft tick *Ornithodoros savignyi*. *Insect Biochemistry and Molecular Biology* 33/6, 623–629. DOI: 10.1016/s0965-1748(03)00047-x.

Mans, B.J., Louw, A.I. and Neitz, A.W. (2003b) The major tick salivary gland proteins and toxins from the soft tick, *Ornithodoros savignyi*, are part of the tick Lipocalin family: Implications for the origins of tick toxicoses. *Molecular Biology and Evolution* 20/7, 1158–1167. DOI: 10.1093/molbev/msg126.

Mans, B.J., Gothe, R. and Neitz, A.W.H. (2004a) Biochemical perspective on paralysis and other forms of toxicoses caused by ticks. *Parasitology* 129, S95–S111.

Mans, B.J., Venter, J.D., Coons, L.B., Louw, A.I. and Neitz, A.W.H. (2004b) A reassessment of argasid tick salivary gland ultrastructure from an immuno-cytochemical perspective. *Experimental and Applied Acarology* 33, 119–129.

Mans, B.J., de Castro, M.H., Pienaar, R., Klerk, D., Gaven, P. *et al.* (2016) Ancestral reconstruction of tick lineages. *Ticks and Tick-Borne Diseases* 7/4, 509–535. DOI: 10.1016/j.ttbdis.2016.02.002.

Mans, B.J., Andersen, J.F., Francischetti, I.M., Valenzuela, J.G., Schwan, T.G. *et al.* (2008) Comparative sialomics between hard and soft ticks: Implications for the evolution of blood-feeding behavior. *Insect Biochemistry and Molecular Biology* 38/1, 42–58.

Mapholi, N.O., Marufu, M.C., Maiwashe, A., Banga, C.B., Muchenje, V. *et al.* (2014) Towards a genomics approach to tick (Acari: Ixodidae) control in cattle: A review. *Ticks and Tick-Borne Diseases* 5, 475–483. DOI: 10.1016/j.ttbdis.2014.04.006.

Marczinke, B.I. and Nichol, S.T. (2002) Nairobi sheep disease virus, an important tick-borne pathogen of sheep and goats in Africa, is also present in Asia. *Virology* 303, 146–151. DOI: 10.1006/viro.2002.1514.

Marendy, D., Baker, K., Emery, D., Rolls, P. and Stutchbury, R. (2019) *Haemaphysalis longicornis*: The life-cycle on dogs and cattle, with confirmation of its vector status for *Theileria orientalis* in Australia. *Veterinary Parasitology* 3, 100022. DOI: 10.1016/j.vpoa.2019.100022.

Maritz, C., Louw, A.I., Gothe, R. and Neitz, A.W.H. (2000) Detection and micro-scale isolation of a low molecular mass paralysis toxin from the tick, *Argas (persicargas) walkerae*. *Experimental & Applied Acarology* 24, 615–630.

Maritz, C., Louw, A.I., Gothe, R. and Neitz, A.W.H. (2001) Neuropathogenic properties of *Argas* (*Persicargas*) *walkerae* larval homogenates. *Comparative Biochemistry and Physiology Part A* 128, 233–239.

Martello, E., Mannelli, A., Ragagli, C., Ambrogi, C., Selmi, M. *et al.* (2014) Range expansion of *Ixodes ricinus* to higher altitude, and co-infestation of small rodents with *Dermacentor marginatus* in the Northern Apennines, Italy. *Ticks and Tick-Borne Diseases* 5/6, 970–974. DOI: 10.1016/j.ttbdis.2014.07.021.

Maruyama, S.R., Anatriello, E., Anderson, J.M., Ribeiro, J.M., Brandão, L.G. *et al.* (2010) The expression of genes coding for distinct types of glycine-rich proteins varies according to the biology of three metastriate ticks, *Rhipicephalus* (boophilus) *microplus*, *Rhipicephalus sanguineus* and *Amblyomma cajennense*. *BMC Genomics* 11, 363. Available at: http://www.biomedcentral.com/1471-2164/11/363 (accessed 18 December 2024).

Masina, S. (1999) The sequence, expression and immunological characterisation of the HT-1 neurotoxin from the Australian paralysis tick ixodes holocyclus. PhD thesis, University of Technology, Sydney, Australia.

Mateos-Hernández, L., Villar, M., Moral, A., GarcíaRodríguez, C., Arias, T.A. *et al.* (2017) Tick–host conflict: Immunoglobulin E antibodies to tick proteins in patients with anaphylaxis to tick bite. *Oncotarget* 8/13, 20630–20644.

Mateos-Hernández, L., Obregón, D., Maye, J., Borneres, J., Versille, N. *et al.* (2020) Anti-tick microbiota vaccine impacts *Ixodes ricinus* performance during feeding. *Vaccines* 8/4, 702. DOI: 10.3390/vaccines8040702.

Mathews-Martin, L., Gonzalez, G., Dheilly, N.M., Amaral-Moraes, R., Dumarest, M. *et al.* (2024) Exposure of cattle to tick-borne encephalitis virus in the historical endemic zone in north-eastern France. *BMC Veterinary Research* 20, 228. DOI: 10.1186/s12917-024-04079-8.

Matthee, S., Meltzer, D.G.A. and Horak, I.G. (1997) Sites of attachment and density assessment of ixodid ticks (Acari: Ixodidae) on impala (*Aepyceros melampus*). *Experimental & Applied Acarology* 21, 179–192.

Michel, A.L. and Bengis, R.G. (2012) The African buffalo: A villain for inter-species spread of infectious diseases in southern Africa. *Onderstepoort Journal of Veterinary Research* 79/2, 453. DOI: 10.4102/ojvr.v79i2.453.

Monti, F., Baratti, M., Viviano, A. and Mori, E. (2023) Ticks in the box: *Argas persicus* occurrence in nest boxes of secondary cavity-nesting bird species in Italy. *European Journal of Wildlife Research* 69, 23. DOI: 10.1007/s10344-023-01656-4.

Moradi-Asl, E. and Jafari, S. (2020) The habitat suitability model for the potential distribution of *Ornithodoros tholozani* (Laboulbène et Mégnin, 1882) and *Ornithodoros lahorensis* (Neumann, 1908) (Acari: Argasidae): the main vectors of tick-borne relapsing fever in Iran. *Annals of Parasitology* 66/3, 357–363. DOI: 10.17420/ap6603.274.

Mount, G.A. and Dunn, J.E. (1983) Economic thresholds for lone star ticks (Acari: Ixodidae) in recreational areas based on a relationship between CO_2 and human subject sampling. *Journal of Economic Entomology* 76/2, 327–329.

Murgia, M.V., Bell-Sakyi, L., de La Fuente, J., Kurtti, T.J., Makepeace, B.L. *et al.* (2019) Meeting the challenge of tick-borne disease control: a proposal for 1000 *Ixodes* genomes. *Ticks and Tick-Borne Diseases* 10/1, 213–218. DOI: 10.1016/j.ttbdis.2018.08.009.

Muto, M., Bazartseren, B., Tsevel, B., Dashzevge, E., Yoshii, K. *et al.* (2015) Isolation and characterization of tick-borne encephalitis virus from *Ixodes persulcatus* in Mongolia in 2012. *Ticks and Tick-Borne Diseases* 6/5, 623–629. DOI: 10.1016/j.ttbdis.2015.05.006.

Nana, P., Maniania, N.K., Maranga, R.O., Kutima, H.L., Boga, H.I. *et al.* (2010) Attraction response of adult *Rhipicephalus appendiculatus* and *Rhipicephalus pulchellus* ticks to extracts from *Calpurnia aurea*. *Veterinary Parasitology* 174/1-2, 124–130. DOI: 10.1016/j.vetpar.2010.08.016.

Naudé, T.W., Heyne, H., Van der Merwe, I.R. and Benic, M.J. (2001) Spinose ear tick, *Otobius megnini* (Dugès, 1884) as the cause of an incident of painful otitis externa in humans. *Journal of the South African Veterinary Association* 72/1, 118–119.

Nava, S., Mangold, A.J. and Guglielmone, A.A. (2008) Aspects of the life cycle of *Amblyomma parvum* (Acari: Ixodidae) under natural conditions. *Veterinary Parasitology* 156, 270–276. DOI: 10.1016/j.vetpar.2008.05.029.

Nava, S., Mangold, A.J. and Guglielmone, A.A. (2009) Field and laboratory studies in a neotropical population of the spinose ear tick, *Otobius megnini*. *Medical and Veterinary Entomology* 23/1, 1–5. DOI: 10.1111/j.1365-2915.2008.00761.x.

Ndhlovu, D.N., Makaya, P.V. and Penzhorn, B.L. (2009) Tick infestation, and udder and teat damage in selected cattle herds of Matabeleland South, Zimbabwe. *Onderstepoort Journal of Veterinary Research* 76, 235–248.

Neitz, A.W.H., Howell, C.J. and Potgieter, D.J.J. (1969) Purification of a toxic component in the oral secretion of the sand tampan *Ornithodoros savignyi* Audouin (1827). *Journal of the South African Chemical Institute* 22, S142–S149.

Neitz, W.O. (1954) *Hyalomma transiens* schulze: A vector of sweating sickness. *Journal of the South African Veterinary Medical Association* 25/1, 19–20.

Nene, V., Lee, D., Kang'a, S., Skilton, R., Shah, T. *et al.* (2004) Genes transcribed in the salivary glands of female *Rhipicephalus appendiculatus* ticks infected with *Theileria parva*. *Insect Biochemistry and Molecular Biology* 34/10, 1117–1128. DOI: 10.1016/j.ibmb.2004.07.002.

Nevill, E.M. (1964) The role of carbon dioxide as stimulant and attractant to the sand tampan, *Ornithodoros savignyi* (Audouin). *Onderstepoort Journal of Veterinary Research* 31, 59.

Noll, M., Wall, R., Makepeace, B.L., Newbury, H., Adaszek, L. *et al.* (2023) Predicting the distribution of *Ixodes ricinus* and *Dermacentor reticulatus* in Europe: A comparison of climate niche modelling approaches. *Parasites & Vectors* 16/1, 384. DOI: 10.1186/s13071-023-05959-y.

Norval, R.A.I. (1974) Copulation and feeding in males of *Ixodes pilosus* Koch 1844 (Acarina: Ixodidae). *Journal of the Entomological Society of Southern Africa* 37/1, 129–133.

Norval, R.A.I., Butler, J.F. and Yunker, C.E. (1989) Use of carbon dioxide and natural or synthetic aggregation-attachment pheromone of the bont tick, *Amblyomma hebraeum*, to attract and trap unfed adults in the field. *Experimental & Applied Acarology* 7, 171–180.

Norval, R.A.I., Perry, B.D., Meltzer, M.I., Kruska, R.L. and Booth, T.H. (1994) Factors affecting the distributions of the ticks *Amblyomma hebraeum* and *A. variegatum* in Zimbabwe: Implications of reduced acaricide usage. *Experimental & Applied Acarology* 18, 383–407.

Numan, M., Alouffi, A., Almutairi, M.M., Tanaka, T., Ahmed, H. *et al.* (2023) First detection of *Theileria sinensis*-like and *Anaplasma capra* in *Ixodes kashmiricus*: With notes on cox1-based phylogenetic position and new locality records. *Animals* 13, 3232. DOI: 10.3390/ani13203232.

Nuttall, G.H.F. (1915) Artificial parthenogenesis in ticks. *Parasitology* 7/4, 457–461. DOI: 10.1017/S0031182000009811.

Nuttall, P.A., Paesen, G.C., Lawrie, C.H. and Wang, H. (2000) Vector–host interactions in disease transmission. *Journal of Molecular Microbiology and Biotechnology* 2/4, 381–386.

Nyangiwe, N. and Horak, I.G. (2007) Goats as alternative hosts of cattle ticks. *Onderstepoort Journal of Veterinary Research* 74, 1–7.

Oliver, J.H. (1971) Parthenogenesis in mites and ticks (Arachnida: Acari). *American Zoologist* 11, 283–299.

Oliver, J.H., Hayes, M.P., Keirans, J.E. and Lavender, D.R. (1993) Establishment of the foreign parthenogenetic tick *Amblyomma rotundatum* (Acari: Ixodidae) in Florida. *Journal of Parasitology* 79/5, 786–790. DOI: 10.2307/3283624.

Ostfeld, R.S., Price, A., Hornbostel, V.L., Benjamin, M.A. and Keesing, F. (2006) Controlling ticks and tick-borne zoonoses with biological and chemical agents. *BioScience* 56/5, 383–394.

Pacheco, I., Mera, I.G.F., Brito, F.F., Torrijos, E.G., Villar, M. *et al.* (2021) Characterization of the anti-α-Gal antibody profile in association with Guillain–Barré syndrome, implications for tick-related allergic reactions. *Ticks and Tick-Borne Diseases* 12, 101651. DOI: 10.1016/j.ttbdis.2021.101651.

Padula, A.M. (2016) Tick paralysis of animals in Australia. In: Gopalakrishnakone, P., Faiz, S.M.A., Gnanathasan, C.A., Habib, A.G., Fernando, R. *et al.* (eds) *Clinical Toxinology in Asia Pacific and Africa*. Springer, Dordrecht, Netherlands. DOI: 10.1007/978-94-007-6288-6_65-1.

Padula, A.M., Leister, E.M. and Webster, R.A. (2020) Tick paralysis in dogs and cats in Australia: Treatment and prevention deliverables from 100 years of research. *Australian Veterinary Journal* 98/1-2, 53–59. DOI: 10.1111/avj.12891.

Pal, U., Yang, X., Chen, M., Bockenstedt, L.K., Anderson, J.F. *et al.* (2004) OspC facilitates *Borrelia burgdorferi* invasion of *Ixodes scapularis* salivary glands. *Journal of Clinical Investigation* 113/2, 220–230. DOI: 10.1172/jci200419894.

Panizza, M.M., Cutullé, C., Primo, M.E., Morel, N., Sebastian, P.S. *et al.* (2022) Assays to evaluate the transovarial transmission of *Anaplasma marginale* by *Rhipicephalus microplus*. *Veterinary Parasitology* 311, 109808. DOI: 10.1016/j.vetpar.2022.109808.

Papadopoulos, B., Morel, P.C. and Aeschlimann, A. (1996) Ticks of domestic animals in the Macedonia region of Greece. *Veterinary Parasitology* 63/1-2, 25–40.

Pegram, R.G. (1976) Ticks (Acarina, Ixodoidea) of the northern regions of the Somali Democratic republic. *Bulletin of Entomological Research* 66/2, 345–363. DOI: 10.1017/S000748530000674X.

Pereira, A., Figueira, L., Nunes, M., Esteves, A., Cotão, A.J. *et al.* (2017) Multiple Phlebovirus (Bunyaviridae) genetic groups detected in *Rhipicephalus*, *Hyalomma* and *Dermacentor* ticks from southern Portugal. *Ticks and Tick-Borne Diseases* 8, 45–52. DOI: 10.1016/j.ttbdis.2016.09.015.

Perkins, I.D. (1987) Use of insecticides to control screw-worm fly strike by *Chrysomya bezziana* in cattle. *Australian Veterinary Journal* 64/1, 17–20. DOI: 10.1111/j.1751-0813.1987.tb06050.x.

Peter, R.J., Van den Bossche, P., Penzhorn, B.L. and Sharp, B. (2005) Tick, fly, and mosquito control – Lessons from the past, solutions for the future. *Veterinary Parasitology* 132/3–4, 205–215. DOI: 10.1016/j.vetpar.2005.07.004.

Pham, M., Underwood, J. and Oliva Chávez, A.S. (2021) Changing the recipe: Pathogen directed changes in tick saliva components. *International Journal of Environmental Research and Public Health* 18, 1806. DOI: 10.3390/ijerph18041806.

Phipps, L.P., Hernández-Triana, L.M., Goharriz, H., Welchman, D. and Johnson, N. (2016) Detection of *Theileria luwenshuni* in sheep from Great Britain. *Parasites & Vectors* 9/1, 203. DOI: 10.1186/s13071-016-1486-5.

Pienaar, R., Neitz, A.W.H. and Mans, B.J. (2018) Tick paralysis: Solving an enigma. *Veterinary Sciences* 5/2, 53. DOI: 10.3390/vetsci5020053.

Probst, J., Springer, A., Fingerle, V. and Strube, C. (2024) Frequency of *Anaplasma phagocytophilum*, *Borrelia* spp., and coinfections in *Ixodes ricinus* ticks collected from dogs and cats in Germany. *Parasites & Vectors* 17, 87. DOI: 10.1186/s13071-024-06193-w.

Qui, Z.-X., Li, Y., Li, M.M., Wang, W.Y., Zhang, T.T. *et al.* (2020) Investigation of three enzymes and their roles in the embryonic development of parthenogenetic *Haemaphysalis longicornis*. *Parasites & Vectors* 13/1, 46. DOI: 10.1186/s13071-020-3916-7.

Rafinejad, J., Choubdar, N., Oshaghi, M.A., Piazak, N., Satvat, T. *et al.* (2011) Detection of *Borrelia persica* infection in *Ornithodoros tholozani* using PCR targeting *rrs* gene and xenodiagnosis. *Iranian Journal of Public Health* 40/4, 138–145.

Rahajarison, P., Arimanana, A.H., Raliniaina, M. and Stachurski, F. (2014) Survival and moulting of *Amblyomma variegatum* nymphs under cold conditions of the Malagasy highlands. *Infection, Genetics and Evolution* 28, 666–675. DOI: 10.1016/j.meegid.2014.06.022.

Rechav, Y. (1991) Some aspects of the life cycle of the tick *Ixodes pilosus* under laboratory conditions. *Journal of the South African Veterinary Association* 62/1, 15–16.

Reid, H.W. and Chianini, F. (2007) Louping-ill. In: Aitken, I.D. (ed.) *Diseases of Sheep*. Blackwell Publishing, Oxford, pp. 250–255.

Rodriguez, M.S.M., Kaier, K., Hehne, M. and Borde, J.P. (2020) Knowledge, habits and attitudes towards TBE and other tick-borne diseases in German forestry trainees. *Ticks and Tick-Borne Diseases* 11, 101307. DOI: 10.1016/j.ttbdis.2019.101307.

Rodriguez-Valle, M., Moolhuijzen, P., Barrero, R.A., Ong, C.T., Busch, G. *et al.* (2018) Transcriptome and toxin family analysis of the paralysis tick, *Ixodes holocyclus*. *International Journal for Parasitology* 48, 71–82. DOI: 10.1016/j.ijpara.2017.07.007.

Rodriguez-Vivas, R.I., Jonsson, N.N. and Bhushan, C. (2020) Strategies for the control of *Rhipicephalus microplus* ticks in a world of conventional acaricide and macrocyclic lactone resistance. *Parasitology Research* 117/1, 3–29. DOI: 10.1007/s00436-017-5677-6.

Rollins, R.E., Margos, G., Brachmann, A., Krebs, S., Mouchet, A. *et al.* (2023) German *Ixodes inopinatus* samples may not actually represent this tick species. *International Journal for Parasitology* 53/13, 751–761. DOI: 10.1016/j.ijpara.2023.06.007.

Rouby, S.R., Hussein, K.H., Aboelhadid, S.M. and El-Sherif, A.M. (2017) Role of *Rhipicephalus annulatus* tick in transmission of lumpy skin disease virus in naturally infected cattle in Egypt. *Advances in Animal and Veterinary Sciences* 5/4, 185–191. DOI: 10.17582/journal.aavs/2017/5.4.185.191.

Rudakov, N., Samoylenko, I., Shtrek, S., Igolkina, Y., Rar, V. *et al.* (2019) A fatal case of tick-borne Rickettsiosis caused by mixed *Rickettsia sibirica* subsp. *sibirica* and 'Candidatus Rickettsia tarasevichiae' infection in Russia. *Ticks and Tick-Borne Diseases* 10/6, 101278. DOI: 10.1016/j.ttbdis.2019.101278.

Rudolf, I., Vojtíšek, J., Kejíková, R., Šikutová, S., Mendel, J. *et al.* (2021) Probable overwintering of adult *Hyalomma rufipes* in central Europe. *Ticks and Tick-Borne Diseases* 12/4, 101718. DOI: 10.1016/j.ttbdis.2021.101718.

Saleem, M.Z., Akhtar, R., Aslam, A. and Rashid, M.I. (2019) Histopathological investigation of skin and hides damage of small and large ruminants due to naturally infested ticks. *Tropical Biomedicine* 36(4), 1081–1086.

Sanogo, Y.O., Zeaiter, Z., Caruso, G., Merola, F., Shpynov, S. *et al.* (2003) *Bartonella henselae* in *Ixodes ricinus Ticks* (Acari: Ixodida) removed from humans, Belluno Province, Italy. *Emerging Infectious Diseases* 9/3, 329–332.

Schnittger, L., Yin, H., Gubbels, M.J., Beyer, D., Niemann, S. *et al.* (2003) Phylogeny of sheep and goat *Theileria* and *Babesia* parasites. *Parasitology Research* 91/5, 398–406. DOI: 10.1007/s00436-003-0979-2.

Schroder, B., Uys, A.C. and Reilly, B.K. (2006) A survey of free-living ixodid ticks on a commercial game farm in the Thabazimbi district, Limpopo Province, South Africa. *Journal of the South African Veterinary Association* 77/3, 141–144.

Schröder, J. (1980) Cattle ticks from the Waterberg district of the Transvaal. *Journal of the South African Veterinary Association* 51/1, 27–30.

Schröder, J. (2023) *Apicomplexa in Livestock*. CAB International, Wallingford, UK.

Schutze, G.E. (2000) Diagnosis and treatment of *Bartonella henselae* infections. *Concise Reviews of Pediatric Infectious Diseases* December 1185–1187.

Senanayake, S.N., Paparini, A., Latimer, M., Andriolo, K., Dasilva, A.J. *et al.* (2012) *Medical Journal of Australia* 196/5, 350–352. DOI: 10.5694/mja11.11378.

Short, N.J., Floyd, R.B., Norval, R.A.I. and Sutherst, R.W. (1989) Survival and behaviour of unfed stages of the ticks *Rhipicephalus appendiculatus*, *Boophilus decoloratus* and *B. microplus* under field conditions in Zimbabwe. *Experimental & Applied Acarology* 6, 215–236.

Sivakumar, T., Tuvshintulga, B., Otgonsuren, D., Batmagnai, E., Ahedor, B. *et al.* (2022) Phylogenetic analyses of the mitochondrial, plastid, and nuclear genes of *Babesia* sp. Mymensingh and its naming as *Babesia naoakii n. sp. Parasites and Vectors* 15, 299. DOI: 10.1186/s13071-022-05374-9.

Sloupenska, K., Dolezilkova, J., Koubkova, B., Hutyrova, B., Racansky, M. *et al.* (2021) Seroprevalence of antibodies against tick-borne pathogens in czech patients with suspected post-treatment lyme disease syndrome. *Microorganisms* 9, 2217. DOI: 10.3390/microorganisms9112217.

Snowball, G.J. (1957) Ecological observations on the cattle tick, *Boophilus microplus* (Canestrini). *Australian Journal of Agricultural Research* 8/4, 394–413.

Sonenshine, D.E., Allan, S.A., Peter, T.F., McDaniel, R. and Burridge, M.J. (2000) Does geographic range affect the attractant-aggregation-attachment pheromone of the tropical bont tick. *Amblyomma Variegatum? Experimental & Applied Acarology* 24, 283–299.

Spernovasilis, N., Markaki, I., Papadakis, M., Mazonakis, N. and Ierodiakonou, D. (2021) Mediterranean spotted fever: Current knowledge and recent advances. *Tropical Medicine and Infectious Diseases* 6, 172. DOI: 10.3390/tropicalmed6040172.

Spickett, A.M. and Heyne, H. (1988) A survey of Karoo tick paralysis in South Africa. *Onderstepoort Journal of Veterinary Research* 55, 89–92.

Spickett, A.M., De Klerk, D., Enslin, C.B. and Scholtz, M.M. (1989a) Resistance of Nguni, Bonsmara and Hereford cattle to ticks in a Bushveld region of South Africa. *Onderstepoort Journal of Veterinary Research* 56, 245–250.

Spickett, A.M., Elliott, E.G.R., Heyne, H. and Neser, J.A. (1989b) Paralysis of laboratory rabbits by nymphae of *Ixodes rubicundus*, Neumann 1904 (Acarina: Ixodidae) and some effects on the life-cycle following feeding under different temperature conditions. *Onderstepoort Journal of Veterinary Research* 56, 59–62.

Spickett, A.M., Horak, I.G., Niekerk, A. and Braack, L.E.O. (1992) The effect of veld-burning on the seasonal abundance of free-living ixodid ticks as determined by drag sampling. *Onderstepoort Journal of Veterinary Research* 59, 285–292.

Stampa, S. (1959) Tick paralysis in the Karoo areas of South Africa. *Onderstepoort Journal of Veterinary Research* 28/2, 169–227.

Stachurski, F. (2000) Invasion of West African cattle by the tick *Amblyomma variegatum*. *Medical and Veterinary Entomology* 14, 391–399.

Stampa, S. and Du Toit, R. (1958) Paralysis of stock due to the Karoo paralysis tick (*Ixodes rubicundus* Neu). *South African Journal of Science September* 241–246.

Stanbury, J.B. and Huyck, J.H. (1945) Tick paralysis: A critical review. *Medicine* 24/3, 129–242.

Steen, N.A., Barker, S.C. and Alewood, P.F. (2006) Proteins in the saliva of the Ixodida (ticks): Pharmacological features and biological significance. *Toxicon* 47/1, 1–20. DOI: 10.1016/j.toxicon.2005.09.010.

Stockman, S. (1916) Louping-ill. *Journal of Comparative Pathology and Therapeutics* 29, 244–264.

Stokowski, M. and Allen, D. (2024) IxPopDyMod: An R package to write, run, and analyze tick population and infection dynamics models. *Parasites & Vectors* 17, 90. DOI: 10.1186/s13071-024-06171-2.

Strydom, T., Lavan, R.P., Torres, S. and Heaney, K. (2023) The economic impact of parasitism from nematodes, trematodes and ticks on beef cattle production. *Animals* 13, 1599. DOI: 10.3390/ani13101599.

Stutzer, C., Mans, B.J., Gaspar, A.R.M., Neitz, A.W.H. and Maritz-Olivier, C. (2009) *Ornithodoros savignyi*: Soft tick apyrase belongs to the 5'-nucleotidase family. *Experimental Parasitology* 122, 318–327. DOI: 10.1016/j.exppara.2009.04.007.

Sugimoto, C. and Fujisaki, K. (2001) Non-transforming *Theileria* parasites of ruminants. In: Dobbelaere, D.A.E. and McKeever, D. (eds) *World Class Parasites. Vol. 3. Theileria*. Theileria. Springer Science+Business Media, New York, pp. 93–106.

Suppan, J., Engel, B., Marchetti-Deschmann, M. and Nürnberger, S. (2018) Tick attachment cement – reviewing the mysteries of a biological skin plug system. *Biological Reviews Cambridge Philosophical Society* 93/2, 1056–1076. DOI: 10.1111/brv.12384.

Sutherst, R.W. (1985) The role of models in tick control. *Australian Veterinary Journal* 62/11, 32–37.

Sutherst, R.W. and Bourne, A.S. (1991) Development, survival, fecundity and behaviour of *Haemaphysalis* (Kaiseriana) *longicornis* (*Ixodidae*) at two locations in southeast Queensland. *International Journal for Parasitology* 21/6, 661–672. DOI: 10.1016/0020-7519(91)90077-K.

Sutherst, R.W. and Maywald, G.F. (1985) A computerised system for matching climates in ecology. *Agriculture, Ecosystems and Environment* 13, 281–299.

Sutherst, R.W., Dallwitz, M.J., Utech, K.B.W. and Kerr, J.D. (1978) Aspects of host finding by the cattle tick *Boophilus microplus*. *Australian Journal of Zoology* 26, 159–174. DOI: 10.1071/ZO9780159.

Swanepoel, A. (1959) Tick paralysis: Regional neurological involvement caused by *Hyalomma truncatum*. *South African Medical Journal* 33/44, 909–911.

Tadesse, F., Abadfaji, G., Girma, S., Kumsa, B. and Jibat, T. (2012) Identification of tick species and their preferred site on cattle's body in and around Mizan Teferi, Southwestern Ethiopia. *Journal of Veterinary Medicine and Animal Health* 4/1, 1–5. DOI: https://doi.org10.5897/JVMAH11.039.

Tatchell, R.J. (1987) Interactions between ticks and their hosts. *International Journal for Parasitology* 17/2, 597–606. DOI: 10.1016/0020-7519(87)90136-6.

Telford, S.R. and Wormser, G.P. (2010) *Bartonella* spp. transmission by ticks not established. *Emerging Infectious Diseases* 16/3, 379–384. DOI: 10.3201/eid1603.090443.

Teo, E.J., Vial, M.N., Hailu, S., Kelava, S., Zalucki, M.P. *et al*. (2021) Climatic requirements of the eastern paralysis tick, *Ixodes holocyclus*, with a consideration of its possible geographic range up to 2090. *International Journal for Parasitology* 51/4, 241–249. DOI: 10.1016/j.ijpara.2020.08.011.

Theiler, G. (1950) Zoological survey of the Union of South Africa. Tick survey-part VI. *Onderstepoort Journal of Veterinary Science and Animal Industry* 24/1-2, 37–52.

Thomas, A.D. (1950) Skin necrosis in dogs caused by the bontpoot tick (*Hyalomma aegyptium*). *Journal of the South African Veterinary Medical Association* 21/3, 114–116.

Tian, Z., Liu, G., Yin, H., Luo, J., Guan, G. *et al*. (2013) Discrimination between ovine *Babesia* and *Theileria* species in China based on the ribosomal protein S8 (RPS8) gene. *Veterinary Parasitology* 197/1–2, 354–359. DOI: 10.1016/j.vetpar.2013.04.033.

Todd, J.L. (1914) Tick paralysis. *Journal of Parasitology* 1/2, 55–64.

Tuppurainen, E.S., Stoltsz, W.H., Troskie, M., Wallace, D.B., Oura, C.A.L. *et al*. (2011) A potential role for ixodid (hard) tick vectors in the transmission of lumpy skin disease virus in cattle. *Transboundary and Emerging Diseases* 58/2, 93–104.

Tuppurainen, E.S., Lubinga, J.C., Stoltsz, W.H., Troskie, M., Carpenter, S.T. *et al*. (2013a) Evidence of vertical transmission of lumpy skin disease virus in *Rhipicephalus decoloratus* ticks. *Ticks and Tick-Borne Diseases* 4, 329–333. DOI: 10.1016/j.ttbdis.2013.01.006.

Tuppurainen, E.S.M., Lubinga, J.C., Stoltsz, W.H., Troskie, M., Carpenter, S.T. *et al*. (2013b) Mechanical transmission of lumpy skin disease virus by *Rhipicephalus appendiculatus* male ticks. *Epidemiology & Infection* 141/2, 425–430. DOI: 10.1017/S0950268812000805.

Uilenberg, G. (1992) Veterinary significance of ticks and tick-borne diseases. In: Fivaz, B., Petney, T. and Horak, I. (eds) *Tick Vector Biology*. Medical and Veterinary Aspects Springer, Heidelberg, pp. 23–33.

Uilenberg, G. (1999) Immunization against diseases caused by *Theileria parva*: A review. *Tropical Medicine and International Health* 4/9, A12–A20.

Uilenberg, G., Hoogstraal, H. and Klein, J.M. (1979) Les tiques (Ixodoidea) de Madagascar et leur rôle vecteur. *Archives de l' Lnstitut Pasteur de Madagascar, Numéro Spécial* 154 pp.

Uilenberg, G., Gray, J. and Kahl, O. (2018) Research on Piroplasmorida and other tick-borne agents: Are we going the right way? *Ticks and Tick-Borne Diseases* 9/4, 860–863. DOI: 10.1016/j.ttbdis.2018.03.005.

Umemiya-Shirafuji, R., Galay, R.L., Maeda, H., Kawano, S., Tanaka, T. *et al.* (2014) Expression analysis of autophagy-related genes in the hard tick *Haemaphysalis longicornis*. *Veterinary Parasitology* 201/1-2, 169–175. DOI: 10.1016/j.vetpar.2014.01.024.

Urquhart, G.M., Armour, J., Duncan, J.L., Dunn, A.M. and Jennings, F.W. (1996) *Veterinary parasitology*, 2nd edn. Blackwell Science, Oxford.

Uys, A.C., Horak, I.G. and Harrison, A. (2015) Questing ixodid ticks on the vegetation of sable antelope and multi-herbivore enclosures in Thabazimbi. *Journal of the South African Veterinary Association* 86/1, 1243. Available at: DOI: 10.4102/jsava.v86i1.1243.

van Nunen, S. (2014) Galactose-alpha-1,3-galactose, mammalian meat and anaphylaxis: A world-wide phenomenon? *Current Treatment Options in Allergy* 1, 262–277. DOI: 10.1007/s40521-014-0022-0.

van Nunen, S. (2015) Tick-induced allergies: Mammalian meat allergy, tick anaphylaxis and their significance. *Asia Pacific Allergy* 5, 3–16. DOI: 10.5415/apallergy.2015.5.1.3.

van Nunen, S.A., O'Connor, K.S., Clarke, L.R., Boyle, R.X. and Fernando, S.L. (2009) An association between tick bite reactions and red meat allergy in humans. *Medical Journal of Australia* 190, 510–511.

Vechtova, P., Fussy, Z., Cegan, R., Sterba, J., Erhart, J. *et al.* (2020) Catalogue of stage-specific transcripts in *Ixodes ricinus* and their potential functions during the tick life-cycle. *Parasites & Vectors* 13/1, 311. DOI: 10.1186/s13071-020-04173-4.

Viljoen, G.J., Bezuidenhout, J.D., Oberem, P.T., Vermeulen, N.M., Visser, L. *et al.* (1986) Isolation of a neurotoxin from the salivary glands of female *Rhipicephalus evertsi evertsi*. *Journal of Parasitology* 72/6, 865–874. Available at: https://www.jstor.org/stable/3281836 (accessed 18 December 2024).

Viljoen, G.J., Van Wyngaardt, S., Gothe, R., Visser, L., Bezuidenhout, J.D. *et al.* (1990) The detection and isolation of a paralysis toxin present in *Argas* (*Persicargas*) *walkerae*. *Onderstepoort Journal of Veterinary Research* 57, 163–168.

Walker, A.R. (2011) Eradication and control of livestock ticks: Biological, economic and social perspectives. *Parasitology* 138, 945–959.

Walker, J.B. and Olwage, A. (1987) The tick vectors of *Cowdria ruminantium* (Ixodoidea, Ixodidae, genus *Amblyomma*) and their distribution. *Onderstepoort Journal of Veterinary Research* 54, 353–379.

Walker, J.B. (1990) Two new species of ticks from southern Africa whose adults parasitize the feet of ungulates: *Rhipicephalus lounsburyi* n. sp., and *Rhipicephalus neumanni* n. sp. (Ixodoidea, ixodidae). *Onderstepoort Journal of Veterinary Research* 57, 57–75.

Walker, J.G., Klein, E.Y. and Levin, S.A. (2014) Disease at the wildlife–livestock interface: Acaricide use on domestic cattle does not prevent transmission of a tick-borne pathogen with multiple hosts. *Veterinary Parasitology* 199/3-4, 206–214. DOI: 10.1016/j.vetpar.2013.11.008.

Wang, J., Chai, Y., Yang, J., Chen, K., Liu, G. *et al.* (2024) Insight into *Hyalomma anatolicum* biology by comparative genomics analyses. *International Journal for Parasitology* 54/3-4, 157–170. DOI: 10.1016/j.ijpara.2023.09.003.

Webster, R.A., Mackie, J.T. and Haskins, S.C. (2013a) Histopathological changes in the lungs from dogs with tick paralysis: 25 cases (2010–2012). *Australian Veterinary Journal* 91/8, 306–311. DOI: 10.1111/avj.12085.

Webster, R.A., Mills, P.C. and Morton, J.M. (2013b) Indications, durations and outcomes of mechanical ventilation in dogs and cats with tick paralysis caused by *Ixodes holocyclus*: 61 cases (2008–2011). *Australian Veterinary Journal* 91/6, 233–239. DOI: 10.1111/avj.12061.

Wechtaisong, W., Bonnet, S.I., Lien, Y.-Y., Chuang, S.-T. and Tsai, Y.-L. (2020) Transmission of *Bartonella henselae* within *Rhipicephalus sanguineus*: Data on the potential vector role of the tick. *PLoS Neglected Tropical Diseases* 14/10, e0008664. DOI: 10.1371/journal.pntd.0008664.

Wilkinson, P.J., Pegram, R.G., Perry, B.D., Lemche, J. and Schels, H.F. (1988) The distribution of African swine fever virus isolated from *Ornithodoros moubata* in Zambia. *Epidemiology and Infection* 101/3, 547–564. DOI: 10.1017/s0950268800029423.

Wilkinson, P.R. (1953) Observations on the sensory physiology and behaviour of larvae of the cattle tick *Boophilus microplus* (can.) (Ixodidae). *Australian Journal of Zoology* 1, 345–356.

Wojan, C., Thrasher, T., Lacey, E. and Clay, K. (2022) Distribution, dynamics, and diversity of questing ticks in the lower midwest. *Journal of Medical Entomology* 59/1, 273–282. DOI: 10.1093/jme/tjab155.

Wright, C.L., Gaff, H.D., Sonenshine, D.E. and Hynes, W.L. (2015) Experimental vertical transmission of *Rickettsia parkeri* in the Gulf Coast tick, *Amblyomma maculatum*. *Ticks and Tick-Borne Diseases* 6, 568–573. DOI: 10.1016/j.ttbdis.2015.04.011.

Wu-Chuang, A., Hodzic, A., Mateos-Hernandez, L., Estrada-Pena, A., Obregon, D. *et al*. (2021) Current debates and advances in tick microbiome research. *Current Research in Parasitology & Vector-Borne Diseases* 1, 100036. DOI: 10.1016/j.crpvbd.2021.100036.

Yin, H., Luo, J., Schnittger, L., Lu, B., Beyer, D. *et al*. (2004) Phylogenetic analysis of *Theileria* species transmitted by *Haemaphysalis qinghaiensis*. *Parasitology Research* 92, 36–42.

Yin, H., Schnittger, L., Luo, J., Seitzer, U. and Ahmed, J.S. (2007) Ovine theileriosis in China: A new look at an old story. *Parasitology Research* 101/S2, 191–195. DOI: 10.1007/s00436-007-0689-2.

Yu, Z.-J., Lu, Y.-L., Yang, X.-L., Chen, J., Wang, H. *et al*. (2014) Cold hardiness and biochemical response to low temperature of the unfed bush tick *Haemaphysalis longicornis* (Acari: Ixodidae). *Parasites & Vectors* 7, 346.

Zintl, A., Mulcahy, G., Skerrett, H.E., Taylor, S.M. and Gray, J.S. (2003) *Babesia divergens*, a bovine blood parasite of veterinary and zoonotic importance. *Clinical Microbiology Reviews* 16/4, 622–636. DOI: 10.1128/CMR.16.4.622-636.2003.

2 Threats to Tick Survival

Abstract

The number of parasitic ticks a host can carry, without its productive and reproductive homeostasis being compromised, is a balance between the tick's reproductive and reinfestation rate, a variety of external factors that can curtail tick survival, and the host's resistance. Hosts play some role in keeping their tick burdens under control by preening and self-grooming. Insectivorous birds such as oxpeckers derive much of their diet from ticks on animals and contribute to moderating tick numbers on a variety of ungulates. Entomo-/acaripathogenic fungi, nematodes and wasps can reduce tick numbers. Some pasture fodder species are reported to suppress tick counts on cattle. Free-living ticks run the risk of predation by ground-dwelling insects, birds and small mammals. The most immediate and dramatic impact on tick numbers on domestic animals thus far has been attributable to the use of chemicals.

'Once the female [tick] has copulated, she climbs with her full count of eight legs to the tip of a protruding branch of any shrub in order either to fall onto small mammals who run by underneath or to let herself be brushed off the branch by larger ones. The eyeless creature finds the way to its lookout with the help of a general sensitivity to light in the skin. The blind and deaf bandit becomes aware of the approach of its prey through the sense of smell. The odour of butyric acid, which is given off by the skin glands of all mammals, gives the tick the signal to leave its watch post and leap off. If it then falls onto something warm – which its fine sense of temperature will tell it – then it has reached its prey, the warm-blooded animal, and needs only use its sense of touch to find a spot as free of hair as possible in order to bore past its own head into the skin tissue of the prey. Now, the tick pumps a stream of warm blood slowly into itself' (Von Uexküll, 1934).

Jakob von Uexküll was a philosopher, with a few misconceptions about a tick's anatomy and life history. But he was clearly fascinated by the concept of a tick population existing as a community within its own environment, having to contend with its own demands for clement weather, a sustainable food supply and a healthy symbiotic microbiome (Brentari, 2015). He would no doubt have been intrigued by reports of maternal behaviour in some soft tick species, such as female egg brooding until hatching or the carrying of larvae to the host, to assist in feeding (Pienaar *et al.*, 2018).

Ticks are no exception to an association with microbiota. In this instance, they modulate arthropod reproductive fitness, survival and vector competence (Narasimhan and Fikrig, 2015; Wu-Chuang *et al.*, 2021). Ticks have been said to coexist with pathogens, endosymbionts and commensal bacteria in an ecological unit referred to as a holobiont (Wu-Chuang *et al.*, 2022).

The balanced coexistence of host and parasite relies on the equilibrium between the parasite's demands and impost on its hosts and the hosts' capacity to cater for these demands without compromising productive and reproductive efficiency, all within a favourable environment that allows this equilibrium to exist. It is a balance between host defences limiting the parasite and the ability of the parasite to modulate, evade or restrict the host response (Tatchell, 1987; Willadsen *et al.*, 1993; Wikel *et al.*, 1994).

Without human intervention, several naturally-occurring phenomena threaten tick survival and can lead to fluctuations in the sizes of their free-living and parasitic populations. Anthropogenic impacts on tick populations can be both chemical and non-chemical.

DOI: 10.1079/9781800625761.0002

2.1 Some Non-chemical Impacts on Ticks

Ticks have to contend with a number of acaripathogenic organisms. Tick innate immunity relies on a variety of small molecules and phagocytosis of invading microbes. The viral, bacterial and protozoal pathogens that ticks transmit (see previous chapter) have to evade these humoral and cellular immune responses to complete their successful transition from midgut to haemolymph, salivary glands or ovaries (Hajdušek *et al.*, 2013).

2.1.1 Preening/grooming

Mammals display a diversity of behaviours concerned with care of the body surface, assigned terms such as grooming or preening. This behaviour can be directed at the animal's own body ('autogrooming'), or that of conspecifics ('allogrooming'), when it forms part of the regulation of social relationships (Spruijt *et al.*, 1992). Host grooming is stimulated by the itch sensation elicited by immunological modulators induced by tick antigens introduced into the skin. It is an important factor in reducing tick burden (Wikel, 1996).

Small antelope groom more frequently than large antelope, which may account for their carrying fewer adult ticks (Gallivan and Horak, 1997). Angora goats are more diligent groomers than Merino sheep (Fourie and Kok, 1992). The impact of self-grooming on tick numbers on cattle is demonstrated easily and dramatically, for example by keeping donor cattle in head stanchions for tick breeding purposes (Schröder 1981–1984, unpublished observations). Cattle with induced infestations of [*B. microplus*] *R. australis* and restrained in harnesses yielded more than three times as many engorged adult female ticks as unharnessed cattle allowed to lick themselves (Snowball, 1956). Cattle showing the greatest increase in tick yield after restraint from grooming were deemed to have been the most 'resistant' (Bennett, 1969), when they were possibly simply more efficient at grooming.

Early domestication and preindustrial animal husbandry would possibly have included manual grooming and removal of visible ticks by stockowners and herders.

2.1.2 Insectivorous birds

Preening, seen as the first line of defence against ectoparasites on birds, makes beak morphology critically important. Altering beak morphology by experimental trimming can lead to a dramatic increase in feather mite numbers on rock pigeons (Clayton *et al.*, 2005). But insectivorous birds do not only preen themselves.

Red-billed oxpeckers (*Buphagus erythrorhynchus*) enjoyed research interest in southern Africa during the last two decades of the previous century when it was realized that they consume roughly their own bodyweight in ixodid ticks from 21 ungulate host species daily (Stutterheim, 1981), examples of which can be seen in Fig. 2.1. This roughly coincided with the appearance of pyrethroid chemicals as cattle acaricides, which were seen to be more 'bird friendly' than the previous more indiscriminately toxic chemicals they were replacing (Stutterheim, 1982). There were great expectations of increasing numbers of oxpeckers on cattle farms using pyrethroid dips, but it was found that oxpecker behaviour on cattle was different and not necessarily to the host's benefit. Oxpeckers on cattle observed in Zimbabwe preferred feeding on blood from open wounds (Weeks, 1999).

Other birds reported to pick ticks from ungulate hosts include black-billed magpies (*Pica pica*), scrub jays (*Aphelocoma coerulescens*) and Galapagos finches (*Geospiza fuliginosa*) (Cooksey and Davey, 1987).

2.1.3 Bushfire

Large tracts of land on different continents burn with such regularity that it is difficult to understand how free-living populations of ticks can survive. There are numerous mentions of the effect of fire but much of it appears to be anecdotal. In southern Africa, it was presumed that veld fires may kill vast numbers of ticks directly, but that there might also be an indirect effect on tick survival by the removal of sheltering plant

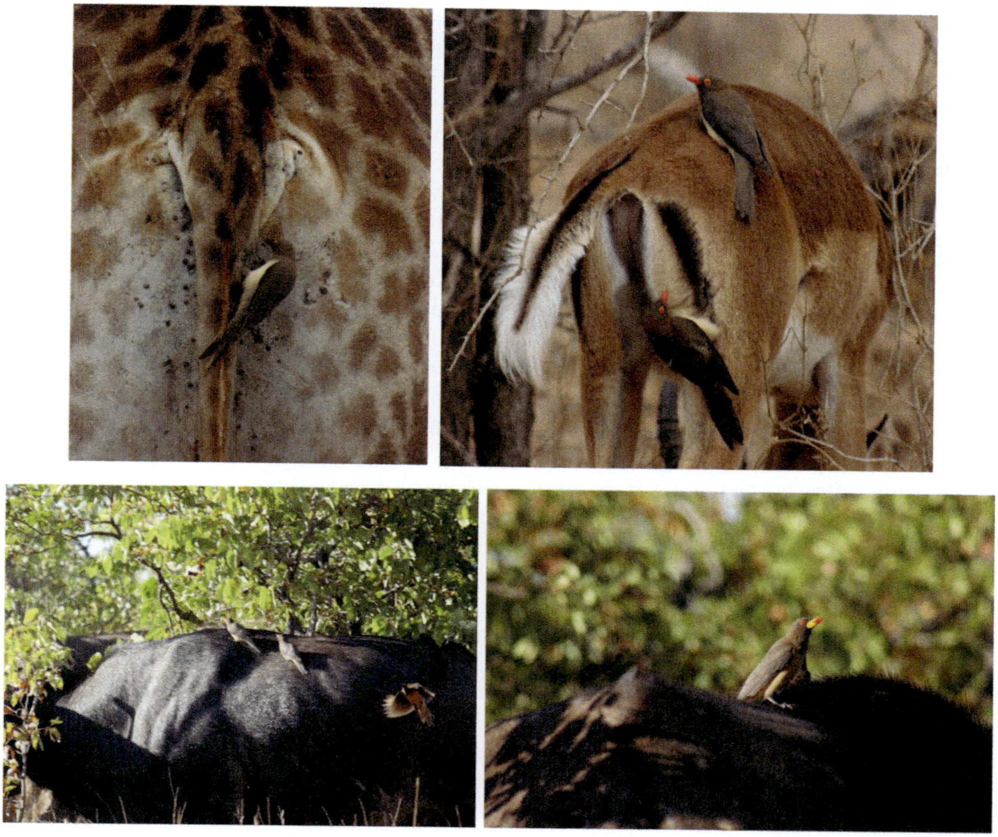

Fig. 2.1. Red-billed oxpeckers (*Buphagus erythrorynchus*) feeding on ticks on (clockwise from top left) giraffe (*Giraffa camelopardus*), impala (*Aepyceros melampus*) and African buffalo (*Syncerus caffer*). Kruger National Park, South Africa. Photos courtesy of Johann Schröder.

material (Stampa and du Toit, 1958; Stampa, 1959; Trollope, 2011; Nieman *et al.*, 2021). In the Ngorongoro Crater and Serengeti grasslands of Tanzania, the prevalence of ticks is high when the grass sward is in a moribund and unacceptable condition for grazing livestock and the grass fuel load exceeds 4000 kg/ha. Maasai communal pastoralists controlled these grasslands by burning (Trollope, 2011). Bushfires lit to find wildfowl in Benin are considered to kill immature ticks in the environment (Adinci *et al.*, 2018).

A number of scientific investigations have shown that bushfire does reduce the numbers of collectable ticks in the environment but that this reduction is temporary (Horak *et al.*, 2006). In Africa, tick abundance was demonstrated to decline for up to 3 years after a fire (Nieman *et al.*, 2021).

Ticks were collected monthly over a period of 2 years in an experiment using a collection method that favoured larvae, in two adjacent areas of the same habitat in the Kruger National Park of South Africa. One area was burnt in September, before the experiment began, and the other was left unburnt. Thirteen tick species were collected and while ten species were more numerous in the unburnt zone, three were more numerous in the burnt zone. Numbers of [*B.*] *Rhipicephalus decoloratus* declined sharply in the burnt zone but increased equally rapidly within 4 months after the fire. There were monthly fluctuations in the numbers of recovered ticks but paired analysis showed no significant difference between the burnt and unburnt zones. Significantly fewer larvae of *Rhipicephalus appendiculatus* were recovered from the burnt zone but there was no significant difference in the numbers of nymphs of the same species collected from the two zones. *R. appendiculatus* adults were not collected from the burnt zone until 7 months after the burn had taken place.

The conclusion was that the temporary and generally short-lived reduction in tick populations after the fire indicated that there was little practical benefit from veld burning in spring as a method of tick control. The unexpectedly quick rebound of some tick numbers after fire could have been due to hatching of tick eggs at ground level that survived the fire, or an influx of tick-infested hosts, attracted by the green sprouting vegetation (Spickett *et al.*, 1992).

2.1.4 Habitat manipulation

Pasture spelling is one of the simplest methods of reducing tick numbers. It deprives questing ticks of a blood meal, with larvae of the oligoxenic species, e.g. *R. annulatus*, *R. decoloratus*, *R. microplus*, being more vulnerable than the unfed nymphs and adults of multihost ticks (Walker, 2011). Dividing a paddock in two and grazing the two halves alternately reduced cattle tick infestation by >90% compared to a similar herd that was set-stocked in an experiment that lasted 18 months (Wilkinson, 1964).

Free-living ticks vary in their ability to survive without a bloodmeal (unfed *Amblyomma hebraeum* larvae, kept in an incubator at 28°C and 70–80% RH, remained responsive to CO_2 for at least 2 years – Schröder 1981–1984, unpublished observations), but keeping cattle away from a paddock will not eradicate the ticks while alternate hosts are available (Laws and Manning, 1910; Laws, 1911; Spickett, 1987).

A system of rotational grazing was investigated in New Caledonia, exploiting natural fluctuations in tick abundance. Cattle were shifted to a new paddock in the afternoon, about 3 weeks after arrival, relying on the fact that engorged adult female *R. microplus* had dropped off earlier that morning. The new paddock had been rested for ca. 45–75 days, depending on the season, allowing the majority of larvae to die off. Based on visual appraisal of the tick burden, the need for acaricidal treatment was reduced by 70.9–82.9% over 2 years (Hüe and Fontfreyde, 2019).

Another form of habitat manipulation is the removal of vegetation cover providing refuge for free-living ticks. Guided by early observations of the preferred habitat and intermediate hosts of *I. rubicundus* (Stampa and du Toit, 1958), Fourie and Kok (1992) and Fourie *et al.* (1996), in an elegant series of experiments, demonstrated that disrupting the natural habitat could reduce the occurrence of Karoo paralysis. The disruptive methods consisted of removing long grass by coarse grazers such as cattle and horses before sheep were introduced to infested paddocks, and relying on Angora goats to browse the undersides of the wild olive trees (*Olea europaea africana*) on the south-facing hillsides which the ticks and their intermediate hosts (scrub hares [*Lepus saxatilis*] and elephant shrews [*Elephantulus* spp.]) normally favour (see Fig. 2.2). A variety of other wild animals serve to sustain *I. rubicundus* in the absence of sheep (Horak *et al.*, 1987).

Removal of invasive honeysuckle from eastern North American forests reduced the number of white-tailed deer (*Odocoileus virginianus*) favouring this habitat, thus reducing the risk of bites from *Amblyomma americanum* infected with *Ehrlichia* spp. (Allan *et al.*, 2010).

A contrary observation was an increase in the population of white-footed mice infested with *I. scapularis* and infected with *Borrelia burgdorferi* as a result of forest fragmentation in New York state in the USA. In this situation, small forest patches favour the mice and increase the risk of tick-borne Lyme disease (Allan *et al.*, 2003).

2.1.5 Acaripathogenic nematodes

Non-parasitic ticks are prone to infestation with ground-dwelling entomopathogenic nematodes. *Heterorhabditis* spp. are regarded as more virulent than *Steinernema* spp. but they seem to be less abundant (Bhat *et al.*, 2023).

Ticks' vulnerability to this infestation seems to vary between tick species and the life cycle stage at the time of infestation. Unfed female [*B.*] *R. annulatus* died sooner than unfed males, that died sooner than engorged females, after *in*

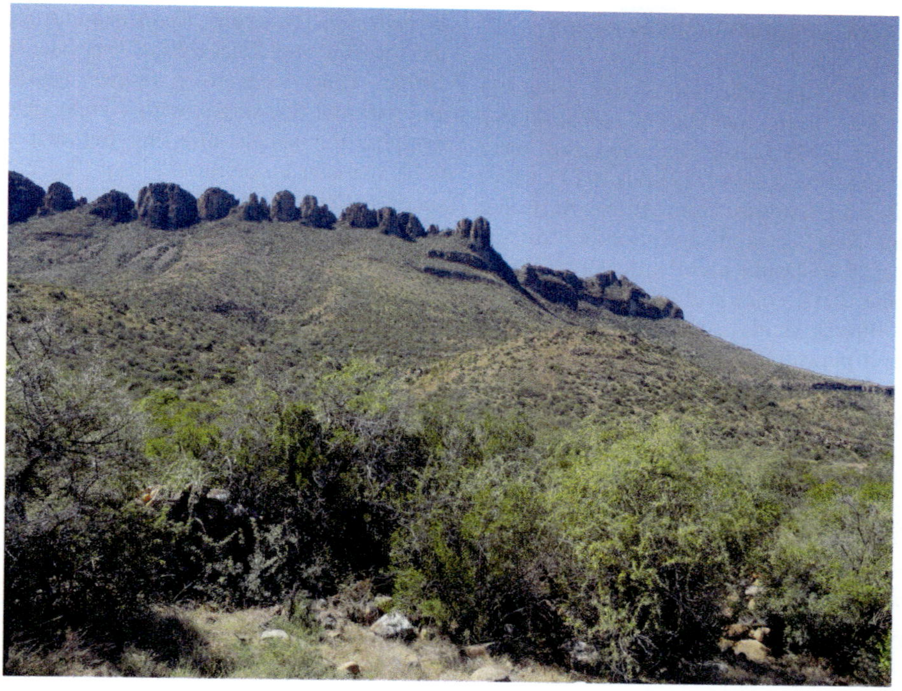

Fig. 2.2. 'Little Teeth Mountain' [Afrikaans: 'Tandjiesberg'] near Graaff Reinet in the area where Stampa did his research on the Karoo paralysis tick. The south-facing slopes of these mountains and hillocks are the preferred habitat for *I. rubicundus*. With acknowledgement of the gracious hospitality of Dr and Mrs M.D. MacFarlane. Photo courtesy of Johann Schröder.

vitro exposure to infestation with *Steinernema carpocapsae*, *Heterorhabditis bacteriophora* and *Heterorhabditis* sp. The nematodes had been reared in final instars of the wax moth *Galleria mellonella*. In the same experiment, replete female *Hyalomma excavatum*, *Rhipicephalus bursa* and *Rhipicephalus sanguineus* took slightly longer to die.

The practical application of this knowledge is as yet unclear but in theory, spraying soil with infective juvenile nematodes where engorged ticks are known to drop off their hosts, in defined ecological niches where nematodes will survive, could serve to reduce the number of females progressing to egg laying (Samish *et al.*, 2000a, b). Engorged female *R. microplus* were released in grassy field plots seeded with cadavers of *Tenebrio molitor* (mealworm beetle) colonised with *H. bacteriophora* 1 week earlier. The numbers of larvae collected from apical grass samples were reduced by up to 73.1% 9 weeks after release of the ticks (Filgueiras *et al.*, 2023).

Although not yet commercialized for ticks, entomopathogenic nematodes are used for controlling insect pests in forests and agricultural and horticultural applications. The nematode infestation is lethal to ticks because of the release of symbiotic bacteria from the nematode microbiome. A number of argasid and ixodid tick species have been shown to be susceptible to nematode infestation (Kocan *et al.*, 1998a, b; Samish and Glazer, 2001; Bhat *et al.*, 2023).

In vitro experiments with engorged female [*B.*] *R. annulatus* assessed nematodes for their 'virulence' according to the exposure time to mortality and the number of nematodes penetrating the ticks. Heterorhabditid isolates were more lethal than steinernematids (Glazer *et al.*, 2001). Unsurprisingly, this host–parasite relationship is also profoundly affected by environmental factors – in this case, factors such as soil type and moisture (Alekseev *et al.*, 2006).

Table 2.1 lists some of the tick species evaluated for their vulnerability to these nematodes.

2.1.6 Acaripathogenic wasps

The first recorded collection of tick parasitoid wasps was from nymphs of *Rhipicephalus sanguineus* in North America, when they were named *Hunterellus hookeri* (Wood, 1911). Other records have stemmed from Africa, Australia, Europe, New Zealand and South America (Fiedler, 1953; Daube and Heath, 1975; Heath and Cane, 2010; Lopes *et al.*, 2012; Ramos *et al.*, 2015; Buczek *et al.*, 2021). There are other genera of parasitoid wasps, but those parasitizing ticks have since been assigned to the genus *Ixodiphagus* and have been found in *Amblyomma, Dermacentor, Hyalomma, Haemaphysalis, Ixodes, Ornithodoros* and *Rhipicephalus* spp. (Hu *et al.*, 1998). They seem to parasitize free-living and parasitic tick stages, with a preference for nymphs, the female inserting her ovipositor to lay her eggs inside the tick host (Fig. 2.3). A survey in Kenya found that 50% of *A. variegatum* nymphs collected from cattle were infested with *I. hookeri* (Mwangi *et al.*, 1994).

The wasp larvae consume the engorged tick's internal organs and emerge as adults 30–57 days after ovipositioning (Ramos *et al.*, 2015, 2023). Much of parasitoid wasp life history still needs to be unravelled, such as the

Table 2.1. Entomopathogenic nematodes killing ticks (author's work).

Tick species	Nematode species	Author
[tb]Dermacentor variabilis	*Steinernema feltiae, S. riobravus*	Kocan *et al.*, 1998b
Rhipicephalus sanguineus	*Steinernema feltiae, S. riobravus*	
Amblyomma maculatum	*S. riobravus*	
Amblyomma cajennense	*S. riobravus*	
Amblyomma americanum	*S. riobravus*	
[B.] Rhipicephalus annulatus	*Steinernema carpocapsae*	Samish *et al.*, 2000b
Hyalomma excavatum	*Heterorhabditis bacteriophora*	
Rhipicephalus bursa	*Heterorhabditis* sp.	
Rhipicephalus sanguineus		
Amblyomma variegatum	*S. carpocapsae*	Samish and Glazer, 2001
[B.] Rhipicephalus decoloratus	*S. riobrave* [sic]	
Hyalomma dromedarii	*Steinernema* sp.	
Ixodes scapularis	*Heterorhabditis megidlis*	
Rhipicephalus appendiculatus	*S. riobrave* [sic]	
Rhipicephalus evertsi	*S. carpocapsae*	
Argas persicus	*Heterorhabditis bacteriophora*	
Ornithodoros moubata	*S. carpocapsae*	
Ornithodoros tholozani	*S. carpocapsae*	
[B.] Rhipicephalus annulatus	*Heterorhabditis bacteriophora*	Glazer *et al.*, 2001
	Heterorhabditis sp.	
	Steinernema carpocapsae	
	Steinernema feltiae	
	Steinernema glaseri	
	Steinernema riobrave	
Ixodes ricinus	*Steinernema carpocapsae*	Hartelt *et al.*, 2008
	Steinernema feltiae	
	Heterorhabditis bacteriophora	

role of *Wolbachia* endosymbionts discovered in *I. hookeri*, indications that *I. hookeri* eggs might overwinter in unfed nymphs of *I. ricinus*, and the possibility that wasp species might have tick species preferences (Ramos *et al.*, 2023). The significance of the detection of *Arsenophonus nasionae*, the male-killing endosymbiont bacterium originally described in the wasp *Nasiona vitripennis*, in *I. hookeri* and parasitized engorged *I. ricinus* nymphs (but not in unparasitized *I. ricinus*) is still to be elucidated (Bohacsova *et al.*, 2016).

A variety of tick species was collected by blanket dragging in southern Italy, but only the *I. ricinus* specimens were found to be infested, and at a low rate, possibly because this collection method favours unfed ticks (Ramos *et al.*, 2015). *I. hookeri* is the most studied but at least ten species in the genus have been described. Attempts to control ticks in the field using this parasitoid have mostly been unsuccessful, but in a small-scale field study, 150,000 *I. hookeri* released over 1 year in a pasture harbouring a small cattle herd reduced the number of *A. variegatum* ticks per animal (Ramos *et al.*, 2023).

In a recent Slovakian study, unfed nymphs of *Haemaphysalis concinna* and *I. ricinus* collected from vegetation during April, May and June were allowed to feed on rabbits. Significant numbers of both tick species yielded *I. hookeri* wasps after the nymphs had become engorged, with the infestation having no apparent effect on the duration of nymph feeding, prior to their demise (Buczek *et al.*, 2021).

Early attempts to rear parasitoid wasps were unsuccessful (Wood, 1911). Deploying them to control ticks will no doubt require consideration of their respective environmental, climatic and host species and density requirements, optimal release methods and numbers, seasonal factors and behaviour (Lopes *et al.*, 2012; Ramos *et al.*, 2023).

2.1.7 Dysbiosis

Arthropods are no exception to the metazoan partnership with a consortium of commensal, symbiotic and pathogenic microorganisms to enhance their health and survival. This microbiome is composed not only of bacteria, but also Archaea, viruses, protozoa, fungi and nematodes. They occur in different parts of the tick's body but the gut microbiota are of special interest, as this is the site of the first encounter between the tick and an incoming pathogen (Narasimhan and Fikrig, 2015). Most argasid and ixodid ticks harbour bacterial endosymbionts. They are transmitted transovarially and are found in unfed tick larvae. Based on their ultrastructure, they have been identified as wolbachiae or rickettsiae, and are closely related to bacterial pathogens transmitted by ticks. They

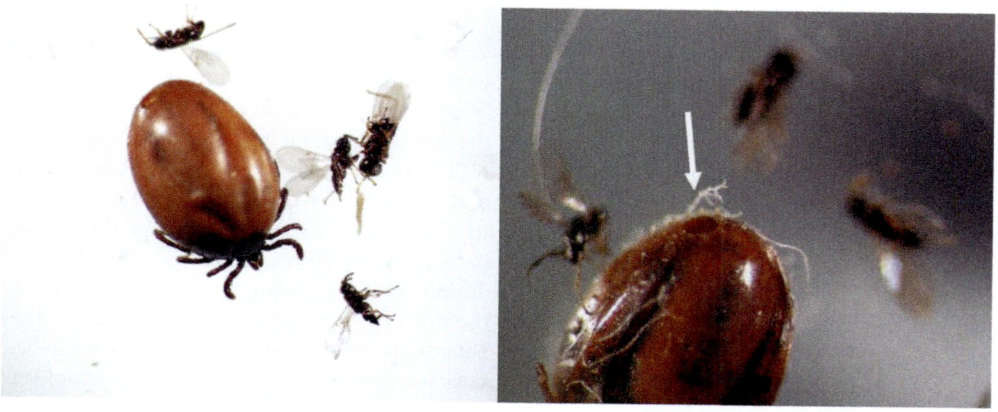

Fig. 2.3. *Ixodes ricinus* nymph with endoparasitoid wasps *Ixodiphagus hookeri* (arrow indicating the aperture in the tick cuticle through which the *I. hookeri* specimens emerged). From Buczek *et al.* (2021) under Creative Commons Attribution 4.0 International License.

were considered to be unrelated to the *Wolbachia* spp. found in insects (Noda *et al.*, 1997).

Symbionts in hard ticks can be obligate, providing the host with essential nutrients for survival, or required for reproductive fitness, or facultative, conferring a broader variety of benefits (Liu *et al.*, 2016). Moulting from one stage to the next is associated with a decline in bacterial diversity (Estrada-Peña and Cabezas-Cruz, 2019).

In what is described as the first culture-independent molecular survey of the bacteriome of *R. microplus*, 121 symbiotic and potentially pathogenic bacterial genera were identified in eggs and adult ticks. PCR amplification of the 16S rRNA gene was followed by pyrosequencing of the amplicons. The ticks were not disinfected prior to DNA extraction, meaning that some of the identified bacteria were probably environmental contaminants (Andreotti *et al.*, 2011). The microbiome of *I. scapularis* was shown by taxa contribution analysis to be highly redundant, with up to 198 bacterial taxa contributing to one functional pathway (Estrada-Peña *et al.*, 2020).

Phylogenetic studies revealed the complexity of *Wolbachia* spp. taxonomy and uncertainty about their role (Hartelt *et al.*, 2003). Depending on the *Wolbachia* strain and arthropod host species, they act as commensalistic or parasitic symbionts (Tijsse-Klasen *et al.*, 2011) and new impacts are regularly discovered, such as altered reproduction, immune response and vector competence (Plantard *et al.*, 2012; Moutailler *et al.*, 2016). The possibility of negative impacts of *Wolbachia* infection on tick survival requires closer scrutiny (Madhav *et al.*, 2020).

Wolbachia infection of *I. ricinus* in The Netherlands has been associated with infestation by the tick parasitoid *Ixodiphagus hookeri* (see section 2.1.8) but other sources of infection might also exist (Tijisse-Klasen *et al.*, 2011), such as coinfestation by filarial nematodes in *A. americanum* (Zhang *et al.*, 2011). The assertion that *Wolbachia pipientis* infection of *I. ricinus* is due to parasitism by *I. hookeri* (Plantard *et al.*, 2012) may need further investigation. *Wolbachia* isolates from mosquitoes and fleas have been grown successfully in cell lines from *I. scapularis*, *I. ricinus* and *R. microplus* (Khoo *et al.*, 2020).

The microbial community of *Hyalomma lusitanicum* in Spain was found to be characterized by an abundance of *Francisella*-like endosymbionts, but the mechanisms underlying this relationship are still to be explored (Díaz-Sánchez *et al.*, 2021).

A number of factors, which include ecology, host characteristics and interactions between microbes, influence the composition of a microbiome (Aivelo *et al.*, 2019). Ticks regulate their own microbiome with their immune system and are vulnerable to a disturbance, known as dysbiosis (Narasimhan and Fikrig, 2015; Budachetri *et al.*, 2016; Dall'Agnol *et al.*, 2021; A. Cabezas-Cruz, Matanzas, Cuba, 2022, personal communication). This disturbance can be caused by, for example, a vectored pathogen (Bonnet *et al.*, 2017; Budachetri *et al.*, 2017; Adegoke *et al.*, 2020; Hamilton *et al.*, 2021), by paratransgenesis, the transgenic manipulation of arthropod vector microbiota or by transfection, for example with *Wolbachia* (Ratcliffe *et al.*, 2022). Antibiotic treatment of the host can disturb tick–microbiota homeostasis, decreasing tick fitness and affecting tick–pathogen interactions (Purnell *et al.*, 1989; Zhong *et al.*, 2007; Wu-Chuang *et al.*, 2022). An immune reaction against key members of the bacterial community of the tick microbiome by host antibodies can cause microbial dysbiosis, with consequences for tick physiology and vector competence (Mateos-Hernández *et al.*, 2020; Wu-Chuang *et al.*, 2022; see section 5.3, this volume).

2.1.8 Bacteria, viruses and fungi

Ticks encounter many potential microbial and viral pathogens during both the parasitic and free-living phases of their life cycles. Pathogens they transmit to their hosts must traverse the gut wall to reach the haemolymph, salivary gland and/or ovaries for the transmission to succeed. In addition, ticks can also be infected by other pathogens (to them), acquired coincidentally during the bloodmeal or from close contact with the microbiota of the host skin. To counter the potentially harmful effects of these infections, ticks have an immune system which is not yet fully understood. It has been shown to contain signalling pathways, antimicrobial peptides, complement-like molecules and regulated cell death (Fogaça *et al.*, 2021).

Bacillus thuringiensis (Bt)

The study of molecular biology has revolutionized much of biological science, from taxonomical identification and classification of living organisms to disease diagnosis, unravelling of life cycles and host–parasite relationships, drug and vaccine development, and forensic medicine, to name but a few.

First discovered in dead silkworms (*Bombyx mori*) in Japan in 1901 and named 'Sottokin' (sudden death), *Bt* was again discovered in Mediterranean flour moths (*Anagasta kuehniella*) in 1915 in the German province of Thüringia (Sanchis, 2011; Sansinenea, 2012) and commercialized as 'Sporéine' in 1938 (Sanchis, 2011). The discovery of a Gram-positive bacterium that produces insecticidal toxins was remarkable in itself, but the ability to clone the *Bt* insecticidal crystal protein gene in 1981 (Palma *et al.*, 2014), and to splice it into a plant's genome, opened the door to unimaginable possibilities. *Bt* cotton was released in the United States and Australia in the late 1990s (Heckel, 2020). *Bt*-based products are considered to be the most successful microbial insecticides to date. *Bt* produces different kinds of proteins with demonstrated toxicity to a wide range of insect orders and mites (Bel *et al.*, 2020).

During sporulation, *Bt* produces a crystalline inclusion which dissolves in the midgut after ingestion by insects, releasing δ-endotoxins (and cytolytic toxins in some isolates) that disrupt epithelium integrity, leading to insect death (Gill *et al.*, 1992; Aronson and Shai, 2001; Bravo *et al.*, 2007). The toxin binds to membrane-bound proteins on the surface of midgut epithelial cells, creating small pores in the membrane, enabling cations and water to flow through, causing the cells to swell and lyse (Bravo *et al.*, 2011; Heckel, 2020). In addition to the crystalline (Cry) proteins, *Bt* also produces surface layer proteins (SLP), vegetative insecticidal toxins (VIP) and secreted insecticidal proteins (SIP) (Mendoza-Almanza *et al.*, 2020; Syed *et al.*, 2020). Variation in the Cry toxin amino acid sequence affects their mechanism of action and can be the result of either spontaneous or directed mutation (Vilchez, 2020). There is also evidence that *Bt* might disrupt vector immunity by causing dysbiosis in the gut microbiota (Li *et al.*, 2020a). *Bt* Cry toxins address different receptors in the midgut of the host insect and *Bt* resistance is linked to loss of the specific receptor for that toxin (Li *et al.*, 2020b).

With this mode of action in mind, it is difficult to imagine how *Bt* could be applied to obligate vertebrate blood-feeding ectoparasites. This point is acknowledged in the case of ticks (Solanke and Narladkar, 2018), but *Bt* has evidently been used successfully against insect pathogen vectors such as *Simulium damnosum* (*Onchocerca volvulus*), *Anopheles* spp. (*Plasmodium* spp.) and *Aedes aegypti* (Dengue fever) (Bravo *et al.*, 2007) and acarines such as mites (Bel *et al.*, 2020).

The effect of *Bt* on several tick species has been evaluated experimentally. Serial dilutions of three commercial strains of *Bt* (*kurstaki* – Dipel 2x®; *israelensis* – Vectobac®; *thuringiensis* – HD703) were applied *in vitro* to engorged and unfed adult *A. persicus* and *H. dromedarii*, at different intervals after ovipositioning, and to batches of newly laid eggs of both species. The strains varied in their lethal potency and were more effective against *A. persicus* than against *H. dromedarii*. Their effect on egg hatchability was comparable and diminished over time (Hassanain *et al.*, 1997).

Rabbits were infested with unfed adult *Hyalomma dromedarii* inside ear bags and sprayed twice 3–5 days later with a commercial formulation of *B. t.* var. *kurstaki*. Detached engorged female ticks were incubated and their ovipositioning and egg hatching observed. This treatment evidently reduced the number of ticks completing their engorgement, but the numbers were too small for an efficacy % calculation, and egg production and hatchability were not recorded (El-Kelesh and El-Refali, 2006).

The hypothetical postingestion fate of *Bt* endotoxins in ticks was studied with intrahaemocoelic injections of *B. t. thuringiensis* H14 δ-endotoxin into engorged female *H. dromedarii*. This produced a dose- and time-dependent response, characterized by death of up to 46.7% of the ticks by 48 hours, and destruction of the haemolymph granular cells due to cell membrane damage (Habeeb and El-Hag, 2008).

Four strains of *Bt* were tested *in vitro* against a multiresistant isolate of *R. microplus* by the engorged adult female immersion method (EAFIM). Exposed ticks were incubated and assessed for up to 20 days for survival and egg production and hatchability. The four strains caused 79–91% tick mortality and significant reductions in egg production and hatchability, but were not significantly different from each other. Ingress of the toxin via the spiracles or genital pore is surmised (Fernández-Ruvalcaba *et al.*, 2010) but was evidently not investigated.

Questing (unfed) adult *I. ricinus* and *Dermacentor reticulatus* were collected from vegetation, immersed for 3 min in different concentrations of four environmental isolates and one commercial strain (*israelensis*) of *Bt*, and observed for mortality over 3 weeks. The strains varied in their potency between tick species and genders. The LC_{50} of the most pathogenic field isolate were 10^6 cfu/ml and 10^{11} cfu/ml for male *D. reticulatus* and female *I. ricinus*, respectively. No lethal effect was observed for the *B. t. israelensis* strain in this experiment (Szczepanska *et al.*, 2018).

In addition to the insecticidal Cry protein produced in small quantities during the sporulation phase, some *Bt* strains also produce SLPs in the vegetative phase, secreted in the bacterial growth medium, enabling mass production (Lormendez *et al.*, 2019; Syed *et al.*, 2020). A *Bt* SLP was first discovered to be insecticidal when tested against the Mexican bean beetle, *Epilachna varivestis* (Peña *et al.*, 2006). Engorged female *R. microplus* were immersed for 5 min in SLP concentrations from 50 to 300 µg/ml, incubated and observed after 14 days for mortality, ovipositioning and egg hatchability. The highest concentration killed 75% of the ticks by 14 days, and the LC_{50} was calculated to be 69.7 µg/ml. The effect on ovipositioning was modest, but all concentrations reduced egg hatchability by more than 80% (Lormendez *et al.*, 2019). The practical applicability of this discovery for livestock tick control remains to be seen.

Acaripathogenic bacteria

The origin or collection of the ticks is not described, but 21 ticks of five species ([*B.*] *R. decoloratus*, *I. holocyclus*, *Amblyomma trigutatum*, *H. longicornis* and *Aponomma fimbriatum*) were washed in disinfectant before being crushed with a mortar and pestle in a 0.5% tryptone solution. Serial dilutions of this suspension were spread on three different growth media and the bacteria cultured. DNA was extracted from the 153 bacterial isolates, PCR performed on the small subunit ribosomal RNA (rRNA) and the amplicons sequenced. Some of the bacteria were considered to have biopesticide potential (Murrell *et al.*, 2003).

The intriguing possibility that the resident microbiome in the healthy bovine haircoat might include organisms potentially useful in curbing tick infestation was investigated in the Probio-TICK initiative of the Australian Government Collaborative Research Centres Project funding scheme. A hand-held vacuum cleaner was used to collect samples off the backs and flanks of 1743 cattle on 25 farms in north-eastern Australia. Extracted DNA was subject to PCR amplification of the 16S rRNA gene, and the amplicons sequenced. Environmental factors (geographic location, solar radiation, rainfall) influenced the microbiome community structure, which was unique for each herd, but several bacterial phyla and families were shared between herds.

Skin probiotic products to ameliorate tick infestations on cattle are under development (Gamage *et al.*, 2022).

Acaripathogenic viruses

Thousands of entomopathogenic viruses have been identified (Harish *et al.*, 2021), but only about 15 of them have been developed commercially for use on crops. Viral biopesticides constituted less than 0.5% of the global pesticide market in 2018 and they all seemed to target insect pests (Smagghe *et al.*, 2023). Baculoviruses (nuclear polyhedrosis viruses) are specific insect pathogens (Assenga *et al.*, 2006). They are not contact active, and often require extended infection periods to kill their host. They have been used as microbial insecticides since the 1970s (Little *et al.*, 2019).

After the discovery of virus-like particles in salivary gland cells of [*B.*] *R. microplus* and mention of the potential role of viruses pathogenic to ticks for biological control (Megaw, 1978), little more seemed to occur until about 20 years later, when it was said that either viruses do not play a role in reducing tick populations or that too little was known about their effect (Samish and Rehacek, 1999), and that only a few virus diseases are known in mites

(Van der Geest *et al.*, 2000), another group of acarine parasites.

There are multiple insect genes encoding chitinase, a moulting enzyme, differentially expressed during development in various insect tissues (Merzendorfer, 2013). After ecdysis, moulting fluid is either resorbed or ingested to avoid inappropriate exposure of the new developing layers of chitin (Arakane and Muthukrishnan, 2009). Chitinases have been used for insect pest control, either in transgenic plants or in genetically modified (GM) entomopathogenic viruses, or expressed and applied directly (Kramer and Muthukrishnan, 1997; Arakane and Muthukrishnan, 2009). Baculoviruses grown in insect cell cultures (so-called 'baculovirus expression vector system' – BEVS) (Druzinec *et al.*, 2013) is one of the expression methods for recombinant proteins, to be used either as antigens in vaccines or in biological pest control.

Ticks also express chitinolytic enzymes subsequent to the end of an instar, to remove old cuticle and allow synthesis of new cuticle for continued growth and development (You *et al.*, 2003).

In 2003, the first report of an insect baculovirus infection in ticks was published. In these experiments, recombinant baculoviruses, constructed to express *H. longicornis* chitinase, were used to infect tick larvae to lethal effect (You *et al.*, 2003). A recombinant baculovirus expressing *H. longicornis* chitinase was lethal to nymphal ticks. This effect could be synergized by the addition of chitinase expressed separately, and mixing the recombinant virus with flumethrin could halve the required dose of this pyrethroid acaricide (Assenga *et al.*, 2006).

Acaripathogenic fungi

A number of entomopathogenic fungi, of which *Metarhizium* and *Beauveria* are the two best-known genera, have also been found to be harmful to ticks. Fungal spores (conidia) germinate on the cuticle of a susceptible arthropod and produce germ tubes which penetrate the body cavity, where the fungus proliferates as hyphae, eventually killing the host (Driver *et al.*, 2000), as shown in Fig. 2.4. Laboratory studies with *Metarhizium anisopliae* and *Beauveria bassiana* against [*B. microplus*] *R. australis* (Leemon, 2009, 2011; Murigu *et al.*, 2016) and *R. microplus* (Bernardo *et al.*, 2018) yielded encouraging results. Fungal spores suspended in oil were more effective than aqueous formulations. *M. anisopliae* outperformed *B. bassiana* when applied to eggs, larvae and engorged adult female *R. microplus* under laboratory conditions in Brazil (Camargo *et al.*, 2012). Different strains of *M. anisopliae* and *B. bassiana* were tested *in vitro* against fed and unfed larvae and nymphs of *I. ricinus* (Hartelt *et al.*, 2008).

However, without some anthropogenic enhancement of ticks' exposure to these fungi (e.g. application of the fungi in large quantities to the host's haircoat), it seems unlikely that this will ever be a significant natural factor in keeping tick numbers in check. Efficacy in pen and field studies in Australia and Kenya was variable (Leemon and Jonsson, 2008; Leemon, 2011, 2012; Murigu *et al.*, 2016; Murigu and Waruiru, 2020), which makes its commercial viability doubtful. In contrast, four treatments by hand-spraying at 15-day intervals reduced tick burdens on Mexican cattle naturally infested with [*B.*] *R. microplus* by 40–91.2% (Alonso-Díaz *et al.*, 2007).

In an unsuccessful alternative approach, a fungal conidial suspension was sprayed onto pasture known to have been contaminated with gravid female *R. microplus*. Efficacy was evaluated on numbers of larvae recovered from the pasture. It was concluded that environmental conditions were probably too harsh to allow survival of sufficient numbers of fungal spores to have an impact on tick numbers (Garcia *et al.*, 2011).

Combining an oil extract of *Calpurnia aurea* (see section 2.2.2) as an attractant with a suspension of *M. anisopliae* conidia in a baited trap, with CO_2 added to extend the range of attraction, adult *R. appendiculatus* and *R. pulchellus* were captured and either incubated for observation or allowed to feed on rabbits. Contaminated trapped males were seen to transfer the fungal infection to coincubated uncontaminated females, leading to the conclusion that this autodissemination might be a viable and environmentally friendly control method in the field (Nana, 2010; Nana *et al.*, 2016). A similar approach was investigated with *M. anisopliae* in semiochemical-baited traps against *A. variegatum*. In this case, the semiochemical was a blend of octenol, butyric acid and attraction-aggregation-attachment

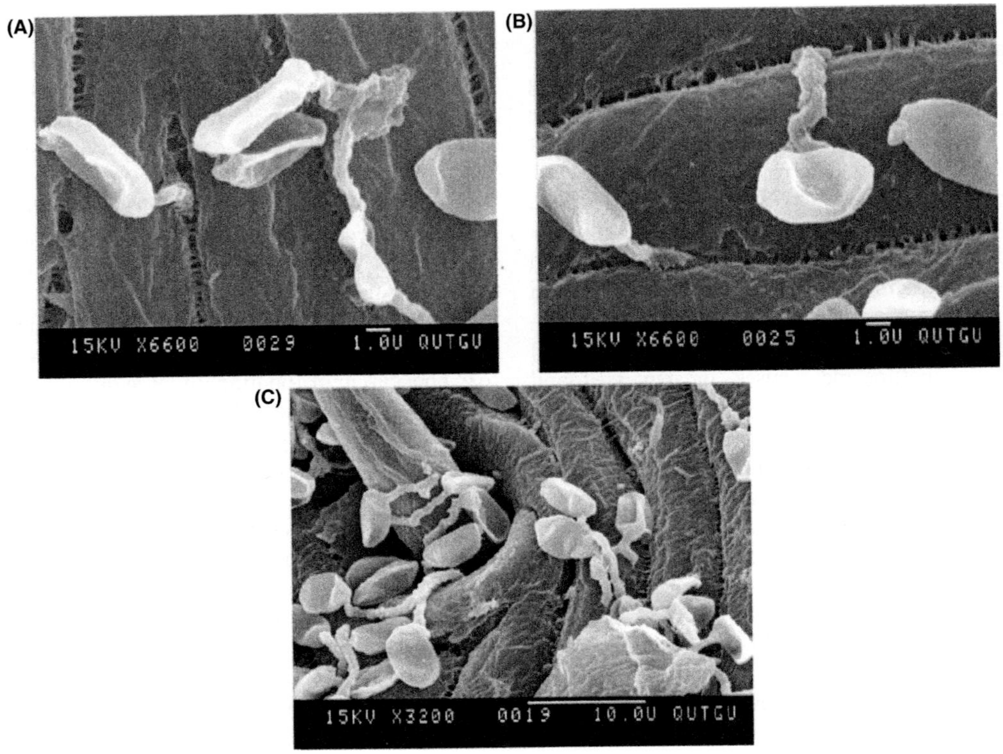

Fig. 2.4. SEM of germinating *M. anisopliae* conidia with germ tubes apparently penetrating the cuticle of [*Boophilus microplus*] *Rhipicephalus australis* after *in vitro* immersion in an oil suspension of fungal spores. From Leemon and Jonsson (2008) with permission of Elsevier.

pheromone (Nchu *et al.*, 2009, 2010). Practical difficulties in the field would be the limit of the attraction distance (5–8m in field experiments), the need for constant replenishment of evaporated semiochemical, and vulnerability to environmental conditions such as wind.

Cattle with daily induced infestations of *R. microplus* 1–24 days old (i.e. larvae, nymphs and engorging adults) were treated with combinations of suspended conidia of *B. bassiana* and an emulsifiable concentrate of *Melia azedarach* green fruit extract. The combination of 0.5% *M. azedarach* extract and 2.4×10^8 *B. bassiana* conidia in 5 litres of water per animal reduced the number of engorged female ticks dropping from days 14 to 20 (larvae at the time of treatment) by 67.4%, which was better than, but not significantly different from, the effect of either the extract or *B. bassiana* conidia alone. None of the treatments had any apparent effect on ovipositioning. The authors surmised that larvae were the most vulnerable life cycle stage due to a thin cuticle and smallest bloodmeal (Sousa *et al.*, 2011).

2.1.9 Predation

Predation is another gauntlet that engorged female ticks have to run after they drop off the host and before they complete their ovipositioning. Vertebrate predators of free-living ticks include birds, lizards and rodents (Cooksey and Davey, 1987; Ostfeld *et al.*, 2006). Field studies with replete [*B. microplus*] *R. australis* females in Queensland demonstrated that mouse predation was higher in winter, while ant predation was more frequent in summer. The authors concluded that this effect would be more noticeable in habitats less favourable for ticks, and that an increase in the predation rate would not result in a proportional decrease in parasitic tick numbers (Sutherst *et al.*, 2000). Shrews seem to be another potential tick predator (Short and Norval, 1982; Durden, 1988). The reports are anecdotal but on small rural properties in Pakistan, cattle cograzing with poultry had four times fewer ticks than where poultry were absent (Rehman *et al.*, 2017).

2.2 Chemicals

Venom systems in mammals are rare and comparatively little is known about them. A number of hypothetical functions have been ascribed to the toxin secreted by the brachial gland in the slow loris (*Loris* spp. and *Nycticebus* spp.), a small primate native to South-east Asia. The observation that they mostly carry no or few ticks gave rise to the notion that the secretion could be acaricidal (Nekaris *et al.*, 2013).

Acaricidal candidate compounds are usually tested *in vitro* first. This allows for rapid screening and titration of test concentrations at much less expense than on-animal tests, either in pens or free range. A number of *in vitro* test methods have been described, mostly using either freshly hatched larvae or newly dropped engorged adult female ticks as the test subjects.

Using larvae yields quick results and requires relatively few laboratory resources. The only criterion evaluated is mortality/survival. Tick larvae (usually hatched *in vitro* from incubated eggs obtained from incubated engorged adult females) are exposed either by immersion (LIM) in serial dilutions of the test material or in filter paper packets saturated with the test solution. The larval packet test (LPT) is more laborious and time-consuming and has in the past been used routinely, for example in surveys for acaricide resistance. A relatively recent innovation has been the larval tarsal test (LTT) which uses multiwell plates and avoids the handling of larvae. The plate is prepared with serial dilutions of the test solution(s). Freshly laid egg clusters are gently dispersed in a rotating bottle with added glass beads and talc before ca. 50 eggs are spooned into each well. The open plate is incubated for 24 hours before being sealed and incubated for a further 3–4 weeks, after which dead or surviving larvae are counted (Lovis *et al.*, 2011, 2013).

Immersing recently detached engorged adult female ticks (EAFIM) in test solutions yields much more information but takes at least 6 weeks to complete and requires more laboratory resources. Criteria of effect are female tick survival and egg production, and egg hatchability (Holdsworth *et al.*, 2006). Another test method used is exposing engorged adult female ticks by incubating them in filter paper envelopes (EFFPE) into which a fixed amount of the test solution has been absorbed (Bagavan *et al.*, 2009). Partially fed *Rhipicephalus turanicus* were exposed to the vapour emanating from different quantities of *Origanum* essential oil soaked into a cotton wick (Cetin *et al.*, 2009). Unfed adult ticks have also been used to assess the contact lethality of 1 μl of test solution applied to the dorsum of each tick (Zorloni *et al.*, 2010).

2.2.1 Synthetic chemicals

The advent of insecticidal chemicals allowed the biggest advance in human management of tick infestations to date. The discovery around the turn of the 19th century that the devastation of East Coast fever in cattle could largely be managed by controlling the tick vector triggered recourse to compounds that today sound desperate in their composition and application methods (Viljoen, 1930). During the 20th century, this became more sophisticated as safer and more potent synthetic molecules were discovered and developed into commercial products (Schröder, 1992). It took some time for alarm about the unintended consequences of indiscriminate and careless release of toxins in the environment to take hold.

The need for judicious application of chemicals to save cost and improve efficacy was mooted after a survey of ticks on cattle in Natal during the 1960s. It was surmised that less chemical might be needed if it were only applied to main tick predilection sites, such as the ears in the case of adult *Rhipicephalus appendiculatus* or relatively hairless areas of the sternum, axilla, belly, groin and perineum for adult *Amblyomma hebraeum*. Chemical could also be conserved by concentrating its application during the season when ticks are most active and prevalent (Baker and Ducasse, 1967). As sound as this advice may seem at face value, it was simply not feasible in large commercial enterprises, where large herds of cattle needed to be mustered at regular intervals and treated in relatively short order to lessen any adverse productivity impact. Predilection site treatment was also mooted for *Amblyomma variegatum* that displays a two-stage infestation pattern, making it vulnerable to chemical footbath exposure (Stachurski, 2000).

The concept of an 'economic threshold' tick count, beyond which chemical application is deemed justifiable, was mooted for *Amblyomma americanum* (Mount and Dunn, 1983) and [*B.*] *Rhipicephalus microplus* (Harley and Wilkinson, 1964; Molento *et al.*, 2013). Replacing organophosphate acaricides with pyrethroids during the 1980s led to reduced plunge dipping frequency for cattle, due to the residual efficacy of the latter chemical group. Pyrethroid treatment of cattle, sheep and goats also reduced tick burdens on sympatric wildlife (Zieger *et al.*, 1998; Horak, 1999).

With sophistication in chemical composition and formulation also came refinements in application methods. Whereas plunge dips and spray races imposed the capital cost of equipment and the management impost of maintaining dipwash/spraywash at an effective concentration, spot-on and pour-on formulations appearing in the 1970s required only an automatic dosing syringe to apply individual dose volumes seldom exceeding 100 ml. But there was still the human resource cost, compounded by the risk of repeat-stress injury if the operator had to treat several hundred animals a day. This cost, in the case of cattle, and the near impossibility of treating wild animal hosts in game reserves, gave rise to the invention of self-medicating applicators dispensing a pour-on formulation (Duncan, 1992; Duncan and Monks, 1992; Burridge *et al.*, 2004). Ear tags impregnated with acaricides was another, but probably less successful, method of chemical tick control. Onset and duration of efficacy were below expectation, and better against ticks attaching near the head (e.g. *R. appendiculatus*) than those preferring the belly and hindquarters for attachment and feeding (e.g. *A hebraeum*) (Owen, 1985; Schröder and van Schalkwyk, 1989).

Acaricidal treatment of cattle for protection against sand tampan is unconventional, due to the soft tick's life history, spending sporadic and very short periods on the host. Treating ivermectin-treated cattle and confining them for 48 hours in pens known to be infested (Fig. 2.5), was shown to be effective in reducing tick numbers in the confined environment by up to 85% (Soll *et al.*, 1984). This is not dissimilar to the notion that ticks on antelopes in small game reserves could be controlled by cograzing with large numbers of tick-susceptible European breed cattle treated with a non-repellent acaricide. The cattle need to be dipped or sprayed at 5-day intervals and introduced in summer, when adult ticks are most abundant (Horak, 1980). The hypothesis was tested and proven in subsequent research (Horak and Knight, 1986).

Acaricide resistance emerging during the past 5–6 decades in different tick species, to most chemicals on most continents, has sharpened the need for reducing reliance on synthetic chemicals as the mainstay of tick management (Baker and Shaw, 1965; Matthewson and Baker, 1975; Nolan and Schnitzerling, 1975, 1976; Baker *et al.*, 1977, 1978, 1979; Solomon *et al.*, 1979; Roulston *et al.*, 1981; Mekonnen *et al.*, 2002; Graf *et al.*, 2004; Cutullé *et al.*, 2009, 2013; Klafke *et al.*, 2010, 2017; Castro-Janer *et al.*, 2010; Alonso-Díaz *et al.*, 2013; Reck *et al.*, 2014; Githaka *et al.*, 2022; Evans *et al.*, 2024). This resistance is heritable and results in a significant increase in the percentage of the population that survives after exposure to a given concentration of that acaricide in comparison with the effective concentration against a susceptible reference strain. It is mostly diagnosed phenotypically, and laboratory confirmation is relatively easily done by the LIM, LPT, LII or EAFIM methods (see above).

Genotypic testing for acaricide resistance requires a molecular marker and several of these have been described for pyrethroids (sodium channel gene mutations), organophosphates (AChE gene variations) and amitraz (β-adrenergic octopamine gene mutations) in *R. microplus* (Rodriguez-Vivas *et al.*, 2018). Using single nucleotide polymorphisms (SNPs) and ribosomal internal transcribed spacer 2 (ITS2) gene fragments, pyrethroid resistance could also be attributed to the carboxylesterase gene (Robbertse *et al.*, 2016). Mutations in the GABA gene are postulated for resistance to dieldrin, fipronil and isoxazolines, but the genomic basis of resistance to MLs in

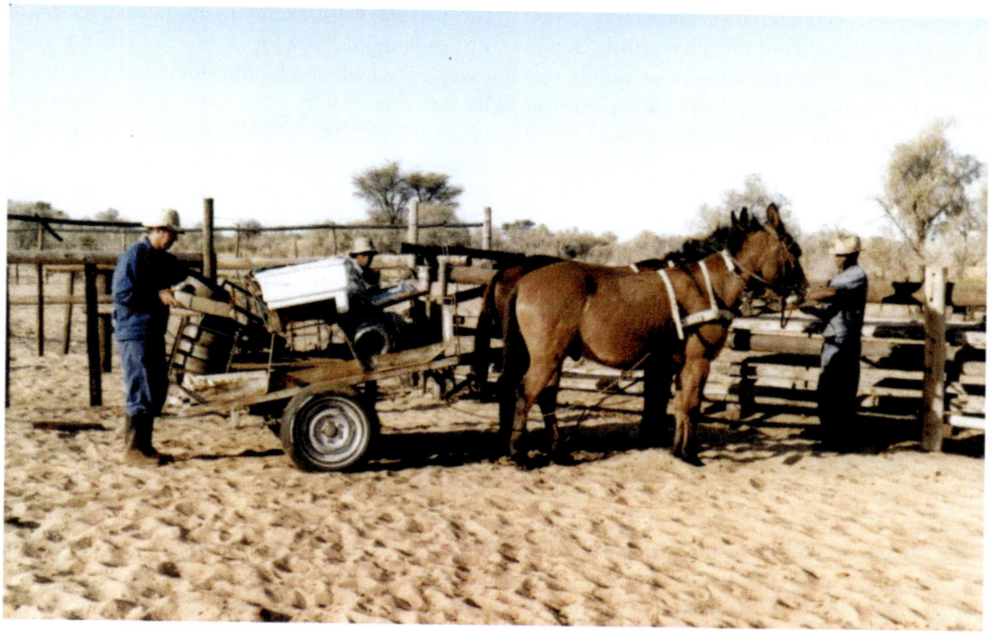

Fig. 2.5. Unconventional transport of material to a remote trial site on the edge of the Kalahari to assess the impact of ivermectin-treated cattle on the *O. savignyi* population in a seldom used sand-bottomed cattle pen. Unpublished private collection, Johann Schröder, 1984.

arthropods has not been clarified (Rodriguez-Vivas *et al.*, 2018). Differentially expressed genes (DEGs) were demonstrated in amitraz-resistant *Rhipicephalus decoloratus* which could identify receptors which enhance neurotransmission and help the ticks survive the effects of the chemical (Baron *et al.*, 2018).

A chemical repellent effect might be preferable to an acaricidal effect in certain circumstances. The insect repellent N,N-diethyl-3-methylbenzamide (DEET) was found to repel nymphs of *A. cajennense* in two different bioassays (Soares *et al.*, 2010b).

2.2.2 Plants

Traditional ethnobotanic medicine has for over a century been overshadowed by pharmaceutical products and pesticides manufactured in vast quantities, offered in convenient formulations and application methods, against a plethora of ailments. Resistance and widespread concern about the environmental impacts and unintended consequences of residues and spillages of synthetic chemicals are the main motivators of renewed interest in phytochemicals. The poorly informed public perception of greater safety, fewer environmental risks and minimal impacts to animal and human health discounts the reality that plants contain some of the most potent toxins known to humanity. Much of the published information is unfortunately anecdotal (e.g. Sanhokwe *et al.*, 2016), with relatively few records of empirical data. Furthermore, mentions of botanical parasiticides seem to be skewed towards anthelmintic rather than acaricidal effects.

There are relatively few descriptions of ticks encountering botanical challenges in the completion of their life cycles. Plant defence mechanisms can be grouped into those forming a physical barrier, for example with hooked trichomes, or with a deterrent effect (Spickett, 1987). Free-living, questing larvae of [B.] *R. microplus* were shown to become trapped and immobilized in the viscous fluid secreted by glandular trichomes of two nutritious varieties of the tropical pasture legume *Stylosanthes*. Within 24 hours the larvae were poisoned by an unidentified vapour from these secretions. Based on the ticks' undeterred negative geotropism, it was concluded that the viscous secretion was not repellent (Sutherst *et al.*, 1982). *Stylosanthes* secretions did not affect nymphal and adult stages of *A. hebraeum*, which are larger (Spickett, 1987). A number of other plants anecdotally reported to be repellent or lethal have been shown not to meet practical expectations for effective tick control (Jonsson and Piper, 2007).

Most literature references to botanical acaricides and tick repellents describe some form of anthropogenic involvement, at least in the form of extraction and application. There is diversity not only in the plant species examined but also the part(s) of the plant, its growth stage and the solvent used for extracting the active principle. Green/dried leaf, flower, seeds, fruit and roots/tubers have all been considered, depending on the plant species. Organic solvents, such as acetone, chloroform, ethyl acetate, hexane and methanol, have been used to this end. There is also a lack of consistency in the test method and tick species, or life cycle stage used in the screening tests.

The chemistry of the active constituent(s) clearly determines the most appropriate solvent to be used for extraction. Whereas acetone and ethanol yielded similar results for some plants, one was clearly superior for others (Fouche *et al.*, 2017, 2021). Previous negative or unconvincing results when only one solvent or extraction method was used may have to be re-examined with this in mind.

Practical questions which would need to be addressed for successful commercialization, such as yield percentage from plant material, toxicity and safety (human, animal, environmental), formulation, residues and price, largely remain unanswered (Jonsson and Piper, 2007). Market failure, lack of a standardized approach and lack of residual efficacy are cited as reasons for failed uptake (Salman *et al.*, 2020).

One review surveyed 238 plant species traditionally used in different formulations for their acaricidal and tick repellent properties. Seven families (Asteraceae, Euphorbiaceae, Fabaceae, Lamiaceae, Meliaceae, Apocynaceae and Solanaceae) represented 46% of the surveyed species (Pavela *et al.*, 2016). Petroleum ether extracts of only two from 42 Rwandan medicinal plants that were examined by the EAFIM were found to be acaricidal (Van Puyvelde *et al.*, 1985). In another review, the morphological and physiological changes in the reproductive system and the salivary gland of a variety of ticks exposed to extracts from eight plant species were assessed by light and electron microscopy and histochemistry (Nwanade *et al.*, 2020).

Acetone extracts of leaves from four tannin-rich plant species were washed with methylene chloride to remove chlorophyll and lipids before being tested *in vitro* against larvae and adults of *R. microplus*. Binding of the tannins with polyethylene glycol (PEG) was done in separate tests to confirm the mode of action. None of the species had any effect on engorged adult tick survival or ovipositioning, but they were all lethal to larvae to some extent, and one reduced egg hatchability (Fernández-Salas *et al.*, 2011).

The acaricidal efficacy of zinc oxide nanoparticles containing ethanolic extracts of neem (*Azadirachta indica*) and lemon grass (*Cymbopogon citratus*) was tested in a variety of *in vitro* bioassays which included the EAFIM and LPT and the less conventional adult packet test, larval immersion test and egg immersion test. Neem nanoparticles outperformed lemon grass in both the EAFIM and LPT, with LC_{90}s of 8.87 and 6.21 mg/l respectively, while nanoparticles containing either plant extract outperformed the plant extract alone (Zaheer *et al.*, 2021).

The systemic efficacy of a neem tree (*A. indica*) tetranortriterpenoid azadirachtin (AZA) extract administered orally to lambs as a feed additive was tested against induced infestations of engorging adult *Dermacentor variabilis*. The highest concentration (0.6% AZA on a dry matter basis) was not lethal to ticks but impaired their feeding. Because AZA affects ticks at moulting, the authors concluded that oligoxenic ticks might be more sensitive than the three-host *D. variabilis* (Landau *et al.*, 2009).

Extracts of mature fruits of *Melia azedarach* tested *in vitro* against larvae and engorged adult females of *R. microplus*, and *in vivo* against induced infestations on calves, showed some effect on tick development but not on reproduction. Green fruit extracts were considered to be more potent, and 5 litres of a 0.5% emulsion concentrate per animal reduced the number of engorged female *R. microplus* dropping 14–20 days later (larvae at the time of treatment) by

54.4%, without any apparent effect on egg production (Sousa *et al.*, 2011).

Gas chromatography/mass spectrometry (GC/MS) of leaf extracts of *Croton sphaerogynus* revealed a variety of constituents, of which the terpenoids were deemed the likeliest candidates responsible for the 99% efficacy in an LPT against *R. microplus* (Righi *et al.*, 2013).

Essential oil was distilled from aerial parts of flowering *Origanum minutiflorum* and fractionated and analysed by GC/MS. Of the eight identified components, carvacrol made up 85.1%. Semi-engorged adult *Rhipicephalus turanicus* were subject to a vapour phase toxicity assay (VPTA), and mortality assessed after 24 hours. Oil concentrations of 5 µl/L required exposure of 120 min to achieve mortalities > 97% (Cetin *et al.*, 2009). Distilled and diluted essential oils of *Pelargonium roseum* and *Eucalyptus globulus* were tested against replete female *R. annulatus* by immersion. *P. roseum* performed best, with a 5% dilution killing 79.2% and 98.3% of ticks by 1 and 6 days respectively post-immersion, and reducing ovipositioning by 87.8% (Pirali-Kheirabadi *et al.*, 2009).

Juice drained from the succulent leaves of *Aloe ferox* in southern Africa has long enjoyed the reputation of medicinal qualities for a variety of ailments. Using a variety of solvents and assay methodologies, powdered plant material was found to contain phenols, flavonoids, flavonols, proanthocyanidins, tannins, alkaloids and saponins, and have potent antioxidant activity (Wintola and Afolayan, 2011). Powdered aloe juice has been commercialized as an additive to maintenance pellets for wildlife, with the advice that it is effective in controlling ticks. Calves with infestations of *R. decoloratus* induced over the previous 25 days were given 5 or 25 mg/kg powdered aloe juice in their ration daily for 22 days. Detached engorged female ticks were collected, weighed and incubated for assessment of fecundity and fertility. The treatment had no effect on the ticks (Fourie *et al.*, 2005).

Garlic (*Allium sativum*) has long had a reputation of arthropodicidal and repellent properties. Three different *in vitro* contact exposure methods were used to investigate the effect of extracts of garlic bulbs on unfed adult *H. m. rufipes* and *R. pulchellus*. Immersion in an aqueous extract was weakly acaricidal. Contact with evaporated dichloromethane extract or direct application of dichloromethane extract in sunflower oil was 100% effective within 24 hours (Nchu *et al.*, 2005).

A bioassay on human volunteers investigated the repellent effect of extracts from ten plant species on unfed nymphs of *A. cajennense*. An amount of 2.75 µl/cm^2 was applied to the proximal phalanx of a volunteer's index finger and one nymph released on the distal phalanx before the finger was inverted, pointing downwards, to stimulate the tick's negative geotropism. Ticks remaining stationary, dropping off or reversing their direction upon contact with the treated skin were considered to have been repelled. The extracts varied in their degree and duration of efficacy (Soares *et al.*, 2010a).

An intriguing idea is to use attractant plant extracts in baited traps to reduce tick numbers on pasture. Extracts of dried *Calpurnia aurea* (Cape laburnum) leaves were compared with an attraction-aggregation-attachment pheromone for their attraction of adult *R. appendiculatus* and *R. pulchellus* ticks *in vitro* by the inverted glass tube bioassay and the dual choice T-olfactometer assay. Extracts were also used to bait traps in pasture plots. Adding CO_2 increased the attraction distance of the oil extract of ca. 50% of the placed ticks from 1 m to 4–5 m (Nana *et al.*, 2010). In a further refinement, conidia of *M. anisopliae* can be added to the trap to kill the captured ticks (see section 2.1.8).

2.3 Host Resistance

Differences in the numbers of ticks carried by different cattle, and differences between breeds of cattle, have been written about for more than a century and yet, scientists remained sceptical well into the twentieth century (Tatchell, 1987). This variation in tick susceptibility has many host-related causes that cannot be directly linked to the immune system.

An intriguing interpretation was that Zebu cattle carry fewer ticks because their skin sebum secretion has a repugnant odour, their skin is tougher and the shorter hair coat provides less shelter for ticks. Curiously, it was also thought that Brahman cattle have a greater ability to perspire and that sweaty cattle, like horses, were repellent to ticks (Kelley, 1932;

Hüe *et al.*, 2014). The greater number of sweat glands in Zebu cattle was confirmed in subsequent research, without alluding to the effect this might have on tick burden (Nay and Hayman, 1956). A short while later, it was stated that no correlation could be found between skin thickness or sweat gland or sebaceous gland concentrations and the degree of resistance, when Zebu and Shorthorn cattle were compared (Riek, 1962).

But the possibility of semiochemical repellence is again raised with regard to benzaldehyde and isobutyric acid which repel *A. sculptum* and which occurs in tick-resistant mammalian hosts (Borges *et al.*, 2015; Ferreira *et al.*, 2020; Bezerra-Santos *et al.*, 2024). Beagles and miniature pinschers are less susceptible to tick infestation than cocker spaniels, thanks to a number of chemicals in their sebum (Zeringóta *et al.*, 2021). Sebum extracts of donkeys contain (*E*)−2-octenal, but not that of horses, which is advanced as the reason for their greater susceptibility to *A. sculptum* infestation (Bezerra-Santos *et al.*, 2024).

Breed differences in host susceptibility to tick infestation, demonstrated by differences in tick burdens, were shown to have a knock-on effect of fewer questing ticks on pasture. There were significantly fewer questing ticks of four species on a paddock grazed by indigenous Nguni than on an adjacent paddock grazed by Bonsmara (a composite breed with ca. 62.5% Zebu content) cattle (Nyangiwe *et al.*, 2011). A comparison of two Zebu (Afrikaner, Drakensberger), one composite (Braford) and one European (Charolais) breeds based on naturally acquired tick numbers in the same habitat and season showed that their tick burdens increased in that sequence, as did their hide thickness and hair coat 'woolliness' (Fourie *et al.*, 2013).

Nguni and Bonsmara heifers exposed to natural infestation with *R. microplus*, *R. decoloratus*, *A. hebraeum*, *R. appendiculatus*, *R. e. evertsi* and *H. marginatum* were compared for their skin thickness, hair length, coat score (smoothness) and tick burdens. Skin thickness was similar in the two breeds but the Nguni had lower coat scores, hair length and tick count values. The authors concluded that a smooth haircoat was an important tick resistance mechanism, but that the genetic basis for this trait needed closer investigation (Marufu *et al.*, 2011).

But there are also individual differences in tick susceptibility within one breed. Heritability for tick burden in cattle is considered sufficient for successful selection for tick resistance (Porto Neto *et al.*, 2011) and estimates of host resistance in various breeds of cattle have been calculated as a tool for breeding selection (Mapholi *et al.*, 2014). Cattle selected for tick resistance within one breed, or selected for breed differences in resistance, were ranked on tick counts after induced infestations on previously exposed Brahman and Shorthorn cattle. Calves from selected cows were significantly more resistant than the progeny of low-resistance cattle (Utech *et al.*, 1978a, b). The proportion of female ticks not engorging after an induced infestation with [*B.*] *R. microplus* larvae was used to estimate resistance in Holstein–Friesian cows in midlactation. Culling the 10% of cattle with the least resistance to ticks could result in removal of 19–21% of ticks from the herd without compromising milk production (Jonsson *et al.*, 2000).

Genome-wide association (GWA) analysis and regional heritability mapping (RHM) analysis have been used to identify SNP markers associated with tick resistance in Nguni cattle. Several genomic regions harbouring quantitative trait loci (QTL) underlying variations in tick burden were identified on 13 different chromosomes. Further analysis was required to identify specific candidate genes with the potential for marker-assisted selection in this breed (Mapholi, 2015). QTL for resistance to *R. microplus* in European and Zebu cattle in Brazil were dispersed over several chromosomes, but their expression was dependent upon the season when the ticks were counted (Gasparin *et al.*, 2007).

Host behaviour, other than self-grooming, has an influence on tick burden, partly explained by the higher tick numbers on browsing ungulates than on grazers (see Chapter 1, this volume; Gallivan and Horak, 1997). This is probably a contributing factor to higher tick numbers seen on European cattle, which frequently seek shade on sunny days, than on Zebu cattle cograzing the same paddock but seemingly less concerned about sunlight exposure (Kelley, 1932; Schröder 1981–1984, unpublished observations). Cattle hosts were seen to detect and avoid high densities of tick larvae on pasture, which would be another population-regulating mechanism (Sutherst *et al.*, 1986).

Although it is regarded as an evolutionary vestige in humans (Naldaiz-Gastesi *et al.*, 2018), fasciculation of the subcutaneous panniculus muscle in cattle and horses is considered a repellent activity against ectoparasites, with Zebu cattle anecdotally displaying more frequent skin twitching than European breeds. No empirical evidence of an effect against ticks was found in this survey.

Adult female [*B.*] *R. decoloratus* removed from six breeds of cattle in the same environment diminished in number in the following sequence: Simmental, Santa Gertrudis, Bonsmara, Afrikaner, Brahman and Nguni (Rechav and Kostrzewski, 1991). It is not possible to say what contribution behaviour, anatomy, physiology, innate or adaptive immunity made to those breed differences.

Transcriptomic analysis identified 53 DEGs, 16 of which were up-/down-regulated between Nelore and Holstein cattle even before tick infestation and may have been indicative of innate tick resistance. An intriguing discovery of this research was that tick-susceptible Holstein cattle attracted more ticks by producing volatile odoriferous compounds, demonstrated *in vitro* with skin rubbings and unfed larvae (Franzin *et al.*, 2017).

Host genetic resistance to ticks and breed differences can be confirmed genomically, but the markers, often consisting of QTLs dispersed over several chromosomes, do not give an indication of the role played by the immune system in this resistance (Gasparin *et al.*, 2007; Porto Neto *et al.*, 2010b, 2012; Mapholi *et al.*, 2014). Tick counts on cattle from seven populations on three continents were correlated with host genotype (based on SNPs) and phenotype (breed) to predict genomic breeding values for the Angus, Brahman, Hereford, Brangus and Braford breeds, using a multitrait approach (Cardoso *et al.*, 2021). Gene expression studies indicate that both non-immune and immune mechanisms have a bearing on tick resistance in cattle (Porto Neto *et al.*, 2010a, 2011). Resistance in cattle to [*R. microplus*] *R. australis* is the result of the interaction of many effector mechanisms, of which innate and adaptive immunity form one component (Jonsson *et al.*, 2014).

Despite the cattle breed differences in susceptibility, the use of tick resistance on its own was considered never to be sufficiently effective to control heartwater vectors, such as *A. hebraeum* (Spickett, 1987). Probably less intensively researched for ticks than is the case for internal parasites, host selection and breeding for parasite resistance and resilience have been shown to come at a production cost, considering the host's finite physiological resources (Laurenson, 2012; Douhard *et al.*, 2022)

Physiological state influences host resistance, for example with pregnant cows carrying more ticks due to the immunosuppression by gestational hormones, and bulls carrying more ticks than heifers and cows, with testosterone suppressing both innate and adaptive immunity (Mapholi *et al.*, 2014).

Innate and naturally acquired adaptive immunity are discussed more extensively in Chapters 3 and 4 respectively.

References

Adegoke, A., Kumar, D., Bobo, C., Rashid, M.I., Durrani, A.Z. *et al.* (2020) Tick-borne pathogens shape the native microbiome within tick vectors. *Microorganisms* 8/9, 1299. DOI: 10.3390/microorganisms8091299.

Adinci, K.J., Akpo, Y., Adoligbe, C., Adehan, S.B., Yessinou, R.E. *et al.* (2018) Preliminary study on the tick population of Benin wildlife at the moment of its invasion by the *Rhipicephalus microplus* tick (Canestrini, 1888). *Veterinary World* 11/6, 845–851.

Aivelo, T., Norberg, A. and Tschirren, B. (2019) Bacterial microbiota composition of *Ixodes ricinus* ticks: The role of environmental variation, tick characteristics and microbial interactions. *PeerJ* 7, e8217. DOI: 10.7717/peerj.8217.

Alekseev, E., Glazer, I. and Samish, M. (2006) Effect of soil texture and moisture on the activity of entomopathogenic nematodes against female *Boophilus annulatus* ticks. *Biocontrol* 51/4, 507–518. DOI: 10.1007/s10526-005-2935-9.

Allan, B.F., Keesing, F. and Ostfeld, R.S. (2003) Effect of forest fragmentation on Lyme Disease risk. *Conservation Biology* 17/1, 267–272.

Allan, B.F., Dutra, H.P., Goessling, L.S., Barnett, K., Chase, J.M. *et al.* (2010) Invasive honeysuckle eradication reduces tick-borne disease risk by altering host dynamics. *Proceedings of the National Academy of Sciences of the USA* 107/43, 18523–18527. DOI: 10.1073/pnas.1008362107.

Alonso-Díaz, M.A., García, L., Galindo-Velasco, E., Lezama-Gutierrez, R., Angel-Sahagún, C.A. *et al.* (2007) Evaluation of *Metarhizium anisopliae* (Hyphomycetes) for the control of *Boophilus microplus* (Acari: Ixodidae) on naturally infested cattle in the Mexican tropics. *Veterinary Parasitology* 147, 336–340. DOI: 10.1016/j.vetpar.2007.03.030.

Alonso-Díaz, M.A., Fernández-Salas, A., Martinez-Ibanez, F. and Osorio-Miranda, J. (2013) *Amblyomma cajennense* (Acari: Ixodidae) tick populations susceptible or resistant to acaricides in the Mexican tropics. *Veterinary Parasitology* 197/1-2, 326–331. DOI: 10.1016/j.vetpar.2013.06.004.

Andreotti, R., Pérez de, A.A., Dowd, S.E., Guerrero, F.D., Bendele, K.G. *et al.* (2011) Assessment of bacterial diversity in the cattle tick *Rhipicephalus* (*Boophilus*) *microplus* through tag-encoded pyrosequencing. *BMC Microbiology* 11, 6. Available at: http://www.biomedcentral.com/1471-2180/11/6 (accessed 29 December 2024).

Arakane, Y. and Muthukrishnan, S. (2009) Insect chitinase and chitinase-like proteins. *Cellular and Molecular Life Sciences* 67/2, 201–216. DOI: 10.1007/s00018-009-0161-9.

Aronson, A.I. and Shai, Y. (2001) Why *Bacillus thuringiensis* insecticidal toxins are so effective: Unique features of their mode of action. *FEMS Microbiology Letters* 195/1, 1–8.

Assenga, S.P., You, M., Shy, C.H., Yamagishi, J., Sakaguchi, T. *et al.* (2006) The use of a recombinant baculovirus expressing a chitinase from the hard tick *Haemaphysalis longicornis* and its potential application as a bioacaricide for tick control. *Parasitology Research* 98, 111–118. DOI: 10.1007/s00436-005-0007-9.

Bagavan, A., Kamaraj, C., Elango, G., Abduz Zahir, A. and Abdul Rahuman, A. (2009) Adulticidal and larvicidal efficacy of some medicinal plant extracts against tick, fluke and mosquitoes. *Veterinary Parasitology* 166/3-4, 286–292. DOI: 10.1016/j.vetpar.2009.09.007.

Baker, J.A.F. and Shaw, R.D. (1965) Toxaphene and lindane resistance in *Rhipicephalus appendiculatus*, the Brown Ear Tick of equatorial and Southern Africa. *Journal of the South African Veterinary Medical Association* 36/3, 321–330.

Baker, J.A.F., Thompson, G.E. and Miles, J.O. (1977) Resistance to toxaphene by the bont tick, *Amblyomma hebraeum* (Koch). *Journal of the South African Veterinary Association* 48/1, 59–65.

Baker, J.A.F., Miles, J.O., Robertson, W.D., Stanford, G.D. and Taylor, R.J. (1978) The current status of resistance to organophosphorus ixodicides by the blue tick, *Boophilus decoloratus* (Koch) in the Republic of South Africa and Transkei. *Journal of the South African Veterinary Association* 49/4, 327–333.

Baker, J.A.F., Jordaan, J.O. and Robertson, W.D. (1979) Ixodicidal resistance in *Boophilus microplus* (Canestrini) in the Republic of South Africa and Transkei. *Journal of the South African Veterinary Association* 50/4, 296–301.

Baker, M.K. and Ducasse, F.B.W. (1967) Tick infestation of livestock in Natal. I. The predilection sites and seasonal variations of cattle ticks. *Journal of the South African Veterinary Association* 38/4, 447–453.

Baron, S., Barrero, R.A., Black, M., Bellgard, M.I., Dalen, E.M. *et al.* (2018) Differentially expressed genes in response to amitraz treatment suggests a proposed model of resistance to amitraz in *R. decoloratus* ticks. *International Journal for Parasitology: Drugs and Drug Resistance* 8, 361–371. DOI: 10.1016/j.ijpddr.2018.06.005.

Bel, Y., Ferré, J. and Hernández-Martínez, P. (2020) *Bacillus thuringiensis* toxins: Functional characterization and mechanism of action. *Toxins* 12, 785. DOI: 10.3390/toxins12120785.

Bennett, G.F. (1969) *Boophilus microplus* (Acarina: Ixodidae): Experimental infestations on cattle restrained from grooming. *Experimental Parasitology* 26, 323–328.

Bernardo, C.C., Barreto, L.P., de Silva, C. d. S.R., Luz, C., Arruda, W. *et al.* (2018) Conidia and blastospores of *Metarhizium* spp and *Beauveria bassiana* s.l.: Their development during the infection process and virulence against the tick *Rhipicephalus microplus*. *Ticks and Tick-Borne Diseases* 9/5, 1334–1342. DOI: 10.1016/j.ttbdis.2018.06.001.

Bezerra-Santos, M.A., Benelli, G., Germinara, G.S., Volf, P. and Otranto, D. (2024) Smelly interactions: Host-borne volatile organic compounds triggering behavioural responses in mosquitoes, sand flies, and ticks. *Parasites & Vectors* 17/1, 227. DOI: 10.1186/s13071-024-06299-1.

Bhat, A.H., Machado, R.A., Abolafia, J., Ruiz-Cuenca, A.N., Askary, T.H. *et al.* (2023) Taxonomic and molecular characterization of a new entomopathogenic nematode species, *Heterorhabditis casmirica* n. sp., and whole genome sequencing of its associated bacterial symbiont. *Parasites & Vectors* 16/1, 383–410. DOI: 10.1186/s13071-023-05990-z.

Bohacsova, M., Mediannikov, O., Kazimirova, M., Raoult, D. and Sekeyova, Z. (2016) *Arsenophonus nasoniae* and Rickettsiae infection of *Ixodes ricinus* due to parasitic wasp *Ixodiphagus hookeri*. *PLoS One* 11/2, e0149950. DOI: 10.1371/journalpone.0149950.

Bonnet, S.I., Binetruy, F., Hernández-Jarguín, A.M. and Duron, O. (2017) The tick microbiome: Why non-pathogenic microorganisms matter in tick biology and pathogen transmission. *Frontiers in Cellular and Infection Microbiology* 7, 236. DOI: 10.3389/fcimb.2017.00236.

Borges, L.M., de Oliveira Filho, J.G., Ferreira, L.L., Louly, C.C., Pickett, J.A. *et al.* (2015) Identification of non-host semiochemicals for the brown dog tick, *Rhipicephalus sanguineus* sensu lato (Acari: Ixodidae), from tick-resistant beagles, *Canis lupus familiaris*. *Ticks and Tick-Borne Diseases* 6/5, 676–682. DOI: 10.1016/j.ttbdis.2015.05.014.

Bravo, A., Gill, S.S. and Soberón, M. (2007) Mode of action of *Bacillus thuringiensis* Cry and Cyt toxins and their potential for insect control. *Toxicon* 49/4, 423–435.

Bravo, A., Likitvivatanavong, S., Gill, S.S. and Soberón, M. (2011) *Bacillus thuringiensis*: A story of a successful bioinsecticide. *Insect Biochemistry and Molecular Biology* 41/7, 423–431. DOI: 10.1016/j.ibmb.2011.02.006.

Brentari, C. (2015) Jakob von Uexküll. The discovery of the umwelt between biosemiotics and theoretical biology. In: Barbieri, M. and Hoffmeyer, J. (eds) *Biosemiotics*, Vol. 9. Springer Science+Business Media, Dordrecht.

Buczek, A., Buczek, W., Bartosik, K., Kulisz, J. and Stanko, M. (2021) *Ixodiphagus hookeri* wasps (Hymenoptera: Encyrtidae) in two sympatric tick species *Ixodes ricinus* and *Haemaphysalis concinna* (Ixodida: Ixodidae) in the Slovak Karst (Slovakia): Ecological and biological considerations. *Scientific Reports* 11, 11310. DOI: 10.1038/s41598-021-90871-7.

Budachetri, K., Crispell, G. and Karim, S. (2017) Amblyomma maculatum SECIS binding protein 2 and putative selenoprotein P are indispensable for pathogen replication and tick fecundity. *Insect Biochemistry and Molecular Biology* 88, 37–47. DOI: 10.1016/j.ibmb.2017.07.006.

Budachetri, K., Gaillard, D., Williams, J., Mukherjee, N. and Karim, S. (2016) A snapshot of the microbiome of *Amblyomma tuberculatum* ticks infesting the gopher tortoise, an endangered species. *Ticks and Tick-Borne Diseases* 7/6, 1225–1229. DOI: 10.1016/j.ttbdis.2016.07.010.

Burridge, M.J., Simmons, L.A., Ahrens, E.H., Naudé, S.A.J. and Malan, F.S. (2004) Development of a novel self-medicating applicator for control of internal and external parasites of wild and domestic animals. *Onderstepoort Journal of Veterinary Research* 71, 41–51.

Camargo, M.G., Golo, P.S., Angelo, I.C., Perinotto, W.M.S., Quinelato, S. *et al.* (2012) Effect of oil-based formulations of acaripathogenic fungi to control *Rhipicephalus microplus* ticks under laboratory conditions. *Veterinary Parasitology* 188, 140–147. DOI: 10.1016/j.vetpar.2012.03.012.

Cardoso, F.F., Matika, O., Djikeng, A., Mapholi, N., Burrow, H.M. *et al.* (2021) Multiple country and breed genomic prediction of tick resistance in beef cattle. *Frontiers in Immunology* 12, 620847. DOI: 10.3389/fimmu.2021.620847.

Castro-Janer, E., Martins, J.R., Mendes, M.C., Namindome, A., Klafke, G.M. *et al.* (2010) Diagnoses of fipronil resistance in Brazilian cattle ticks (*Rhipicephalus* (*Boophilus*) *microplus*) using *in vitro* larval bioassays. *Veterinary Parasitology* 173, 300–306. DOI: 10.1016/j.vetpar.2010.06.036.

Cetin, H., Cilek, J.E., Aydin, L. and Yanikoglu, A. (2009) Acaricidal effects of the essential oil of *Origanum minutiflorum* (*Lamiaceae*) against *Rhipicephalus turanicus* (Acari: Ixodidae). *Veterinary Parasitology* 160, 359–361. DOI: 10.1016/j.vetpar.2008.11.009.

Clayton, D.H., Moyer, B.R., Bush, S.E., Jones, T.G., Gardiner, D.W. *et al.* (2005) Adaptive significance of avian beak morphology for ectoparasite control. *Proceedings of the Royal Society B*272/1565, 811–817. DOI: 10.1098/rspb.2004.3036.

Cooksey, L.M. and Davey, R.B. (1987) Predation of cattle fever ticks by hispid cotton rats in south Texas. *Journal of Parasitology* 73/6, 1272–1273.

Cutullé, C., Jonsson, N.N. and Seddon, J. (2009) Population structure of Australian isolates of the cattle tick *Rhipicephalus* (*Boophilus*) microplus. *Veterinary Parasitology* 161/3-4, 283–291. DOI: 10.1016/j.vetpar.2009.01.005.

Cutullé, C., Lovis, L., D'Agostino, B.I., Balbiani, G.G., Morici, G. *et al.* (2013) *In vitro* diagnosis of the first case of amitraz resistance in *Rhipicephalus microplus* in Santo Tome (Corrientes), Argentina. *Veterinary Parasitology* 192/1-3, 296–300. DOI: 10.1016/j.vetpar.2012.10.014.

Dall'Agnol, B., McCulloch, J.A., Mayer, F.Q., Souza, U., Webster, A. *et al.* (2021) Molecular characterization of bacterial communities of two neotropical tick species (*Amblyomma aureolatum* and *Ornithodoros brasiliensis*) using rDNA 16S sequencing. *Ticks and Tick-Borne Diseases* 12, 101746. DOI: 10.1016/j.ttbdis.2021.101746.

Daube, B.M. and Heath, A.C.G. (1975) Observations on the biology and seasonal abundance of an encyrtid wasp, a parasite of ticks in Queensland. *Journal of Medical Entomology* 12/4, 443–447. DOI: 10.1093/jmedent/12.4.443.

Díaz-Sánchez, S., Fernández, A.M., Habela, M.A., Calero-Bernal, R., Mera, I.G.F. *et al.* (2021) Microbial community of *Hyalomma lusitanicum* is dominated by *Francisella*-like endosymbiont. *Ticks and Tick-Borne Diseases* 12/2, 101624. DOI: 10.1016/j.ttbdis.2020.101624.

Douhard, F., Doeschl-Wilson, A.B., Corbishley, A., Hayward, A.D., Marcon, D. *et al.* (2022) The cost of host genetic resistance on body condition: Evidence from divergently selected sheep. *Evolutionary Applications* 15/9, 1374–1389. DOI: 10.1111/eva.13442.

Driver, F., Milner, R.J. and Trueman, J.W.H. (2000) A taxonomic revision of *Metarhizium* based on a phylogenetic analysis of rDNA sequence data. *Mycological Research* 104/2, 134–150. DOI: 10.1017/S0953756299001756.

Druzinec, D., Salzig, D., Brix, A., Kraume, M., Vilcinskas, A. *et al.* (2013) Optimization of insect cell based protein production processes – online monitoring, expression systems, scale up. *Advances in Biochemical Engineering/Biotechnology* 136, 65–100. DOI: 10.1007/10_2013_205.

Duncan, I.M. (1992) Tick control on cattle with flumethrin pour-on through a Duncan applicator. *Journal of the South African Veterinary Association* 63/3, 125–127.

Duncan, I.M. and Monks, N. (1992) Tick control on eland (*Taurotragus oryx*) and buffalo (*Syncerus caffer*) with flumethrin 1% pour-on through a Duncan applicator. *Journal of the South African Veterinary Association* 63/1, 7–10.

Durden, L.A. (1988) Predation of ticks by shrews. *Journal of Parasitology* 74/4, 740.

El-Kelesh, E.A.M. and El-Refali, M.A.H. (2006) Insecticidal effect of *Bacillus thuringiensis* var *kurstaki* against *Hyalomma dromedarii* on experimentally infested rabbits. *Egyptian Journal of Agricultural Research* 84/3, 993–1000.

Estrada-Peña, A. and Cabezas-Cruz, A. (2019) Towards the integrative analysis of tick microbiome. *Ticks and Tick-Borne Diseases* 10/1, 34–35. DOI: 10.1016/j.ttbdis.2018.08.017.

Estrada-Peña, A., Cabezas-Cruz, A. and Obregon, D. (2020) Behind taxonomic variability: The functional redundancy in the tick microbiome. *Microorganisms* 8/11, 1829. DOI: 10.3390/microorganisms8111829.

Evans, A., Madder, M., Fourie, J., Halos, L., Kumsa, B. *et al.* (2024) Acaricide resistance status of livestock ticks from East and West Africa and *in vivo* efficacy of acaricides to control them. *International Journal for Parasitology: Drugs and Drug Resistance* 25, 100541. DOI: 10.1016/j.ijpddr.2024.100541.

Fernández-Ruvalcaba, M., Peña-Chora, G., Romo-Martínez, A., Hernández-Velázquez, V., Parra, A.B.D.L. *et al.* (2010) Evaluation of *Bacillus thuringiensis* pathogenicity for a strain of the tick, *Rhipicephalus microplus*, resistant to chemical pesticides. *Journal of Insect Science* 10, 186.

Fernández-Salas, A., Alonso-Díaz, M.A., Acosta-Rodríguez, R., Torres-Acosta, J.F.J., Sandoval-Castro, C.A. *et al.* (2011) *In vitro* acaricidal effect of tannin-rich plants against the cattle tick *Rhipicephalus* (*Boophilus*) *microplus* (Acari: Ixodidae). *Veterinary Parasitology* 175/1-2, 113–118. DOI: 10.1016/j.vetpar.2010.09.016.

Ferreira, L.L., Oliveira Filho, J.G., Oliveira Silva, F., Lacerda Ferraz, A.L. and Mascarin, G.M. (2020) Attract or repel *Amblyomma sculptum* ticks: Screening of semiochemicals. *Veterinary Parasitology* 278, 109036. DOI: 10.1016/j.vetpar.2020.109036.

Fiedler, O.G.H. (1953) A new African tick parasite, *Hunterellus theilerae* sp. n. *Onderstepoort Journal of Veterinary Research* 26/1, 61–64.

Filgueiras, M.D.G., Matos, R.S., Barreto, L.P., Mascarin, G.M., Rizzo, P.V. *et al.* (2023) From the laboratory to the field: efficacy of entomopathogenic nematodes to control the cattle tick. *Pest Management Science* 79/1, 216–225. DOI: 10.1002/ps.7190.

Fogaça, A.C., Sousa, G., Pavanelo, D.B., Esteves, E., Martins, L.A. *et al.* (2021) Tick immune system: What is known, the interconnections, the gaps, and the challenges. *Frontiers in Immunology* 12, 628054. DOI: 10.3389/fimmu.2021.628054.

Fouche, G., Sakong, B.M., Adenubi, O.T., Dzoyem, J.P., Naidoo, V. *et al.* (2017) Investigation of the acaricidal activity of the acetone and ethanol extracts of 12 South African plants against the adult ticks of

Rhipicephalus turanicus. *Onderstepoort Journal of Veterinary Research* 84/1, a1523. DOI: 10.4102/ojvr.v84i1.1523.

Fouche, G., Sakong, B.M., Adenubi, O.T., Dzoyem, J.P., Naidoo, V. *et al.* (2021) Corrigendum: investigation of the acaricidal activity of the acetone and ethanol extracts of 12 South African plants against the adult ticks of *Rhipicephalus turanicus*. *Onderstepoort Journal of Veterinary Research* 88(1), a1950. DOI: 10.4102/ojvr.v88i1.1950.

Fourie, L.J. and Kok, O.B. (1992) The role of host behaviour in tick-host interactions: A domestic host-paralysis tick model. *Experimental & Applied Acarology* 13, 213–225.

Fourie, J.J., Fourie, L.J. and Horak, I.G. (2005) Efficacy of orally administered powdered aloe juice (*Aloe ferox*) against ticks on cattle and ticks and fleas on dogs. *Journal of the South African Veterinary Association* 76/4, 193–196.

Fourie, L.J., Kok, D.J., Krugel, L., Snyman, A. and Van der Lingen, F. (1996) Control of Karoo paralysis ticks through vegetation management. *Medical and Veterinary Entomology* 10, 39–43.

Fourie, P.J., Foster, L.A. and Neser, F.W.C. (2013) Differences in physical traits such as coat score and hide thickness, together with tick burden and body condition score, in four cattle breeds in the south-eastern Free State province of South Africa. *Journal for New Generation Sciences* 11/1, 66–73.

Franzin, A.M., Maruyama, S.R., Garcia, G.R., Oliveira, R.P., Ribeiro, J.M.C. *et al.* (2017) Immune and biochemical responses in skin differ between bovine hosts genetically susceptible and resistant to the cattle tick *Rhipicephalus microplus*. *Parasites & Vectors* 10/1, 51. DOI: 10.1186/s13071-016-1945-z.

Gallivan, G.J. and Horak, I.G. (1997) Body size and habitat as determinants of tick infestations of wild ungulates in South Africa. *South African Journal of Wildlife Research* 27/2, 63–70.

Gamage, H.K., Vuong, D., Minns, S.A., Chen, R., Piggott, A.M. *et al.* (2022) The composition and natural variation of the skin microbiota in healthy Australian cattle. DOI: 10.21203/rs.3.rs-2207709/v1.

Garcia, M.V., Monteiro, A.C., Szabó, M.P.J., Mochi, D.A., Simi, L.D. *et al.* (2011) Effect of *Metarhizium anisopliae* fungus on off-host *Rhipicephalus* (*Boophilus*) *microplus* from tick-infested pasture under cattle grazing in Brazil. *Veterinary Parasitology* 181/2-4, 267–273. DOI: 10.1016/j.vetpar.2011.04.031.

Gasparin, G., Miyata, M., Coutinho, L.L., Martinez, M.L., Teodoro, R.L. *et al.* (2007) Mapping of quantitative trait loci controlling tick [*Riphicephalus* [sic] (*Boophilus*) *microplus*] resistance on bovine chromosomes 5, 7 and 14. *Animal Genetics* 38, 453–459. DOI: 10.1111/j.1365-2052.2007.01634.x.

Gill, S.S., Cowles, E.A. and Pietrantonio, P.V. (1992) The mode of action of *Bacillus thuringiensis* endotoxins. *Annual Review of Entomology* 37/1, 615–634.

Githaka, N.W., Kanduma, E.G., Wieland, B., Darghouth, M.A. and Bishop, R.P. (2022) Acaricide resistance in livestock ticks infesting cattle in Africa: Current status and potential mitigation strategies. *Current Research in Parasitology & Vector-Borne Diseases* 2, 100090. DOI: 10.1016/j.crpvbd.2022.100090.

Glazer, I., Alekseev, E. and Samish, M. (2001) Factors affecting the virulence of entomopathogenic nematodes to engorged female *Boophilus annulatus* ticks. *Journal of Parasitology* 87/4, 808–812.

Graf, J.F., Gogolewski, R., Leach-Bing, N., Sabatini, G.A., Molento, M.B. *et al.* (2004) Tick control: An industry point of view. *Parasitology* 129, S427–S442. DOI: 10.1017/S0031182004006079.

Habeeb, S.M. and El-Hag, H.A.A. (2008) Ultrastructural changes in hemocyte cells of hard tick (*Hyalomma dromedarii*: Ixodidae): A model of *Bacillus thuringiensis* var. *thuringiensis* H14 δ-endotoxin mode of action. *American-Eurasian Journal of Agricultural & Environmental Science* 3/6, 829–836.

Hajdušek, O., Šíma, R., Ayllón, N., Jalovecká, M., Perner, J. *et al.* (2013) Interaction of the tick immune system with transmitted pathogens. *Frontiers in Cellular and Infection Microbiology* 3, 26. DOI: 10.3389/fcimb.2013.00026.

Hamilton, P.T., Maluenda, E., Sarr, A., Belli, A., Hurry, G. *et al.* (2021) *Borrelia afzelii* infection in the rodent host has dramatic effects on the bacterial microbiome of *Ixodes ricinus* ticks. *Applied and Environmental Microbiology* 87, e00641-21. DOI: 10.1128/AEM.00641-21.

Harish, S., Murugan, M., Kannan, M., Parthasarathy, S., Prabhukarthikeyan, S.R. *et al.* (2021) Entomopathogenic viruses. In: Omkar (ed.) *Microbial Approaches for Insect Pest Management*. Springer Nature, Singapore. DOI: 10.1007/978-981-16-3595-3_1.

Harley, K.L.S. and Wilkinson, P.R. (1964) A comparison of cattle tick control by 'conventional' acaricidal treatment, planned dipping, and pasture spelling. *Australian Journal of Agricultural Research* 15/5, 841–853. DOI: 10.1071/AR9640841.

Hartelt, K., Wurst, E., Collatz, J., Zimmermann, G., Kleespies, R.G. *et al.* (2008) Biological control of the tick *Ixodes ricinus* with entomopathogenic fungi and nematodes: Preliminary results from laboratory experiments. *International Journal of Medical Microbiology* 298/S1, 314–320.

Hartelt, K., Oehme, R., Frank, H., Brockmann, S.O., Hassler, D. and Kimmig, P. (2003) Pathogens and symbionts in ticks: Prevalence of *Anaplasma phagocytophilum* (Ehrlichia sp.), *Wolbachia* sp., *Rickettsia* sp., *and Babesia* sp. in southern Germany. *International Journal of Medical Microbiology* 293(Suppl 37), 86–92.

Hassanain, M.A., El Garhy, M.F., Abdel-Ghaffar, F.A., El-Sharaby, A. and Megeed, K.N.A. (1997) Biological control studies of soft and hard ticks in Egypt. The effect of *Bacillus thuringiensis* varieties on soft and hard ticks (Ixodidae). *Parasitology Research* 83, 209–213. DOI: 10.1007/s004360050235.

Heath, A.C.G. and Cane, R.P. (2010) A new species of *Ixodiphagus* (Hymenoptera: Chalcidoidea: Encyrtidae) parasitizing seabird ticks in New Zealand. *New Zealand Journal of Zoology* 37/2, 147–155. DOI: 10.1080/03014223.2010.482973.

Heckel, D.G. (2020) How do toxins from *Bacillus thuringiensis* kill insects? An evolutionary perspective. *Archives of Insect Biochemistry and Physiology* 104/2, e21673. DOI: 10.1002/arch.21673.

Holdsworth, P.A., Kemp, D., Green, P., Peter, R.J., Bruin, C. *et al.* (2006) World association for the advancement of veterinary parasitology (W.A.A.V.P.) guidelines for evaluating the efficacy of acaricides against ticks (Ixodidae) on ruminants. *Veterinary Parasitology* 136/1, 29–43. DOI: 10.1016/j.vetpar.2005.11.011.

Horak, I.G. (1980) The control of parasites in antelope in small game reserves. *Journal of the South African Veterinary Association* 51/1, 17–19.

Horak, I.G. (1999) Parasites of domestic and wild animals in South Africa. XXXVII. Ixodid ticks on cattle on Kikuyu grass pastures and in Valley Bushveld in the Eastern Cape Province. *Onderstepoort Journal of Veterinary Research* 66, 175–184.

Horak, I.G. and Knight, M.M. (1986) A comparison of the tick burdens of wild animals in a nature reserve and on an adjacent farm where tick control is practised. *Journal of the South African Veterinary Association* 57/4, 199–203.

Horak, I.G., Moolman, L.C. and Fourie, L.J. (1987) Some wild hosts of the Karoo paralysis tick, *Ixodes rubicundus* Neumann, 1904 (Acari: Ixodidae). *Onderstepoort Journal of Veterinary Research* 54, 49–51.

Horak, I.G., Gallivan, G.J., Spickett, A.M. and Potgieter, A.L.F. (2006) Effect of burning on the numbers of questing ticks collected by dragging. *Onderstepoort Journal of Veterinary Research* 73/3, 163–174.

Hu, R., Hyland, K.E. and Oliver, J.H. (1998) A review on the use of Ixodiphagus wasps (Hymenoptera: Encyrtidae) as natural enemies for the control of ticks (Acari: Ixodidae). *Systematic and Applied Acarology* 3/1, 19–28. DOI: 10/11158/saa.3.1.3.

Hüe, T. and Fontfreyde, C. (2019) Development of a new approach of pasture management to control *Rhipicephalus microplus* infestation. *Tropical Animal Health and Production* 51, 1989–1995. DOI: 10.1007/s11250-019-01899-x.

Hüe, T., Hurlin, J.-C., Teurlai, M. and Naves, M. (2014) Comparison of tick resistance of crossbred Senepol x Limousin to purebred Limousin cattle. *Tropical Animal Health and Production* 46/2, 447–453. DOI: 10.1007/s11250-013-0512-2.

Jonsson, N.N. and Piper, E.K. (2007) *Integrated Control Programs for Ticks on Cattle*. University of Queensland, Australia.

Jonsson, N.N., Matschoss, A.L., Pepper, P., Green, P.E. and Ansell, J. (2000) Resistance of Holstein-Friesian cows to infestation by the cattle tick (*Boophilus microplus*). *Veterinary Parasitology* 89, 297–305.

Jonsson, N.N., Piper, E.K. and Constantinoiu, C.C. (2014) Host resistance in cattle to infestation with the cattle tick *Rhipicephalus microplus*. *Parasite Immunology* 36/11, 553–559. DOI: 10.1111/pim.12140.

Kelley, R.B. (1932) *Zebu (Brahman) Cross Cattle and Their Possibilities in North Australia*. Council for Scientific and Industrial Research, Melbourne, Australia.

Khoo, J.J., Kurtti, T.J., Husin, N.A., Beliavskaia, A., Lim, F.S. *et al.* (2020) Isolation and propagation of laboratory strains and a novel flea-derived field strain of *Wolbachia* in tick cell lines. *Microorganisms* 8, 988. DOI: 10.3390/microorganisms8070988.

Klafke, G.M., de Albuquerque, T.A., Miller, R.J. and Schumaker, T.T.S. (2010) Selection of an ivermectin-resistant strain of *Rhipicephalus microplus* (Acari: Ixodidae) in Brazil. *Veterinary Parasitology* 168/1-2, 97–104. DOI: 10.1016/j.vetpar.2009.10.003.

Klafke, G., Webster, A., Agnol, B.D., Pradel, E., Silva, J. *et al.* (2017) Multiple resistance to Acaricides in field populations of *Rhipicephalus microplus* from Rio rande do Sul state, Southern Brazil. *Ticks and Tick-Borne Diseases* 8/1, 73–80. DOI: 10.1016/j.ttbdis.2016.09.019.

Kocan, K.M., Blouin, E.F., Pidherney, M.S., Claypool, P.L., Samish, M. *et al.* (1998a) Entomopathogenic nematodes as a potential biological control method for ticks. *Annals of the New York Academy of Sciences* 849/1, 355–364. DOI: 10/1111/j.1749-6632.1998.tb11070.x.

Kocan, K.M., Pidherney, M.S., Blouin, E.F., Claypool, P.L., Samish, M. *et al.* (1998b) Interaction of entomopathogenic nematodes (*Steinernematidae*) with selected species of Ixodid ticks (Acari: Ixodidae). *Journal of Medical Entomology* 35/4, 514–520.

Kramer, K.J. and Muthukrishnan, S. (1997) Insect chitinases: Molecular biology and potential use as biopesticides. *Insect Biochemistry and Molecular Biology* 27/11, 887–900. DOI: 10.1016/S0965-1748(97)00078-7.

Landau, S.Y., Provenza, F.D., Gardner, D.R., Pfister, J.A., Knoppel, E.L. *et al.* (2009) Neem-tree (*Azadirachta indica* Juss.) extract as a feed additive against the American dog tick (*Dermacentor variabilis*) in sheep (*Ovis aries*). *Veterinary Parasitology* 165, 311–317. DOI: 10.1016/j.vetpar.2009.07.047.

Laurenson, Y.C.S.M. (2012) Modelling nematode infections in sheep and parasite control strategies. PhD thesis, University of Edinburgh, Edinburgh, UK.

Laws, H.E. (1911) Note on eradication of ticks by the starvation method. *Agricultural Journal of the Union of South Africa* 1/4, 570–579.

Laws, H.E. and Manning, B. (1910) Eradication of ticks by the starvation method. *Agricultural Journal of the Cape of Good Hope* 37/1, 9–17.

Leemon, D.M. (2009) Evaluation of *Metarhizium anisopliae* for biopesticide control of livestock ectoparasites. PhD thesis, University of Queensland, Brisbane, Australia.

Leemon, D.M. (2011) Fungal biopesticide for cattle tick control. Final report: MLA project B.AHE.0020. Available at: https://www.mla.com.au (accessed 29 May 2022).

Leemon, D.M. (2012) Fungal biopesticide for cattle tick and buffalo fly control. Final report: MLA project B.AHE.0193. Available at: https://www.mla.com.au (accessed 29 May 2022).

Leemon, D.M. and Jonsson, N.N. (2008) Laboratory studies on Australian isolates of *Metarhizium anisopliae* as a biopesticide for the cattle tick *Boophilus microplus*. *Journal of Invertebrate Pathology* 97, 40–49. DOI: 10.1016/j.jip.2007.07.006.

Li, S., Mandal, S., Xu, X. and Jin, F. (2020a) The tripartite interaction of host immunity – *Bacillus thuringiensis* infection – gut microbiota. *Toxins* 12/8, 514. DOI: 10.3390/toxins12080514.

Li, X., Miyamoto, K., Takasu, Y., Wada, S., Iizuka, T. *et al.* (2020b) Functional receptor for *Bacillus thuringiensis* Cry2A toxins in *Bombyx mori*, but not for Cry1A, Cry1C, Cry1D, Cry1F, or Cry9A toxins. *Toxins* 12/2, 104. DOI: 10.3390/toxins12020104.

Little, N.S., Luttrell, R.G., Mullen, R.M., Allen, K.C. and Parys, K.A. (2019) Comparative activity of commercial baculovirus formulations against heliothine pests of cotton. *Southwestern Entomologist* 44/1, 105–115.

Liu, L., Li, J., Liu, J., Yu, Z., Yang, X. *et al.* (2016) Population dynamics of multiple symbionts in the hard tick, *Dermacentor silvarum* Olenev (Acari: Ixodidae). *Ticks and Tick-Borne Diseases* 7/1, 188–192. DOI: 10.1016/j.ttbdis.2015.10.002.

Lopes, A.J.O., Nascimento-Júnior, J.R.S., Silva, C.G., Prado, A.P., Labruna, M.B. *et al.* (2012) Parasitism by *Ixodiphagus* wasps (Hymenoptera: Encyrtidae) in *Rhipicephalus sanguineus* and *Amblyomma* ticks (Acari: Ixodidae) in three regions of Brazil. *Journal of Economic Entomology* 105/6, 1979–1981. DOI: 10.1603/EC12012.

Lormendez, C.C., Fernandez-Ruvalcaba, M., Adames-Mancebo, M., Hernandez-Velazquez, V.M., Zuñiga-Navarrete, F. *et al.* (2019) Mass production of a S-layer protein of *Bacillus thuringiensis* and its toxicity to the cattle tick *Rhipicephalus microplus*. *Scientific Reports* 9, 17586. DOI: 10.1038/s41598-019-53854-3.

Lovis, L., Perret, J.L., Bouvier, J., Fellay, J.M., Kaminsky, R. *et al.* (2011) A new *in vitro* test to evaluate the resistance level against acaricides of the cattle tick, *Rhipicephalus* (*Boophilus*) *microplus*. *Veterinary Parasitology* 182/2-4, 269–280. DOI: 10.1016/j.vetpar.2011.06.004.

Lovis, L., Mendes, M.C., Perret, J.L., Martins, J.R., Bouvier, J. *et al.* (2013) Use of the Larval Tarsal Test to determine acaricide resistance in *Rhipicephalus* (*Boophilus*) *microplus* Brazilian field populations. *Veterinary Parasitology* 191/3-4, 323–331. DOI: https://10.1016/j.vetpar.2012.09.011.

Madhav, M., Baker, D., Morgan, J.A.T., Asgari, S. and James, P. (2020) *Wolbachia*: A tool for livestock ectoparasite control. *Veterinary Parasitology* 288, 109297. DOI: 10.1016/j.vetpar.2020.109297.

Mapholi, N.O. (2015) Exploring genetic architecture of tick resistance in South African Nguni cattle. PhD thesis, Stellenbosch University, Stellenbosch.

Mapholi, N.O., Marufu, M.C., Maiwashe, A., Banga, C.B., Muchenje, V. *et al.* (2014) Towards a genomics approach to tick (Acari: Ixodidae) control in cattle: A review. *Ticks and Tick-Borne Diseases* 5, 475–483. DOI: 10.1016/j.ttbdis.2014.04.006.

Marufu, M.C., Qokweni, L., Chimonyo, M. and Dzama, K. (2011) Relationships between tick counts and coat characteristics in Nguni and Bonsmara cattle reared on semiarid rangelands in South Africa. *Ticks and Tick-Borne Diseases* 2/3, 172–177. DOI: 10.1016/j.ttbdis.2011.07.001.

Mateos-Hernández, L., Obregón, D., Maye, J., Borneres, J., Versille, N. *et al.* (2020) Anti-tick microbiota vaccine impacts *Ixodes ricinus* performance during feeding. *Vaccines* 8/4, 702. DOI: 10.3390/vaccines8040702.

Matthewson, M.D. and Baker, J.A.F. (1975) Arsenic resistance in species of multi-host ticks in the Republic of South Africa and Swaziland. *Journal of the South African Veterinary Association* 48/4, 341–344.

Megaw, M.W. (1978) Virus-like particles pathogenic to salivary glands of the tick *Boophilus microplus*. *Nature* 271/5644, 483–484. DOI: https://10.1038/271483a0.

Mekonnen, S., Bryson, N.R., Fourie, L.J., Peter, R.J., Spickett, A.M. *et al.* (2002) Acaricide resistance profiles of single- and multi-host ticks from communal and commercial farming areas in the Eastern Cape and North-west provinces of South Africa. *Onderstepoort Journal of Veterinary Research* 69/2, 99–105.

Mendoza-Almanza, G., Esparza-Ibarra, E.L., Ayala-Luján, J.L., Mercado-Reyes, M., Godina-González, S. *et al.* (2020) The cytocidal spectrum of *Bacillus thuringiensis* toxins: From insects to human cancer cells. *Toxins* 12/5, 301. DOI: 10.3390/toxins12050301.

Merzendorfer, H. (2013) Insect-derived chitinases. *Advances in Biochemical Engineering/Biotechnology* 136, 19–50. DOI: 10.1007/10_2013_207.

Molento, M.B., Fortes, F.S., Buzatti, A., Kloster, F.S., Sprenger, L.K. *et al.* (2013) Partial selective treatment of *Rhipicephalus microplus* and breed resistance variation in beef cows in Rio Grande do Sul, Brazil. *Veterinary Parasitology* 192/1-3, 234–239. DOI: 10.1016/j.vetpar.2012.10.021.

Mount, G.A. and Dunn, J.E. (1983) Economic thresholds for lone star ticks (Acari: Ixodidae) in recreational areas based on a relationship between CO_2 and human subject sampling. *Journal of Economic Entomology* 76/2, 327–329.

Moutailler, S., Valiente Moro, C., Vaumourin, E., Michelet, L., Tran, F.H. *et al.* (2016) Coinfection of ticks: The rule rather than the exception. *PLoS Neglected Tropical Diseases* 10/3, e0004539. DOI: 10.1371/journal.pntd.0004539.

Murigu, M.M. and Waruiru, R.M. (2020) Comparative efficacy of *Metarhizium anisopliae* and amitraz in control of *Rhipicephalus decoloratus* on cattle under field conditions in Kenya. *Alexandria Journal of Veterinary Sciences* 66/1, 52–59. DOI: 10.5455/ajvs.89391.

Murigu, M.M., Nana, P., Waruiru, R.M., Nga'nga, C.J., Ekesi, S. *et al.* (2016) Laboratory and field evaluation of entomopathogenic fungi for the control of amitraz-resistant and susceptible strains of *Rhipicephalus decoloratus*. *Veterinary Parasitology* 225, 12–18. DOI: 10.1016/j.vetpar.2016.05.026.

Murrell, A., Dobson, S.J., Yang, X., Lacey, E. and Barker, S.C. (2003) A survey of bacterial diversity in ticks, lice and fleas from Australia. *Parasitology Research* 89/4, 326–334. DOI: 10.1007/s00436-002-0722-4.

Mwangi, E.N., Kaaya, G.P., Essuman, S.U. and Kimondo, M.G. (1994) Parasitism of *Amblyomma variegatum* by a hymenopteran parasitoid in the laboratory, and some aspects of its basic biology. *Biological Control* 4/2, 101–104. DOI: 10.1006/bcon.1994.1017.

Naldaiz-Gastesi, N., Bahri, O.A., Munain, A., McCullagh, K.J.A. and Izeta, A. (2018) The *Panniculus carnosus* muscle: An evolutionary enigma at the intersection of distinct research fields. *Journal of Anatomy* 233/3, 275–288. DOI: 10.1111/joa.12840.

Nana, P. (2010) Potential of integrating *Calpurnia aurea* with entomopathogenic fungus *Metarhizium anisopliae* for the control of *Rhipicephalus appendiculatus* and *Rhipicephalus pulchellus*. PhD thesis, Jomo Kenyatta University of Agriculture and Technology, Nairobi, Kenya.

Nana, P., Maniania, N.K., Maranga, R.O., Kutima, H.L., Boga, H.I. *et al.* (2010) Attraction response of adult *Rhipicephalus appendiculatus* and *Rhipicephalus pulchellus* ticks to extracts from *Calpurnia aurea*. *Veterinary Parasitology* 174/1-2, 124–130. DOI: 10.1016/j.vetpar.2010.08.016.

Nana, P., Ekesi, S., Nchu, F. and Maniania, N.K. (2016) Compatibility of *Metarhizium anisopliae* with *Calpurnia aurea* leaf extracts and virulence against *Rhipicephalus pulchellus*. *Journal of Applied Entomology* 140/8, 590–597. DOI: 10.1111/jen.12289.

Narasimhan, S. and Fikrig, E. (2015) Tick microbiome: The force within. *Trends in Parasitology* 31/7, 315–323. DOI: 10.1016/j.pt.2015.03.010.

Nay, T. and Hayman, R.H. (1956) Sweat glands in Zebu (*Bos indicus* L.) and European (*B. taurus* L.) cattle. I. Size of individual glands, the denseness of their population, and their depth below the skin surface. *Australian Journal of Agricultural Research* 7/5, 482–492.

Nchu, F., Magano, S.R. and Eloff, J.N. (2005) *In vitro* investigation of the toxic effects of extracts of *Allium sativum* bulbs on adults of *Hyalomma marginatum rufipes* and *Rhipicephalus pulchellus*. *Journal of the South African Veterinary Association* 76/2, 99–103.

Nchu, F., Maniania, N.K., Toure, A., Hassanali, A. and Eloff, J.N. (2009) The use of a semiochemical bait to enhance exposure of *Amblyomma variegatum* (Acari: Ixodidae) to *Metarhizium anisopliae* (Ascomycota: Hypocreales). *Veterinary Parasitology* 160, 279–284. DOI: 10.1016/j.vetpar.2008.11.005.

Nchu, F., Maniania, N.K., Hassanali, A. and Eloff, J.N. (2010) Performance of a *Metarhizium anisopliae*-treated semiochemical-baited trap in reducing *Amblyomma variegatum* populations in the field. *Veterinary Parasitology* 169, 367–372. DOI: 10.1016/j.vetpar.2010.01.020.

Nekaris, K.A.-I., Moore, R.S., Rode, E.J. and Fry, B.G. (2013) Mad, bad and dangerous to know: The biochemistry, ecology and evolution of slow loris venom. *Journal of Venomous Animals and Toxins Including Tropical Diseases* 19, 21. Available at: http://www.jvat.org/content/19/1/21 (accessed 29 December 2024).

Nieman, W.A., Wilgen, B.W. and Leslie, A.J. (2021) A review of fire management practices in African savanna-protected areas. *Koedoe* 63/1, a1655. DOI: 10.4102/koedoe.v63i1.

Noda, H., Munderloh, U.G. and Kurtti, T.J. (1997) Endosymbionts of ticks and their relationship to *Wolbachia* spp. and tick-borne pathogens of humans and animals. *Applied and Environmental Microbiology* 63/10, 3926–3932.

Nolan, J. and Schnitzerling, H.J. (1975) Characterization of acetylcholinesterases of acaricide-resistant and susceptible strains of the cattle tick *Boophilus microplus* (Can.): I. Extraction of the critical component and comparison with enzyme from other sources. *Pesticide Biochemistry and Physiology* 5/2, 178–188.

Nolan, J. and Schnitzerling, H.J. (1976) Characterization of acetylcholinesterases of acaricide-resistant and susceptible strains of the cattle tick *Boophilus microplus* (can.): II. The substrate specificity and catalytic efficiency of the critical enzyme component. *Pesticide Biochemistry and Physiology* 6/2, 142–147.

Nwanade, C.F., Yu, Z. and Liu, J. (2020) Botanical acaricides induced morphophysiological changes of reproductive and salivary glands in tick: A mini-review. *Research in Veterinary Science* 132, 285–291. DOI: 10.1016/j.rvsc.2020.07.008.

Nyangiwe, N., Goni, S., Hervé-Claude, L.P., Ruddat, I. and Horak, I.G. (2011) Ticks on pastures and on two breeds of cattle in the Eastern Cape province, South Africa. *Onderstepoort Journal of Veterinary Research* 78/1, 320. DOI: 10.4102/ojvr.v78i1.320.

Ostfeld, R.S., Price, A., Hornbostel, V.L., Benjamin, M.A. and Keesing, F. (2006) Controlling ticks and tick-borne zoonoses with biological and chemical agents. *BioScience* 56/5, 383–394.

Owen, I.L. (1985) Field efficacy of ear tags impregnated with insecticide against the cattle tick *Boophilus microplus*. *Australian Veterinary Journal* 62/1, 24–25. DOI: 10.1111/j.1751-0813.1985.tb06036.x.

Palma, L., Muñoz, D., Berry, C., Murillo, J. and Caballero, P. (2014) *Bacillus thuringiensis* toxins: An overview of their biocidal activity. *Toxins* 6, 3296–3325. DOI: 10.3390/toxins6123296.

Pavela, R., Canale, A., Mehlhorn, H. and Benelli, G. (2016) Application of ethnobotanical repellents and acaricides in prevention, control and management of livestock ticks: A review. *Research in Veterinary Science* 109(1), 9. DOI: 10.1016/j.rvsc.2016.09.001.

Peña, G., Miranda-Rios, J., Riva, G., Pardo-Lopez, L., Soberon, M. *et al.* (2006) A *Bacillus thuringiensis* S-layer protein involved in toxicity against *Epilachna varivestis* (Coleoptera: Coccinellidae). *Applied and Environmental Microbiology* 72/1, 353–360. DOI: 10.1128/AEM.72.1.353–360.2006.

Pienaar, R., de Klerk, D.G., Putterill, J.F. and Mans, B.J. (2018) Notes on maternal behaviour in soft ticks: specifically observed in *Argas* (*Argas*) *striatus* Bedford, 1932 and *Argas* (*Secretargas*) *transgariepinus* White, 1846. *Ticks and Tick-Borne Diseases* 9, 889–895. DOI: 10.1016/j.ttbdis.2018.03.020.

Pirali-Kheirabadi, K., Razzaghi-Abyaneh, M. and Halajian, M. (2009) Acaricidal effect of *Pelargonium roseum* and *Eucalyptus globulus* essential oils against adult stage of *Rhipicephalus* (*Boophilus*) *annulatus in vitro*. *Veterinary Parasitology* 162, 346–349. DOI: 10.1016/j.vetpar.2009.03.015.

Plantard, O., Bouju-Albert, A., Malard, M.A., Hermouet, A., Capron, G. *et al*. (2012) Detection of *Wolbachia* in the tick *Ixodes ricinus* is due to the presence of the Hymenoptera endoparasitoid *Ixodiphagus hookeri*. *PLoS One* 7/1, e30692. DOI: 10.1371/journal.pone.0030692.

Porto Neto, L.R., Bunch, R.J., Harrison, B.E. and Barendse, W. (2010a) DNA variation in the gene ELTD1 is associated with tick burden in cattle. *Animal Genetics* 42/1, 50–55. DOI: 10.1111/j.1365-2052.2010.02120.x.

Porto Neto, L.R., Bunch, R.J., Harrison, B.E., Prayaga, K.C. and Barendse, W. (2010b) Haplotypes that include the *integrin alpha* 11 gene are associated with tick burden in cattle. *BMC Genetics* 11, 55. DOI: 10.1186/1471-2156-11-55.

Porto Neto, L.R., Jonsson, N.N. and d'Occhio, M.J. (2011) Molecular genetic approaches for identifying the basis of variation in resistance to tick infestation in cattle. *Veterinary Parasitology* 180, 165–172. DOI: 10.1016/j.vetpar.2011.05.048.

Porto Neto, L.R., Jonsson, N.N., Ingham, A., Bunch, R.J., Harrison, B.E. *et al*. (2012) The RIPK2 gene: A positional candidate for tick burden supported by genetic associations in cattle and immunological response of knockout mouse. *Immunogenetics* 64/5, 379–388. DOI: 10.1007/s00251-012-0601-9.

Purnell, R.E., Gunter, T.D. and Schröder, J. (1989) Development of a prophylactic regime using long-acting tetracycline for the control of redwater and heartwater in susceptible cattle moved into an endemic area. *Tropical Animal Health and Production* 21, 11–19.

Ramos, R.A.N., Campbell, B.E., Whittle, A., Lia, R.P., Montarsi, F. *et al*. (2015) Occurrence of *Ixodiphagus hookeri* (Hymenoptera: Encyrtidae) in *Ixodes ricinus* (Acari: Ixodidae) in Southern Italy. *Ticks and Tick-Borne Diseases* 6, 234–236. DOI: 10.1016/j.ttbdis.2015.01.001.

Ramos, R.A.N., de Macedo, L.O., Bezerra-Santos, M.A., Carvalho, G.A., Verocai, G.G. *et al*. (2023) The role of parasitoid wasps, *Ixodiphagus* spp. (Hymenoptera: Encyrtidae) in tick control. *Pathogens* 12, 676. DOI: 10.3390/pathogens12050676.

Ratcliffe, N.A., Furtado Pacheco, J.P., Dyson, P., Castro, H.C., Gonzalez, M.S. *et al*. (2022) Overview of paratransgenesis as a strategy to control pathogen transmission by insect vectors. *Parasites & Vectors* 15(1), 112. DOI: 10.1186/s13071-021-05132-3.

Rechav, Y. and Kostrzewski, M.W. (1991) Relative resistance of six cattle breeds to the tick *Boophilus decoloratus* in South Africa. *Onderstepoort Journal of Veterinary Research* 58, 181–186.

Reck, J., Klafke, G.M., Webster, A., Agnol, B.D., Scheffer, R. *et al*. (2014) First report of fluazuron resistance in *Rhipicephalus microplus*: A field tick population resistant to six classes of acaricides. *Veterinary Parasitology* 201/1-2, 128–136. DOI: 10.1016/j.vetpar.2014.01.012.

Rehman, A., Nijhof, A.M., Sauter-Louis, C., Schauer, B., Staubach, C. *et al*. (2017) Distribution of ticks infesting ruminants and risk factors associated with high tick prevalence in livestock farms in the semi-arid and arid agro-ecological zones of Pakistan. *Parasites & Vectors* 10/1, 190. DOI: 10.1186/s13071-017-2138-0.

Riek, R.F. (1962) Studies on the reactions of animals to infestation with ticks. VI. resistance of cattle to infestation with the tick *Boophilus microplus* (Canestrini). *Australian Journal of Agricultural Research* 13/3, 532–550. DOI: 10.1071/AR9620532.

Righi, A.A., Motta, L.B., Klafke, G.M., Pohl, P.C., Furlan, C.M. *et al*. (2013) Chemical composition and efficacy of dichloromethane extract of *Croton sphaerogynus* Baill. (Euphorbiaceae) against the cattle tick *Rhipicephalus microplus* (Acari: Ixodidae). *Veterinary Parasitology* 192, 292–295. DOI: 10.1016/j.vetpar.2012.11.005.

Robbertse, L., Baron, S., Merwe, N.A., Madder, M., Stoltsz, W.H. *et al*. (2016) Genetic diversity, acaricide resistance status and evolutionary potential of a *Rhipicephalus microplus* population from a disease-controlled cattle farming area in South Africa. *Ticks and Tick-Borne Diseases* 7/4, 595–603. DOI: 10.1016/j.ttbdis.2016.02.018.

Rodriguez-Vivas, R.I., Jonsson, N.N. and Bhushan, C. (2018) Strategies for the control of *Rhipicephalus microplus* ticks in a world of conventional acaricide and macrocyclic lactone resistance. *Parasitology Research* 117/1, 3–29. DOI: 10.1007/s00436-017-5677-6.

Roulston, W.J., Wharton, R.H., Nolan, J., Kerr, J.D., Wilson, J.T. *et al*. (1981) A survey for resistance in cattle ticks to acaricides. *Australian Veterinary Journal* 57/8, 362–371.

Salman, M., Abbas, R.Z., Israr, M., Abbas, A., Mehmood, K. *et al*. (2020) Repellent and acaricidal activity of essential oils and their components against *Rhipicephalus* ticks in cattle. *Veterinary Parasitology* 283, 109178. DOI: 10.1016/j.vetpar.2020.109178.

Samish, M. and Glazer, I. (2001) Entomopathogenic nematodes for the biocontrol of ticks. *Trends in Parasitology* 17/8, 368–184.

Samish, M. and Rehacek, J. (1999) Pathogens and predators of ticks and their potential in biological control. *Annual Review of Entomology* 44, 159–182. DOI: 10.1146/annurev.ento.44.1.159.

Samish, M., Alekseev, E. and Glazer, I. (2000a) Biocontrol of ticks by entomopathogenic nematodes. Research Update. *Annals of the New York Academy of Sciences* 916/1, 589–594. DOI: 10/1111/j.1749-6632.2000.tb05341.x.

Samish, M., Alekseev, E. and Glazer, I. (2000b) Mortality rate of adult ticks due to infection by entomopathogenic nematodes. *Journal of Parasitology* 86/4, 679–684.

Sanchis, V. (2011) From microbial sprays to insect-resistant transgenic plants: History of the biospesticide *Bacillus thuringiensis*. A review. *Agronomy for Sustainable Development* 31/1, 217–231. DOI: 10.1051/agro/2010027.

Sanhokwe, M., Mupangwa, J., Masika, P.J., Maphosa, V. and Muchenje, V. (2016) Medicinal plants used to control internal and external parasites in goats. *Onderstepoort Journal of Veterinary Research* 83/1, a1016. DOI: 10.4102/ojvr.v83i1.1016.

Sansinenea, E. (ed.) (2012) Discovery and description of *Bacillus thuringiensis*. In: *Bacillus Thuringiensis Biotechnology*. Springer, Dordrecht, pp. 3–18.

Schröder, J. (1992) Chemical control of ticks on cattle. In: Fivaz, B., Petney, T. and Horak, I. (eds) *Tick Vector Biology*. Medical and Veterinary Aspects Springer, Heidelberg, pp. 175–233.

Schröder, J. and van Schalkwyk, P.C. (1989) [Die doeltreffendheid van alfametrien-deurweekte oorplaatjies teen beesbosluise] The efficacy of alphamethrin-impregnated ear tags as a method to control cattle ticks. *Journal of the South African Veterinary Association* 60/2, 79–82.

Short, N.J. and Norval, R.A.I. (1982) Tick predation by shrews in Zimbabwe. *Journal of Parasitology* 68/6, 1052. DOI: 10.2307/3281090.

Smagghe, F., Spooner-Hart, R., Chen, Z.H. and Donovan-Mak, M. (2023) Biological control of arthropod pests in protected cropping by employing entomopathogens: Efficiency, production and safety. *Biological Control* 25, 105337. DOI: 10.1016/j.biocontrol.2023.105337.

Snowball, G.J. (1956) The effect of self-licking by cattle on infestations of cattle tick *Boophilus microplus* (Canestrini). *Australian Journal of Agricultural Research* 7, 227–232.

Soares, S.F., Borges, L.M.F., de Sousa Braga, R., Ferreira, L.L., Louly, C.C.B. *et al.* (2010a) Repellent activity of plant-derived compounds against *Amblyomma cajennense* (Acari: Ixodidae) nymphs. *Veterinary Parasitology* 167/1, 67–73. DOI: 10.1016/j.vetpar.2009.09.047.

Soares, S.F., Braga, R.D.S., Ferreira, L.L., Louly, C.C.B., Sousa, L.A.D.D. *et al.* (2010b) Repellent activity of DEET against amblyomma cajennense (acari: ixodidae) nymphs submitted to different laboratory bioassays. *Revista Brasileira de Parasitologia Veterinária* 19/1, 12–16. DOI: 10.4322/rbpv.01901003.

Solanke, P.B. and Narladkar, B.W. (2018) Status of bacterial biocontrol agents against cattle tick *Rhipicephalus (B.) microplus* (Acarina: Ixodidiae [sic]): Review. *Journal of Entomology and Zoology Studies* 6/5, 720–726.

Soll, M.D., Swan, G.E., Schröder, J. and Bezuidenhout, J.D. (1984) Efficacy of ivermectin against the sand tampan (*Ornithodoros savignyi*). *Veterinary Record* 114, 70.

Solomon, K.R., Baker, M.K., Heyne, H. and van Kleef, J. (1979) The use of frequency diagrams in the survey of resistance to pesticides in ticks in southern Africa. *Onderstepoort Journal of Veterinary Research* 46, 171–177.

Sousa, L.A.D., Júnior, H.B.P., Soares, S.F., Ferri, P.H., Ribas, P. *et al.* (2011) Potential synergistic effect of *Melia azedarach* fruit extract and *Beauveria bassiana* in the control of *Rhipicephalus* (*Boophilus*) *microplus* (Acari: Ixodidae) in cattle infestations. *Veterinary Parasitology* 175, 320–324. DOI: 10.1016/j.vetpar.2010.10.012.

Spickett, A.M. (1987) The natural control of heartwater vectors. *Onderstepoort Journal of Veterinary Research* 54, 535–539.

Spickett, A.M., Horak, I.G., Niekerk, A. and Braack, L.E.O. (1992) The effect of veld-burning on the seasonal abundance of free-living ixodid ticks as determined by drag sampling. *Onderstepoort Journal of Veterinary Research* 59, 285–292.

Spruijt, B.M., van Hooff, J.A.R.A.M. and Gispen, W.H. (1992) Ethology and neurobiology of grooming behaviour. *Physiological Reviews* 72/3, 825–852. DOI: 10.1152/physrev.1992.72.3.825.

Stachurski, F. (2000) Invasion of West African cattle by the tick *Amblyomma variegatum*. *Medical and Veterinary Entomology* 14, 391–399.

Stampa, S. (1959) Tick paralysis in the Karoo areas of South Africa. *Onderstepoort Journal of Veterinary Research* 28/2, 169–227.

Stampa, S. and du Toit, R. (1958) Paralysis of stock due to the Karoo paralysis tick (*Ixodes rubicundus* Neu.). *South African Journal of Science September* 241–246.

Stutterheim, C.J. (1981) The feeding behaviour of the redbilled oxpecker. *South African Journal of Zoology* 16/4, 267–269. DOI: 10.1080/02541858.1981.11447767.

Stutterheim, C.J. (1982) Past and present ecological distribution of the redbilled oxpecker (*Buphagus erythrorhynchus*) in South Africa. *South African Journal of Zoology* 17/4, 190–196. DOI: 10.1080/02541858.1982.11447802.

Sutherst, R.W., Jones, R.J. and Schnitzerling, H.J. (1982) Tropical legumes of the genus *Stylosanthes* immobilise and kill cattle ticks. *Nature* 295, 320–321.

Sutherst, R.W., Floyd, R.B., Bourne, A.S. and Dallwitz, M.J. (1986) Cattle grazing behavior regulates tick populations. *Experientia* 42, 194–196. DOI: 10.1007/BF01952465.

Sutherst, R.W., Wilson, L.J. and Cook, I.M. (2000) Predation of the cattle tick, *Boophilus microplus* (Canestrini) (Acarina: Ixodidae), in three Australian pastures. *Australian Journal of Entomology* 39/2, 70–77.

Syed, T., Askari, M., Meng, Z., Li, Y., Abid, M.A. *et al.* (2020) Current insights on vegetative insecticidal proteins (Vip) as next generation pest killers. *Toxins* 12, 522. DOI: 10.3390/toxins12080522.

Szczepanska, A., Kiewra, D. and Guz-Regner, K. (2018) Sensitivity of *Ixodes ricinus* (L., 1758) and *Dermacentor reticulatus* (Fabr., 1794) ticks to *Bacillus thuringiensis* isolates: Preliminary study. *Parasitology Research* 117/12, 3897–3902. DOI: 10.1007/s00436-018-6096-z.

Tatchell, R.J. (1987) Interactions between ticks and their hosts. *International Journal for Parasitology* 17/2, 597–606. DOI: 10.1016/0020-7519(87)90136-6.

Tijsse-Klasen, E., Braks, M., Scholte, E.-J. and Sprong, H. (2011) Parasites of vectors – *Ixodiphagus hookeri* and its *Wolbachia* symbionts in ticks in the Netherlands. *Parasites & Vectors* 4, 228.

Trollope, W.S.W. (2011) Personal perspectives on commercial versus communal African fire paradigms when using fire to manage rangelands for domestic livestock and wildlife in Southern and East Arican ecosystems. *Fire Ecology* 7/1, 57–73. DOI: 10.4996/fireecology.0701057.

Utech, K.B.W., Seifert, G.W. and Wharton, R.H. (1978a) Breeding Australian Illawarra Shorthorn cattle for resistance to *Boophilus microplus*, I Factors affecting resistance. *Australian Journal of Agricultural Research* 29/2, 411–422. DOI: 10.1071/AR9780411.

Utech, K.B.W., Wharton, R.H. and Kerr, J.D. (1978b) Resistance to *Boophilus microplus* (Canestrini) in different breeds of cattle. *Australian Journal of Agricultural Research* 29, 885–895.

Van der Geest, L.P.S., Elliot, S.L., Breeuwer, J.A.J. and Beerling, E.A.M. (2000) Diseases of mites. *Experimental & Applied Acarology* 24, 497–560.

Van Puyvelde, L., Geysen, D., Ayobangira, F.-X., Hakizamungu, E., Nshimiyimana, A. *et al.* (1985) Screening of medicinal plants of Rwanda for acaricidal activity. *Journal of Ethnopharmacology* 13/2, 209–215. DOI: 10.1016/0378-8741(85)90008-X.

Vilchez, S. (2020) Making 3D-Cry toxin mutants: Much more than a tool of understanding toxins mechanism of action. *Toxins* 12/9, 600. DOI: 10.3390/toxins12090600.

Viljoen, P.R. (1930) The East Coast fever problem in the Union. *Papers Veterinary Section, No. 15*. Available at: https://repository.up.ac.za/bitstream/handle/2263/133 42/15_paper15_viljoen.pdf?sequence=1 (accessed 10 April 2023).

Von Uexküll, J. (1934) Translated by J. D. O'Neil. *[Streifzüge durch die Umwelten von Tieren und Menschen: Ein Bilderbuch unsichtbarer Welten] Forays into the Worlds of Animals and Humans: A Picture Book of Invisible Worlds*. University of Minnesota Press, Minneapolis.

Walker, A.R. (2011) Eradication and control of livestock ticks: Biological, economic and social perspectives. *Parasitology* 138, 945–959.

Weeks, P. (1999) Interactions between red-billed oxpeckers, *Buphagus erythrorhynchus*, and domestic cattle, *Bos taurus*, in Zimbabwe. *Animal Behaviour* 58, 1253–1259.

Wikel, S.K. (1996) Host immunity to ticks. *Annual Review of Entomology* 41/1, 1–22. DOI: 10.1146/annurev.en.41.010196.000245.

Wikel, S.K., Ramachandra, R.N. and Bergman, D.K. (1994) Tick induced modulation of the host immune response. *International Journal for Parasitology* 24/1, 59–66.

Wilkinson, P.R. (1964) Pasture spelling as a control measure for cattle ticks in southern Queensland. *Australian Journal of Agricultural Research* 15, 822–840. DOI: 10.1017/AR9640822.

Willadsen, P., Eisemann, C.H. and Telham, R.L. (1993) 'Concealed' antigens: Expanding the range of immunological targets. *Parasitology Today* 9/4, 132–135. DOI: 10.1016/0169-4758(93)90177-H.

Wintola, O.A. and Afolayan, A.J. (2011) Phytochemical constituents and antioxidant activities of the whole leaf extract of *Aloe ferox* Mill. *Pharmacognosy Magazine* 7/28, 325–333. DOI: 10.4103/0973-1296.90414.

Wood, H.P. (1911) Notes on the life history of the tick parasite *Hunterellus hookeri* Howard. *Journal of Economic Entomology* 4, 425–431.

Wu-Chuang, A., Hodzic, A., Mateos-Hernandez, L., Estrada-Pena, A., Obregon, D. *et al.* (2021) Current debates and advances in tick microbiome research. *Current Research in Parasitology & Vector-Borne Diseases* 1, 100036. DOI: 10.1016/j.crpvbd.2021.100036.

Wu-Chuang, A., Obregon, D., Mateos-Hernandez, L. and Cabezas-Cruz, A. (2022) Anti-tick microbiota vaccines: How can this actually work? *Biologia* 77/6, 1555–1562. DOI: 10.1007/s11756-021-00818-6.

You, M., Xuan, X., Tsuji, N., Kamio, T., Taylor, D. *et al.* (2003) Identification and molecular characterization of a chitinase from the hard tick *Haemaphysalis longicornis*. *Journal of Biological Chemistry* 278/10, 8556–8563. DOI: 10.1074/jbc.M206831200.

Zaheer, T., Imran, M., Pal, K., Sajid, M.S., Abbas, R.Z. *et al.* (2021) Synthesis, characterization and acaricidal activity of green-mediated ZnO nanoparticles against *Hyalomma* ticks. *Journal of Molecular Structure* 1227, 129652. DOI: 10.1016/j.molstruc.2020.129652.

Zeringóta, V., Pereira-Junior, R.A., Sarria, A.L.F., Henrique, A.C.C., Birkett, M.A. *et al.* (2021) Identification of a non-host semiochemical from miniature pinscher, *Canis lupus familiaris*, that repels *Rhipicephalus sanguineus* sensu lato (Acari: Ixodidae). *Ticks and Tick-Borne Diseases* 12/1, 101582. DOI: 10.1016/j.ttbdis.2020.101582.

Zhang, X., Norris, D.E. and Rasgon, J.L. (2011) Distribution and molecular characterization of *Wolbachia* endosymbionts and filarial nematodes in Maryland populations of the lone star tick (*Amblyomma americanum*). *FEMS Microbiology and Ecology* 77/1, 50–056. DOI: 10.1111/j.1574-6941.2011.01089.x.

Zhong, J., Jasinskas, A. and Barbour, A.G. (2007) Antibiotic treatment of the tick vector *Amblyomma americanum* reduced reproductive fitness. *PLoS One* 2/5, e405. DOI: 10.1371/journal.pone.0000405.

Zieger, U., Horak, I.G., Cauldwell, A.E., Uys, A.C. and Bothma, J. du P. (1998) The effect of chemical tick control on cattle on free-living ixodid ticks and on ticks parasitic on sympatric impala in the Central Province, Zambia. *South African Journal of Wildlife Research* 28/1, 10–15.

Zorloni, A., Penzhorn, B.L. and Eloff, J.N. (2010) Extracts of *Calpurnia aurea* leaves from southern Ethiopia attract and immobilise or kill ticks. *Veterinary Parasitology* 168/1-2, 160–164. DOI: 10.1016/j.vetpar.2009.10.026.

3 Innate Resistance to Ticks

Abstract

Some animals are innately more resistant to tick infestation than others. This resistance can result from differences in behaviour and phenotype but the important contributor is innate immunity, which does not require prior exposure to the pathogen. The innate immune system is complex and relies on receptors that can recognize pathogens and set in motion a network of signals that activate effector cells and protective mechanisms. First exposure to a pathogen activates the innate immune response, which then transitions to adaptive immunity against subsequent exposures. Tick saliva contains a multitude of proteins, many of which aim to ensure successful completion of the bloodmeal by inhibiting haemostasis and inflammation.

Protective immunity is the result of interaction between antigen-non-specific innate immunity (this chapter) and antigen-specific adaptive immunity (Chapter 4, this volume) (Palucka and Banchereau, 1999).

This chapter is largely based on a comprehensive review of the innate immune system, published more than 10 years ago (Meeusen *et al.*, 2013). Innate resistance is the first line of defence against infections and infestations, requiring no prior exposure of the host to the pathogen and playing a key role in the activation and orientation of adaptive immunity (de Veer *et al.*, 2007; Bottazzi *et al.*, 2010). All metazoans have a well-conserved innate immune system that relies on interactions between non-clonally distributed pattern recognition receptors in the host and molecular patterns in microbes. *Drosophila* has been an attractive model organism for studying the innate immune system (Goto *et al.*, 2008a, b).

Innate immunity has been described as 'the ability to (i) recognize structures that are present in large groups of microorganisms and are distinct from self, (ii) activate effector mechanisms that will destroy within hours most microorganisms encountered in life, and (iii) activate and orientate an adaptive immune response that, through clonal expansion of lymphocytes, will be aimed specifically at persistent microorganisms' (Vasselon and Detmers, 2002). The innate response to infection instructs and controls the subsequent adaptive immune response (Vasselon and Detmers, 2002).

The components of the innate and adaptive immune systems are illustrated in the simplistic graphic form of a mind map in Fig. 3.1.

3.1 Components of Innate Immunity

The innate immune system is primitive and conserved evolutionarily, and is mostly present and constant, independent of pathogen exposure. It involves resident immune cells such as macrophages and dendritic cells. These act in consort with physical barriers (epithelium), chemicals (inflammatory and anti-inflammatory cytokines) and receptors that recognize pathogens and patterns. Discovery of the dendritic cell and the activation of innate immunity was rewarded with the 2011 Nobel Prize in Physiology or Medicine (Meeusen *et al.*, 2013).

Innate immunity has cellular and humoral components. Humoral elements include pantrexins, complement components, correctins and ficolins. In response to microorganisms and tissue damage, neutrophils, macrophages and dendritic cells produce fluid phase pattern recognition molecules (PRMs) of different molecular classes. Humoral PRMs interact with and

DOI: 10.1079/9781800625761.0003

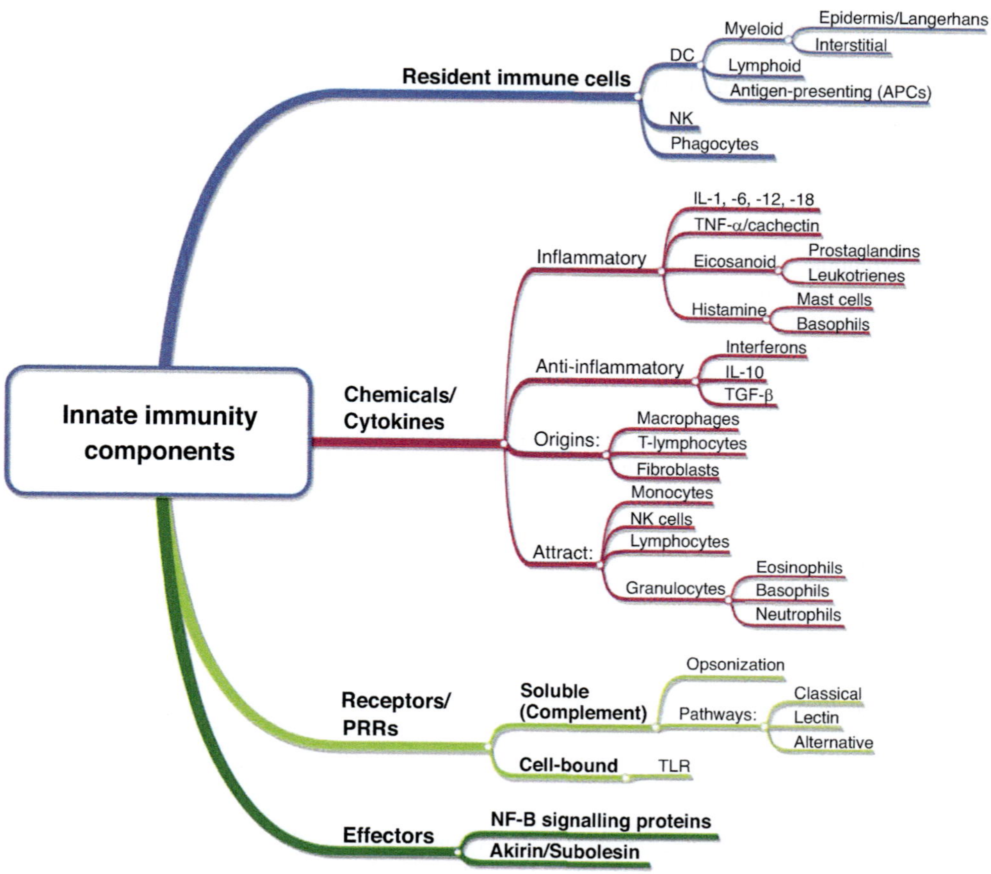

Fig. 3.1. Graphic representation of the components of the innate immune system, drawn from cited references, using MindMapper 21 Pro© software. Abbreviations in the illustration are explained in the text. Photo courtesy of Johann Schröder.

regulate cellular effectors. The humoral arm of innate immunity consists of different molecules, sharing functional outputs with antibodies (Bottazzi *et al.*, 2010).

Innate immunity generates a rapid inflammatory response to an invading pathogen (Hertzog *et al.*, 2011b). An effective immune response requires the ordered, sequential expression and secretion of inflammatory cytokines by the appropriate cells (Hertzog *et al.*, 2011b). Inflammation is characterized by the cardinal signs of redness (*rubor*), swelling (*tumor*), heat (*calor*), pain (*dolor*) and loss of function (*laesa functio*). These are the result of increased blood flow, vascular permeability and cell infiltration, and chemicals released from stimulated innate immune cells. After an inflammatory innate immune stimulus is received, dendritic cells induce the antigen-specific proliferation of T- and B-cells of adaptive immunity (Meeusen *et al.*, 2013).

Mobilization of mast cells and eosinophils as part of a type II (allergic type) immune response, greatly influencing the final outcome of the adaptive immune response, is the principal characteristic ascribed to the innate immune system, referring specifically to gastrointestinal nematodes (de Veer *et al.*, 2007). These are probably equally relevant to other macroparasites, such as ticks.

3.1.1 Resident immune cells

The cells of the innate immune system, which include dendritic cells (DC), natural killer (NK) and phagocytic cells, recognize non-processed antigens, using pattern recognition receptors (PRRs). DC are distributed as sentinels throughout the body, to capture antigen, migrate to draining lymphoid organs and present the antigen to selected antigen-specific lymphocytes, thus initiating the immune response. DC were first observed in 1868 in the epidermis and called Langerhans cells. DC are now believed to comprise three distinct subpopulations within the myeloid (Langerhans cells and interstitial DC) and lymphoid lineages (Palucka and Banchereau, 1999).

Tick salivary antigens were found to be associated with discrete dendritic cells in the epidermis. This provided evidence that they were Langerhans cells, occurring as a network that may entrap antigenic material and play a role in the primary immune response. Evidence suggested that they may present the retained antigens to lymphocytes in either the skin or the lymph nodes (Allen *et al.*, 1979). Langerhans cell numbers in the epidermis decrease during primary tick infestation and increase at tick attachment sites in the early phase of secondary infestation (Wikel, 1996).

3.1.2 Chemicals

Cytokines are a large and diverse group of small proteins acting as signalling molecules to regulate inflammation and modulate cellular activities. Chemokines are a group of secreted proteins within the cytokine family whose function is to induce cell migration. These 'chemotactic cytokines' are expressed either constitutively, to maintain homeostasis in immune surveillance and haemopoiesis, or in response to an inflammatory stimulus, targeting cells of the innate and adaptive immune system.

A cytokine or chemokine ligand ('any molecule or atom that . . . binds to a receiving protein molecule, otherwise known as a receptor' (Cuffari, 2022)) binds with its cognate receptor, which is activated, triggering a cascade of signalling events. These events regulate functions such as cell adhesion, phagocytosis, cytokine secretion, cell activation, proliferation, survival and death, and angiogenesis and proliferation (Ramesh *et al.*, 2013).

Inflammatory cytokines include interleukin (IL)−1 and IL-6 and tumour necrosis factor α (TNF-α), formerly known as cachectin. IL-1 and TNF-α are pyrogens, whereas IL-6 also has an anti-inflammatory role, depending on the cell context and stimulus. Examples of anti-inflammatory cytokines are interferons (IFNs), IL-10 and transforming growth factor (TGF) β. They prevent the perpetuation of chronic inflammation. TGF-β can also be proinflammatory, depending on whether it is regulating adaptive (pro-) or innate (anti-) cells (Meeusen *et al.*, 2013).

When first discovered in the 1950s, IFN was considered to be an antiviral protein but it is now known to be a big family, grouped into three types, with diverse functions. In 2011, nearly 2000 interferon-regulated genes (IRGs) had been identified in the human genome. The proteins encoded by these IRGs can be nuclear, cytoplasmic, membrane bound, ribosomal, lysosomal or localized in mitochondria or the Golgi apparatus. They can be structural, signal transduction adaptors, enzymes, metabolic factors, membrane and secreted proteins. Interferons influence effector cells of the innate and adaptive immune responses by regulating cell proliferation, cell cycle (survival and apoptosis), cell differentiation and migration. Keeping the interferon response in check is the negative feedback loop of more than 400 IFN-repressed genes that mediate gene expression. Data enabling the definition of IRGs, signalling pathways, regulatory networks and tissue specificities are assimilated in the INTERFEROME database (Hertzog *et al.*, 2011a).

Interferon (IFN) γ is a proinflammatory cytokine (Robbertse *et al.*, 2017) that stimulates production by various cells of the chemokine CXCL10 that promotes recruitment of $CD8^+$ and Th1-type $CD4^+$ effector T cells (see section 4.1.2, this volume) to infected or inflamed non-lymphoid tissues (Peperzak *et al.*, 2013).

The cells from which these cytokines originate include macrophages, T-lymphocytes and fibroblasts. The cytokines attract monocytes, NK cells, lymphocytes and granulocytes (eosinophils, neutrophils and basophils) (Meeusen *et al.*, 2013).

Eicosanoid inflammatory mediators partly develop from the metabolism of arachidonic acid through either the cyclo-oxygenase or the lipoxygenase pathway. The former gives rise to prostaglandins while the latter leads to the production of leukotrienes (Loick and Theissen, 1994). Leukotrienes induce microcirculatory alterations in response to noxious stimuli, such as short-lived vasoconstriction of arterioles followed by extravasation of macromolecules or adhesion of leucocytes to the endothelium in postcapillary venules (Dahlén *et al.*, 1981). Leukotriene B4 (LTB4) is one of the most potent leucotactic substances known (Salmon and Higgs, 1987). Production of LTB4 is increased by inflammatory mediators such as endotoxin, complement fragments, TNF and interleukins. LTB4 induces recruitment of neutrophils, monocytes and eosinophils, and stimulates the production of proinflammatory cytokines to augment and prolong tissue inflammation (Crooks and Stockley, 1998).

In addition to the eicosanoid leukotrienes and prostaglandins, histamine is also a mediator of inflammation. It is a vasodilator, smooth muscle constrictor and stimulator of vascular permeability and secretion of respiratory mucus and gastric acid. Histamine is synthesized in the Golgi apparatus of mast cells and basophils and is released when allergens bind to IgE antibodies on these cells, or when tissue is damaged. T-lymphocytes (see ection 4.1.3, this volume) may also play a role in mast cell degranulation (White, 1999).

The phenotypic resemblance of basophils, least abundant granulocyte and less than 1% of peripheral blood leucocytes to mast cells often leads to the former being considered as the blood-circulating precursors of the tissue-resident mast cells. The phenotypic resemblance is based on the basophilic granules, expression of the high-affinity FceRI IgE receptor on the cell surface and the release of histamine in response to a variety of stimuli. But non-redundant roles of basophils in immunity to parasitic infections, allergic inflammation and regulation of innate and adaptive immunity seem to indicate functional involvement of basophils in acquired tick resistance (Karasuyama *et al.*, 2020).

3.1.3 Receptors

Pathogen recognition receptors (PRRs) are either soluble (e.g. complement) or cell bound (e.g. Toll-like receptor – TLR) proteins. These receptors recognize pathogen-associated (PAMPs) and danger-associated molecular patterns (DAMPs) and once activated, they can result in an innate immune response, characterized by cytokine- and chemokine-mediated inflammation, increased phagocytosis and/or lysis of infectious agents (Swain *et al.*, 2012; Meeusen *et al.*, 2013).

The complement system contains more than 30 proteins, either circulating in the blood or present as membrane-associated proteins. They assist or 'complement' the immune system by opsonizing pathogens for removal by phagocytes. Initially identified as playing a major role in innate immunity, complement is also recognized as an important participant in adaptive immunity (maintaining immunological memory) and is also involved in tissue regeneration.

Complement is activated via three different pathways involving proteins that are sequentially cleaved and activated. The *classical* pathway is initiated by the formation of immune complexes when IgG or IgM binds to pathogens or non-self antigens (Sarma and Ward, 2011). The *lectin* pathway is activated when mannose-binding lectin (MBL) or ficolin binds to surfaces of pathogens such as yeasts, bacteria, viruses and parasites (Van Asbeck *et al.*, 2008; Sarma and Ward, 2011). The *alternative* pathway is triggered by carbohydrates, lipids and proteins found on foreign surfaces. The pathways converge at C3, the most abundant complement protein (Sarma and Ward, 2011).

The first member of the Toll receptor family was discovered in a *Drosophila melanogaster* (fruit fly) mutant, followed by identification of mammalian homologues (TLRs) and recognition of its homology with the interleukin cytokine family, implying a role in the immune response. TLRs are conserved and able to recognize a diverse array of divergent pathogen ligands.

They play a central role in the initiation of cellular innate immune responses, providing the transmembrane molecules that link the extracellular, where contact with the pathogen occurs, and intracellular, where signalling cascades are initiated, compartments. Expression of TLR endows cells with the ability to activate, e.g. NF-κB in response to lipopolysaccharide (Vasselon and Detmers, 2002).

A plethora of other receptors form part of the innate immune system but their relevance to tick infestation is unclear or unknown. They include RIG-I-like helicases (RLH), cytoplasmic RNA and DNA sensors, NOD-like receptors (NLR), C-type lectins (CTLs), pentraxins and alarmins (Meeusen *et al.*, 2013). Although NLRs were acknowledged for their role in signal transduction in innate immune responses, their molecular mode of action was largely unknown (Proell *et al.*, 2008). This multiprotein inflammasome complex is now known to play a pivotal role in regulating the innate immune system and inflammatory signalling. The NLRs include the NLRP3, expressed by macrophages, glial cells, neurons and endothelial cells. After activation by PAMPs and DAMPs, the NLRP3 inflammasome leads to release of the IL-1β and IL-18 proinflammatory cytokines (Swanson *et al.*, 2019; Söderbom and Zeng, 2020; Blevins *et al.*, 2022).

Receptors for the Fc portion of immunoglobulins (see ection 4.1.3, this volume) are found on all cell types of the immune system (Fridman, 1991).

3.1.4 Effectors

Effector mechanisms of the humoral innate immune system include activation and regulation of the complement cascade, agglutination and neutralization, facilitation of recognition via cellular receptors (opsonization) and regulation of inflammation (Bottazzi *et al.*, 2010).

Stimuli from the external environment set in train signalling patterns, read by downstream effectors of cellular behaviour, such as gene expression. One such effector leading to proinflammatory gene synthesis is the nuclear factor κ-B (NF-κB) family of signalling proteins or transcription factors regulating the expression of genes intrinsic to inflammation (Janssen *et al.*, 1995; Goto *et al.*, 2008a, b; Yu *et al.*, 2009; Meeusen *et al.*, 2013; Maity and Wollman, 2020).

Akirin is a nuclear transcription cofactor involved in innate immunity and conserved in insects such as *Anopheles* mosquitoes. It regulates NF-κB-dependent gene expression in the IMD (immune deficiency) antibacterial defence response pathway (Letinic *et al.*, 2021). Its orthologue in ticks is subolesin (Artigas-Jerónimo *et al.*, 2018; see section 5.2.5, this volume).

3.2 Innate Immunity Genetics and Heritability

The genetic determinants of (breed) variability in susceptibility/resistance are deemed not to be the genes involved in acquired immunity but rather the genes of the innate immune response at the start of an infection or vaccination. The innate immune system and its receptors seem to account for most of the host variability in resistance or susceptibility to parasite infestations. Genetic lesions or polymorphisms in genes of innate immune pathways are revealed in subtle phenotypes of impaired resistance to a family of pathogens (Meeusen *et al.*, 2013).

Genetically controlled variation in tick numbers occurs within breeds and is said to be more than 40% heritable. Tick resistance is a composite trait with many non-immune components (see section 2.3, this volume). Variation in the immune components could relate to hypersensitivity and humoral and cellular responses. Proteomic analysis might enable the discovery of biomarkers with which resistant cattle could be selected (see *Histological and molecular changes* below) (Raza *et al.*, 2021, 2023).

3.3 Innate Immunity to Ticks

Cattle that are resistant to ticks can be selected genomically but the identified genomic markers cannot be assumed to indicate stronger innate immunity. Breed genetic differences in susceptibility to ticks (see section 2.3, this volume) might be attributable to factors other than immunity, such as hair length, coat thickness, smoothness and colour, body size and physiological status (Mapholi *et al.*, 2014; Mapholi, 2015).

Histamine released in response to a tick bite not only impairs the tick's attachment but also diminishes its feeding and reproductive success (Paesen *et al.*, 2000). An alternative interpretation is that in susceptible cattle, a chronic state of inflammation is beneficial to the tick through increased capillary permeability, thus facilitating tick feeding and survival (Piper, 2010) (see section 3.5 below).

Extracts of larvae of [*B. microplus*] *R. australis* were shown to contain allergens able to elicit an immediate hypersensitivity reaction but also the production of antibodies. Both reactions were found to be significantly correlated with resistance to ticks (Willadsen *et al.*, 1978). Resistance to ticks has both innate and adaptive immune components and the relative importance of each seems to differ between cattle breeds. The resistance seems to have its biggest effect against attaching tick larvae, thwarting their attempts to feed (Jonsson *et al.*, 2014).

3.3.1 Manifestation

To the naked eye, resistance to ticks is manifest in the smaller numbers of ticks that resistant animals carry. European breed cattle can carry 5–10 times as many ticks as Zebu facing the same infestation challenge (Jonsson *et al.*, 2014). Engorged dropped adult female ticks that are collected and examined reveal that their engorgement is impaired, as are their fecundity (egg production) and fertility (egg hatchability).

There is thus host variation – some animals carry more ticks than others. This variation is either visible, in the phenotypic distinction between different breeds of livestock, or invisible, as in individual genetic variation which can be determined by quantitative genetics and expressed as an estimated predictive breeding value, or genomically, where the responsible gene(s) sequences are known (Gasparin *et al.*, 2007; Mapholi *et al.*, 2014; Mapholi, 2015).

On naïve, previously unexposed cattle infested with between 500 and 20,000 larvae, there is no difference in the percentage of ticks maturing. Where a higher tick density might be expected to lead to competition for feeding sites or an enhanced host response, this appeared not to be the case, with tick mortality being density independent. This was true for both European and Zebu cattle used in the experiments (Sutherst *et al.*, 1978).

A possible 'knock-on' manifestation of resistance to ticks might be reduced transmission of tick-borne pathogens. Cross-bred cattle exposed to the same [*B. microplus*] *R. australis* tick infestation challenge were 1.5 times as likely to become infected with *Anaplasma marginale* as were their Brahman cograzers (Bock *et al.*, 1999a). A similar tendency was seen when Queensland laboratory records were analysed for *Babesia* spp. prevalence and the number of cases in European (taurine) cattle were found to be 10–12 times greater than in Zebu cattle (Bock *et al.*, 1999b).

Resistance to ticks might also be inferred from the fact that Zebu cattle seemed to require far fewer acaricidal treatments than European breed cattle in a survey conducted in the tick-infested areas of Queensland during 1977–78. In the same survey, 97.8% of producers were engaged in controlling [*B. microplus*] *R. australis* on their cattle, more than half of producers had switched to pure-bred or cross-bred Zebu cattle in the preceding 10 years and up to 45% had done so on account of resistance to ticks (Elder *et al.*, 1980a, b, c).

Histamine-mediated cutaneous inflammation is one of the innate immune reactions mounted by host animals against blood-feeding ticks. It adversely affects attachment of ticks to the skin but also diminishes their feeding and reproductive success (Paesen *et al.*, 2000).

3.3.2 Differences in tick resistance

The phenotypical differences between European and Zebu cattle, one of which is their susceptibility to tick infestation, have been described extensively and are frequently alluded to in this volume. Larvae and nymphs of induced infestations of [*B. microplus*] *R. australis* grew more slowly on Brahman than on Shorthorn cattle (Wagland, 1978). The immunological basis for this difference was not understood (Constantinoiu *et al.*, 2010) and is the subject of ongoing research.

A bit of background information on this distinction is the explanation of the division of prehistoric cattle into the Auroch type (with long hair, unpigmented skin, short horns, found mainly north and south of the respective 30° latitudes) and the Indian type (short-haired, pigmented skin, long-horned, found within the equatorial belt). Foci of Auroch-type cattle uncharacteristically occurring within the equatorial belt were to be found at altitudes of 1200m and above. Historians at the time of Julius Caesar evidently noted the difference in appearance of cattle in Italy and northern Gaul. Texan cattle breeders discovered that, as they introduced more of the European genotype into their original Zebu herds originating from Mexico, the less resistant they became to ectoparasites and Texan fever (babesiosis) (Anon., 1932; Kelley, 1932).

A potentially controversial question has been whether breed differences in tick susceptibility are a function of innate or adaptive immunity. Based on the outcome of large single induced infestations of (presumably) [*B. microplus*] *R. australis* on previously unexposed cattle, the assumption has been that breed differences do not become evident until animals had been infested with ticks at least three times. It was acknowledged that while a degree of resistance developed within 8 days, individual differences did not stabilize until approximately 30 days after infestation (Hewetson, 1972).

A comprehensive analysis was performed of the peripheral blood mononuclear cell (PBMC) population, cytokine and gene expression by peripheral blood leucocytes, and levels of tick-specific immunoglobulin G1 (IgG1) antibodies in the peripheral circulation of tick-susceptible Holstein and tick-resistant Brahman cattle previously exposed to natural *R. microplus* infestation (Piper *et al.*, 2009). The immune response of the European cattle was based on a type I hypersensitivity reaction and a sustained inflammatory response (Constantinoiu *et al.*, 2010), which characterizes innate immunity. The Zebu cattle developed a T-cell-mediated response and the related leucocyte cytokine spectrum (see Chapter 4, this volume). This greater ability of European cattle to recognize and respond to tick salivary antigens possibly sets up a chronic inflammation which benefits the tick with increased capillary permeability, creating a suitable environment for tick feeding and survival (Piper, 2010).

Tick burdens

European cattle were reported to carry 10.5 times as many engorged [*B. microplus*] *R. australis* as Droughtmaster (a hybrid developed in Australia by crossing Brahman bulls with cows of European breeds) cattle grazing under the same conditions (Francis and Ashton, 1967).

The Nguni breed is a subtype of African Sanga cattle and a genetic mixture of Indian and European breeds, with smaller cervicothoracic humps than Zebu cattle. They are renowned for their hardiness and resistance to ticks and tick-borne disease (Anon., 2002). Archaeological evidence suggests their presence in southern Africa (south of the Congo, the Democratic Republic of Congo and Tanzania) from the late Stone Age (AD 253–453) (Lander and Russell, 2018). Over a 2-year period of exposure to natural infestation, Nguni cattle carried significantly fewer *A. hebraeum*, [*B.*] *R. decoloratus* and *Hyalomma* spp. than either Hereford or Bonsmara cattle simultaneously grazing the same paddock (Spickett *et al.*, 1989).

Originating from the West Indies but with N'Dama genetic content, Senepol is regarded as a tropically adapted taurine beef breed. Its superior tick resistance had been suspected but was proven in a trial comparing one-sided counts of 4.5–8 mm engorging adult *R. microplus* on pure-bred Limousin and Limousin × Senepol cattle exposed to natural infestation on the same pastures in New Caledonia. The Limousin cattle carried 6.4 times as many ticks as the Limousin × Senepol (Hüe *et al.*, 2014).

The tick loads resulting from induced infestation of tick-naïve Nelore (a breed originating from Andhra Pradesh in India) and Holstein calves with *R. microplus* larvae were compared after 21 days. The Holstein calves, chosen for tick susceptibility, displayed significantly more ticks than the Nelore breed (Franzin *et al.*, 2017). Nellore cattle in the Cerrado biome in Brazil were found to carry fewer *R. microplus* ticks than Brangus cattle over a 12-month period (Martins *et al.*, 2022). In the latter part of the 20th century, virtually all beef producers in northern Australia used cattle with >37.5% Zebu/indicine genetic content (Bock *et al.*, 1997).

More larvae from an induced infestation of [*B. microplus*] *R. australis* survived on European than on Zebu cattle. The rate of survival was not affected by tick density, regardless of whether they were challenged with 500 or 20,000 larvae (Sutherst *et al.*, 1978). Variable proportions of larvae, nymphs and female *H. longicornis* matured on naturally infested, previously unexposed cattle, indicating different levels of resistance to each instar (Sutherst *et al.*, 1979).

Histological and molecular changes

When cattle with high and low tick burdens in each group were compared, the latter were shown to have a higher frequency of the amylase B gene. The mean tick count of both Droughtmaster and European cattle carrying the amylase B allele was 37% lower than the number of ticks on those not carrying this allele (Francis and Ashton, 1967). In contrast, cattle of 25 populations of diverse breeds carrying significantly more ticks were of the amylase C phenotype (Ashton *et al.*, 1968). Amylase is expressed at high levels in the pancreas (all vertebrates) and salivary glands (some primates, rodents, lagomorphs and chiropterans) (Samuelson *et al.*, 1996) and catalyses the first step in the digestion of dietary starch and glycogen. Amylase-encoding genes are not known to interfere with any defence system of the host (Hynes *et al.*, 2014). The relevance, if any, of the amylase B gene to tick resistance could not be established, but it is tempting to surmise about the potential role of circulating amylase in neutralizing glycoproteins in tick saliva.

The inflammatory chemokine CXCL10 is upregulated in response to tick infestation, to a greater degree in susceptible than in resistant cattle breeds (Robbertse *et al.*, 2017).

Skin biopsies were collected from susceptible (Holstein) and resistant (Nelore) calves before, and 2 and 9 days after (by which time the larvae had moulted to nymphs) a single induced *R. microplus* infestation. Feeding larvae and nymphs were also collected for examination of their gene expression profiles. The skin samples were subject to comprehensive examination of gene expression and histological appearance of tick bite wounds. The allergic contact-like dermatitis leading to production of IL-6 and expression of proinflammatory cytokines and chemokines that recruit granulocytes and T-lymphocytes was delayed in susceptible hosts. Transcripts encoding secreted molecules modulating host immunity were more abundant in the salivary glands of larvae and nymphs feeding on susceptible hosts. In genetically tick-resistant animals, the inflammatory reaction destabilized the tick cement cone. Tick-resistant hosts significantly affected the expression of genes encoding secreted immunomodulatory proteins (see section 3.4 below) in tick salivary glands. The interpretation was that resistant hosts deal with the infestation earlier, by way of the inflammatory response, which means that ticks are less able to express those proteins that suppress host immunity, inflammation and coagulation (Franzin *et al.*, 2017).

Differential abundance analyses of the protein profiles from serum samples revealed significant differences for 28 proteins in naïve Santa Gertrudis cattle. The animals were subsequently classified as resistant or susceptible, based on their tick counts. In tick-resistant cattle, 21 of these proteins were more abundant. They were involved in the regulation of immune responses and included aerpin-A10, α1-acid glycoprotein, coagulation factor V and three complement proteins (Raza *et al.*, 2021).

3.4 Modulation of Innate Immunity

Innate immunity is moderated by endogenous prophylactic and therapeutic modulators, some stimulatory and others suppressive. Although the inflammatory response to a pathogen forms the basis of innate immunity, its effects of fever and pain (*calor, dolor*) can be clinically unacceptable, which has given rise to the development of anti-inflammatory drugs with different modes of action (Meeusen *et al.*, 2013). Inappropriate complement activation can be pathological or injurious, needing modulation. This is achieved by a variety of endogenous mechanisms, such as cleavage enzymes, clearance of immune complexes by phagocytosis and preventing the assembly or activity of complement C3 convertase (Sarma and Ward, 2011).

Exogenous enhancement of the initial inflammation of the innate immune response can be beneficial, such as when it improves the immunogenicity of a vaccine. The use of adjuvants is discussed in section 5.5.1 (this volume).

In order to complete their life cycles and transmit their pathogens, ticks have evolved sophisticated mechanisms to evade and modulate the host's innate immune (inflammation, in primary infestations) defence, and both innate and adaptive immunity during secondary or subsequent infestations, with a pharmacopoeia of bioactive lipids and proteins in their saliva (Mans, 2005; Mans *et al.*, 2008; Francischetti *et al.*, 2009; Chmelař *et al.*, 2016, 2017; Denisov and Dijkgraaf, 2021). With a mixture of tick species often found infesting the same animal, it seems plausible that they utilize universally conserved proteins, such as calreticulin (CRT), to regulate and facilitate feeding (Kim *et al.*, 2015a). Comparative analysis of the sialome (salivary gland secretory proteome) has indicated that the major protein families are conserved in soft and hard ticks (Mans and Ribeiro, 2008).

Proteolytic enzymes (proteases, proteinases, peptidases) are ubiquitous enzymes participating in a range of physiological processes, such as extracellular digestion, protein degradation and tissue development. They often function in proteolytic cascades, as in the case of coagulation of plasma, and each step activates another downstream protease, with endogenous inhibitors to balance the system.

Protease inhibitors are widely distributed in nature and serine protease inhibitors (serpins) form the largest, most studied superfamily. They are important constituents of the proteins secreted into the host in tick saliva. They are grouped into Kunitz inhibitors, serpins and components and exert their effects not only against blood coagulation but also the host's immune response. Serpins are abundant in ticks from a variety of species and they perform various functions (Chmelař *et al.*, 2017).

The Kunitz inhibitors contain a structure known as the Kunitz fold (Corral-Rodríguez *et al.*, 2009) and they are ubiquitous, from microbes to mammals. They can have single or multiple Kunitz inhibitory domains, characterized by its peptide chain with a conserved spacing between cysteine residues and a typical disulfide bonding pattern. Bovine pancreatic trypsin inhibitor (BPTI) was the first one to be described in 1936 (Ranasinghe and McManus, 2013).

Based on their ultrastructure, there are four types of acini in tick salivary glands. Types I–III occur in female ticks and one is agranular in appearance, while two are granular. The fourth type of acinus occurs in male ixodid ticks and is involved in the transfer of the spermatophore from the male to the female. Early publications assigned function to the various salivary gland acini based on their morphology (Neelakanta and Sultana, 2022) but it has been acknowledged that proteome expression analysis might be a more reliable indicator in the case of haemostatic proteins (Mans *et al.*, 2004).

It would be expected that the minute quantities injected by a tick larva, weighing about 20 μg unfed, would be rapidly dispersed into the host's systemic circulation. But the intriguing aspect of ticks' ability to remain attached despite the host's immune response seems to be that some of the salivary components become bound to the host's tissue around the attachment site. Two tick antigens, one an esterase and the other a proteinase inhibitor, displaying this polymerization behaviour were described (Willadsen and McKenna, 1983) but it has since been suggested that most of the saliva components remain in the immediate vicinity of the feeding lesion to prevent coagulation, inflammation and immune reactions (Steen *et al.*, 2006).

3.4.1 Anticoagulant effects

A crucial element in the host response to vascular injury is thrombocytes, activated by adenosine diphosphate (ADP) released from damaged endothelial cells. Antihaemostatic effects, allowing uninterrupted feeding, are some of the first manifestations of tick interference with the host's defence (Stutzer *et al.*, 2009). Anticoagulants in tick saliva have been grouped as factor Xa inhibitors, tissue factor pathway inhibitors and direct thrombin inhibitors (Hovius *et al.*, 2008).

Apyrases (ATP: diphosphohydrolases) form part of the arthropod anticoagulant repertoire and degrade ATP and ADP to AMP and inorganic phosphate. *Apyrase* activity was ascribed to *Ornithodoros moubata*, *Ornithodoros savignyi* and *Ixodes scapularis* in 1985, when sequence data were not yet available (Stutzer *et al.*, 2009).

One of the families identified from the group of haemostatic protein enzymes by proteome expression analysis (Mans *et al.*, 2004) are the *5'-nucleotidases*, found in *O. savignyi* and [*B.*] *R. microplus* (Stutzer *et al.*, 2009).

Ornithodoros savignyi secretes a number of *savignygrins* that inhibit platelet aggregation, thus allowing parasitism on a wide host range (Mans *et al.*, 2002, 2003a). The tick *lipocalin* family is big and groups phylogenetically in genus-specific clades, suggesting that functional divergence occurred after evolutionary speciation. *Moubatin* is a lipocalin and an inhibitor of collagen-induced platelet aggregation in *O. moubata* (Mans *et al.*, 2003b), due to scavenging of thromboxane (Mans and Ribeiro, 2008).

Salp14 delays blood coagulation by inhibiting factor Xa, has been identified in *I. scapularis* and has been described as the prototypic tick saliva anticoagulant (Narasimhan *et al.*, 2002, 2004; Denisov *et al.*, 2021). RNAi was used to silence the expression of Salp14 and reduced the ability of *I. scapularis* to feed, measured by a 50–70% decline in engorgement weights. This was attributed to a 60–80% reduction in antifactor Xa activity (Narasimhan *et al.*, 2004).

Prostaglandins have divergent roles in the regulation of immune responses. Known to occur in salivary glands of [*B.*] *R. microplus*, *I. scapularis* and *A. americanum*, salivary prostaglandins E_2 and I_2 are vasodilators and inhibitors of platelet aggregation (Brossard and Wikel, 2004).

Metalloproteases (MPs) constitute 79% of the 5.7% proteases contained in saliva from *I. scapularis* (Kim *et al.*, 2016b). They fulfill diverse biological functions, such as preventing blood clotting, degrading extracellular matrix proteins and antiangiogenic activity, thereby inhibiting host tissue repair. They are considered essential for successful completion of a bloodmeal, preventing haemostasis by breaking down fibrin and fibrinogen. Their involvement in tick feeding has been confirmed by upregulation of MP transcription in salivary glands. Inhibition of MP expression in *I. ricinus* by RNAi inhibits fibrinogen breakdown and prevents completion of the bloodmeal (Ali *et al.*, 2015).

Calreticulins (CRT) are conserved calcium-binding proteins, shown to be secreted in the saliva of several tick species to regulate and facilitate feeding (Kim *et al.*, 2015a; Zheng *et al.*, 2022). CRT binds factor Xa, an important protease in the blood-clotting cascade (Kim *et al.*, 2015a).

Several *serpins* feature in the coagulation cascade and they are abundant in tick saliva. They can reduce platelet aggregation and delay plasma clotting time (Chmelař *et al.*, 2017; Costa *et al.*, 2021). *Iris* (*I. ricinus* immunosuppressor; Narasimhan *et al.*, 2002) has antihaemostatic properties which include suppression of coagulation and fibrinolysis (Chmelař *et al.*, 2017). It has been identified in *I. ricinus* and *Ixodes persulcatus* (Toyomane *et al.*, 2016; Pham *et al.*, 2021). *Amblyomma americanum* serpin 19 (AAS19) is highly conserved and inhibits five of the eight serine protease factors in the coagulation cascade (Kim *et al.*, 2015b, 2016a). A recombinant serpin-15 from [*R. microplus*] *R. australis* (RmS15) expressed by *Pichia pastoris* was demonstrated to inhibit thrombin and delay plasma coagulation (Rodriguez-Valle *et al.*, 2015; Xu *et al.*, 2016). Because it shares 89.58% amino acid identity with RmS15 and is expressed in the salivary gland, RhS8 from *R. haemaphysaloides* is assumed to have the same effect on haemagglutination. But RhS8 is also expressed in the tick's fat body and ovary (not in the midgut). Gene silencing with RNAi demonstrated that RhS8 is involved in vitellogenesis (Xu *et al.*, 2020). Serpins identified in *A. sculptum* saliva did not inhibit coagulation and are assumed to play another role in haematophagy (Costa *et al.*, 2021).

Techniques such as nuclear magnetic resonance (NMR) and X-ray crystallography have revealed structural differences between the Kunitz domains from BPTI and tick anticoagulant protein (TAP) (Antuch *et al.*, 1994; St Charles *et al.*, 2000). Their inhibitory specificity varies with the particular amino acids at the reactive sites (Ranasinghe and McManus, 2013). BPTIs act as thrombin, factor Xa and platelet aggregation inhibitors in soft ticks, and inhibit the factor VII a:tissue factor (fVIIa/TF) complex in hard ticks (Mans and Ribeiro, 2008), such as *R. microplus*, but not thrombin (Corral-Rodríguez *et al.*, 2009). In blood-sucking arthropods, several of them also defend against microbial pathogen invasion (Ranasinghe and McManus, 2013).

Several two-domain Kunitz inhibitors have been isolated from both soft ticks (e.g. *ornithodorin* from *O. moubata*) and hard ticks (e.g. *boophilin* from [*B.*] *R. microplus*) (Corral-Rodríguez *et al.*, 2009). Boophilin was cloned and overexpressed in *E. coli* and found not only to inhibit the procoagulant enzyme thrombin but to also interfere with other serpins, such as trypsin and plasmin (Macedo-Ribeiro *et al.*, 2008).

Sequential secretion of functionally similar but chemically different salivary proteins during blood feeding is thought to protect tick feeding from the host's immune system. Host immune responses to tick salivary proteins secreted 24 hours after attachment will not be effective at later feeding stages. Another finding was that fibrinogen was highly abundant in tick saliva at the time of detachment, allowing healing of the bite wound when the tick detaches (Kim *et al.*, 2016b).

3.4.2 Inhibition of complement activation

Tick-mediated immunosuppressive countermeasures include inhibition of complement activation and antibody responses (Wikel, 1999).

Calreticulin (CRT) was the first molecularly cloned tick salivary gland protein, shown to be secreted in *Amblyomma* and *Dermacentor* saliva. Known as a major endoplasmic reticulum (ER) calcium-binding protein, tick-secreted CRT lacks the ER retention signal (Jaworski *et al.*, 1995). CRT has since been reported to sequester C1q in the classical complement pathway (see section 3.1.3 above) but recombinant *A. americanum* CRT did not inhibit this pathway, nor did it affect plasma clotting or platelet aggregation, and may be functionally different (Kim *et al.*, 2015a).

Lipocalins in tick saliva function as anti-complement factors and inhibitors of platelet aggregation and toxins in soft ticks, such as *O. moubata* complement inhibitor (OMCI) in moubatin (Mans *et al.*, 2008; Mans and Ribeiro, 2008).

Salp14, in addition to delaying thrombin generation and blood coagulation, also contributes to delaying the lectin complement pathway through interaction with mannan-binding lectin-associated serine proteases (Denisov *et al.*, 2021).

3.4.3 Anti-inflammatory effects

Several micro-RNAs (miRNAs) and non-coding RNAs (ncRNAs) have been discovered in tick saliva that could target host genes involved in inflammation and regulation of tick infestation (Boulanger and Wikel, 2021).

Lipocalins occur in all living organisms, play important roles in immune responses and transport of hydrophobic molecules, and have low amino acid sequence similarity, but share a highly conserved protein tertiary structure in the form of a barrel with a central pocket. More than 300 lipocalins are known to occur in ticks and those from saliva or salivary glands are only assigned to the lipocalin family based on their structural similarity (Cheng *et al.*, 2010).

Tick histamine-binding proteins are *lipocalins* ('calyces for lipophilic ligands') with two binding pockets (Paesen *et al.*, 2000), and there are estimated to be several hundred molecules (Guizzo *et al.*, 2023). Four lipocalins have been found in *I. persulcatus* saliva, and their histamine-binding activity confirmed *in vitro* (Konnai *et al.*, 2011). In hard ticks, lipocalins scavenge histamine and serotonin (Mans *et al.*, 2008). They bind histamine by sequestering it in a binding cavity in the lipocalin fold (Paesen *et al.*, 2000; Mans, 2005). *R. appendiculatus* secretes histamine-binding proteins into the wound site during early feeding, addressing the pain and itch response at the infestation site by sequestering the locally released histamine molecules and preventing them from reaching their target cells (Paesen *et al.*, 2000). Another histamine-binding lipocalin was identified in the salivary glands of *Hyalomma asiaticum* (Aounallah *et al.*, 2020).

Leukotriene mediators of inflammation are also bound by some tick lipocalins (Beaufays *et al.*, 2008a, b; Mans and Ribeiro, 2008), and lipocalins also play a role in modulating the adaptive immune response (see section 4.6, this volume).

Three recombinant *R. microplus* serine protease inhibitors (*serpins*) were shown to inhibit proinflammatory and procoagulant proteases (Tirloni *et al.*, 2016). Ticks can alleviate the itch and pain of their bites, caused by mast cell and basophil degranulation and release of histamine and serotonin, with salivary components that

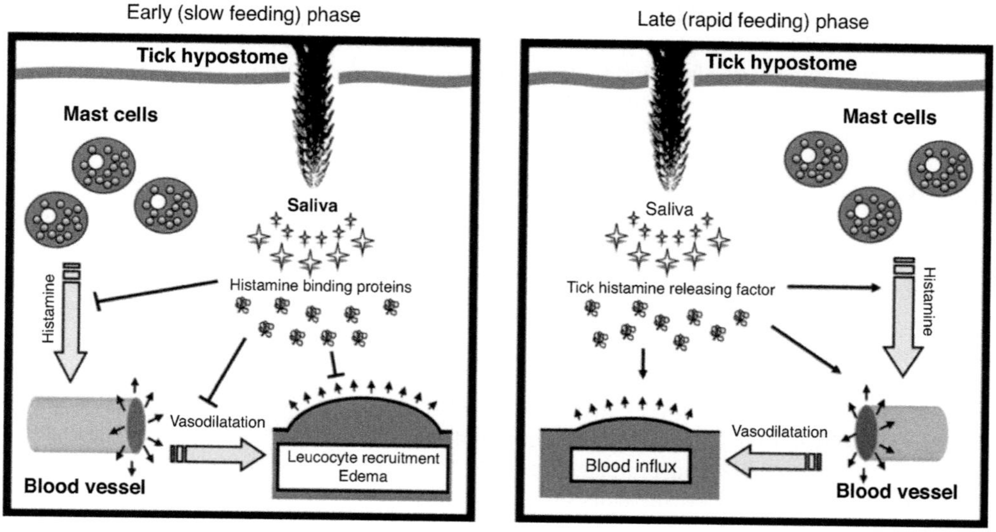

Fig. 3.2. Modulation of histamine dynamics during tick feeding. Histamine release is initially opposed by tick salivary histamine-binding proteins, and then encouraged by tick histamine-releasing factor. From Chmelař *et al.* (2012) with permission of Elsevier.

sequester these molecules or modulate mast cell function. *R. microplus* saliva contains serpins (Bouton *et al.*, 2023) that modulate mast cell function by inhibiting chymase and vascular permeability in acute inflammation. IRS-2, the second serpin to be characterized in *I. ricinus*, displayed inhibitory activity against mast cell chymase and cathepsin G, two proteases involved in inflammatory responses. It also inhibited the production of proinflammatory IL-6 in DC, impairing the signalling of T-helper cells, inhibiting the maturation of proinflammatory Th17 lymphocytes (Chmelař *et al.*, 2017). Tryptogalinin is a Kunitz serpin, isolated from *I. scapularis* and displaying flexibility in its high affinity for several serine proteases involved in inflammation and vertebrate immunity, which may facilitate tick blood feeding (Valdes *et al.*, 2013).

Transcriptomic analysis revealed the temporal expression of 44 *A. americanum* salivary genes (Bullard *et al.*, 2016). Fig. 3.2 provides a graphic representation of the way in which tick saliva orchestrates the role of the host's histamine release. In the early feeding phase, histamine-binding proteins suppress the inflammatory response, while tick histamine-releasing factor encourages a blood influx in the late feeding phase, when rapid engorgement occurs (Chmelař *et al.*, 2012).

The pharmacopoeia of bioactive compounds in secreted tick saliva raises the question of exploiting their possible therapeutic benefit. Tick histamine-binding lipocalins might be useful against, for example, conjunctivitis, allergic rhinitis and rheumatoid arthritis (Mans, 2005).

3.4.4 Immunosuppression

Lymphocytes from tick-infested hosts have a reduced ability to proliferate *in vitro* in response to T-lymphocyte mitogens, macrophages produce less IL-1 and TNF-α, while T-lymphocytes produce less IL-2 and IFN-γ (Wikel *et al.*, 1994).

Sialostatins identified in the saliva of *I. persulcatus* were orthologues of sialostatins from *I. scapularis*. They are expressed in the salivary glands of the tick throughout its life, from before they start feeding and during engorgement. They exert their immunosuppressant effects by inhibiting cathepsin L and S, and the production of IFN-γ inducible protein 10 (IP-10), TNF-α and IL-6 by bone marrow-derived dendritic cells (BMDCs) (Sajiki *et al.*, 2020). Cathepsins L and S play important roles in MHC II antigen processing and presentation (see section 4.1.1, this volume; Pham *et al.*, 2021). IP-10 is a chemokine that induces chemotaxis, apoptosis, cell growth and angiostasis after binding to its receptor. It is a biomarker for predicting the severity of various diseases and an alteration in its expression is associated with immune dysfunction (Liu *et al.*, 2011).

3.4.5 Enhanced pathogen transmission

Tick saliva prepares the site of inoculation, making it tolerant of inoculated pathogens. This preparation is quick for viruses, whose transmission starts within minutes of commencement of the bloodmeal. Bacteria and protozoa face a delay of 12–24 hours before inoculation is observed. Tick modulation of the host's defence allows *B. burgdorferi* to multiply and persist in the skin for months. Hypodermal adipocytes have been shown to play a role in the case of *Plasmodium* (malaria) and *Trypanosoma* (sleeping sickness) infections, but their role has not yet been defined for tick-borne diseases (Boulanger and Wikel, 2021). More discussion of this immunomodulatory effect of ticks is provided in section 4.5.5, this volume.

3.5 Transition to Adaptive Immunity

Complement plays a major role in the robust and rapid innate immune response to invading pathogens, but it is also important in adaptive immunity involving T- and B-cells that help in the elimination of pathogens (Sarma and Ward, 2011). Dendritic cells also form a link between innate and adaptive immunity, in their role as antigen-presenting cells (APC) (Palucka and Banchereau, 1999; Burster *et al.*, 2010). DC are the most potent APC in priming naïve T-cells (see section 4.1.2, this volume) (Mejri and Brossard, 2007). The major histocompatibility complex (MHC; see section 4.1.1, this volume) is another 'bridging' link ensuring the presentation of foreign antigens for activation of the adaptive immune response (Janeway *et al.*, 2001).

The transition from innate to adaptive immunity could be studied in previously naïve cattle infested seven times at weekly intervals with larvae of [*R. microplus*] *R australis*. The dynamics of leucocyte (T-cells, B-cells, MHC class II-expressing cells and granulocytes) infiltrations in the skin near tick mouth parts were compared for European (Holstein-Friesian) and Zebu (Brahman) cattle. Granulocytes and MHC class II-expressing cells infiltrated closest to the mouthparts of larvae, and granulocyte infiltrations increased more rapidly and numerously from the day after infestation in European cattle. There was no difference between the breeds in the infiltration of T-cells ($CD3^+$, $CD4^+$, $CD8^+$, $\gamma\delta$), which increased substantially at 7 weeks after the first infestation. There were more of all cell types except granulocytes in the skin of Zebu cattle but this difference was only significant for $\gamma\delta$ T-cells (Constantinoiu *et al.*, 2010).

Tick-susceptible (European) cattle respond to infestation with [*B. microplus*] *R. australis* with an apparently non-protective antibody intense inflammatory response, whereas tick-resistant (Zebu) cattle demonstrate different structural responses in the skin at the tick attachment site. The susceptibility of European breeds may be due to their heightened ability to recognize and respond to tick salivary antigens introduced during the blood-feeding process. This ability may act to set up a chronic state of inflammation that is beneficial to the tick through increased capillary permeability providing a suitable environment for tick feeding and survival (Piper, 2010). In other words, it is probable that the transition to adaptive immunity to ticks is less successful in European than in Zebu cattle.

References

Ali, A., Parizi, L.F., Guizzo, M.G., Tirloni, L., Seixas, A. *et al.* (2015) Immunoprotective potential of a *Rhipicephalus* (*Boophilus*) *microplus* metalloprotease. *Veterinary Parasitology* 207, 107–114. DOI: 10.1016/j.vetpar.2014.11.007.

Allen, J.R., Khalil, H.M. and Wikel, S.K. (1979) Langerhans cells trap tick salivary gland antigens in tick-resistant guinea pigs. *Journal of Immunology* 122/2, 563–565. DOI: 10.4049/jimmunol.122.2.563.

Anon. (1932) The development of a new breed of cattle for a tropical environment. *Australian Veterinary Journal* 8/2, 64–67. DOI: 10.1111/j.1751-0813.1932.tb06243.x.

Anon. (2002) Nguni: The breed from the past for the future. *Embryo Plus*. Available at: https://web.archive.org/web/20060223035015/http://www.embryoplus.com/cattle_nguni.html (accessed 24 March 2024).

Antuch, W., Güntert, P., Billeter, M., Hawthorne, T., Grossenbacher, H. *et al.* (1994) NMR solution structure of the recombinant tick anticoagulant protein (rTAP), a factor Xa inhibitor from the tick *Ornithodoros moubata*. *FEBS Letters* 352, 251–257.

Aounallah, H., Bensaoud, C., M'ghirbi, Y., Faria, F., Chmelař, J. *et al.* (2020) Tick salivary compounds for targeted immunomodulatory therapy. *Frontiers in Immunology* 11, 583845. DOI: 10.3389/fimmu.2020.583845.

Artigas-Jerónimo, S., Villar, M., Cabezas-Cruz, A., Valdés, J.J., Estrada-Peña, A. *et al.* (2018) Functional evolution of subolesin/akirin. *Frontiers in Physiology* 9, 1612. DOI: 10.3389/fphys.2018.01612.

Ashton, G.C., Seifert, G.W. and Francis, J. (1968) An association between serum amylase phenotype and tick infestation in cattle. *Australian Journal of Biological Science* 21, 303–308. DOI: 10.1071/BI9680303.

Beaufays, J., Adam, B., Decrem, Y., Prévôt, P.P., Santini, S. *et al.* (2008a) *Ixodes ricinus* tick lipocalins: Identification, cloning, phylogenetic analysis and biochemical characterization. *PLoS One* 3/12, e3941. DOI: 10.1371/journal.pone.0003941.

Beaufays, J., Adam, B., Menten-Dedoyart, C., Fievez, L., Grosjean, A. *et al.* (2008b) Ir-LBP, an *Ixodes ricinus* tick salivary LTB4-binding lipocalin, interferes with host neutrophil function. *PLoS One* 3/12, e3987. DOI: 10.1371/journal.pone.0003987.

Blevins, H.M., Xu, Y., Biby, S. and Zhang, S. (2022) The NLRP3 inflammasome pathway: A review of mechanisms and inhibitors for the treatment of inflammatory diseases. *Frontiers in Aging Neuroscience* 14, 879021. DOI: 10.3389/fnagi.2022.879021.

Bock, R.E., de Vos, A.J., Kingston, T.G. and McLellan, D.J. (1997) Effect of breed of cattle on innate resistance to infection with *Babesia bovis, B. Bigemina and Anaplasma marginale*. *Australian Veterinary Journal* 75/5, 337–340. DOI: 10.1111/j.1751-0813.1997.tb15706.x.

Bock, R.E., Kingston, T.G. and de Vos, A.J. (1999a) Effect of breed of cattle on innate resistance to infection with *Anaplasma marginale* transmitted by *Boophilus microplus*. *Australian Veterinary Journal* 77/11, 748–751.

Bock, R.E., Kingston, T.G. and de Vos, A.J. (1999b) Effect of breed of cattle on transmission rate and innate resistance to infection with *Babesia bovis* and *B. bigemina* transmitted by *Boophilus microplus*. *Australian Veterinary Journal* 77/7, 461–464.

Bottazzi, B., Doni, A., Garlanda, C. and Mantovani, A. (2010) An integrated view of humoral innate immunity: Pentraxins as a paradigm. *Annual Review of Immunology* 28, 157–183.

Boulanger, N. and Wikel, S. (2021) Induced transient immune tolerance in ticks and vertebrate host: A keystone of tick-borne diseases? *Frontiers in Immunology* 12, 625993. DOI: 10.3389/fimmu.2021.625993.

Bouton, M.C., Geiger, M., Sheffield, W.P., Irving, J.A., Lomas, D.A. *et al.* (2023) The under-appreciated world of the serpin family of serine proteinase inhibitors. *EMBO Molecular Medicine* 15, e17144. DOI: 10.15252/emmm.202217144.

Brossard, M.L. and Wikel, S.K. (2004) Tick immunobiology. *Parasitology* 129, S161–S176. DOI: 10.1017/S0031182004004834.

Bullard, R.L., Williams, J. and Karim, S. (2016) Temporal gene expression analysis and RNA silencing of single and multiple members of gene family in the Lone Star tick *Amblyomma americanum*. *PLoS One* 11/2, e0147966. DOI: 10.1371/journal.pone.0147966.

Burster, T., Macmillan, H., Hou, T., Boehm, B.O. and Mellins, E.D. (2010) Cathepsin G: Roles in antigen presentation and beyond. *Molecular Immunology* 47/4, 658–665. DOI: 0.1016/j.molimm.2009.10.003.

Cheng, P.H., Mans, B.J., Neitz, A.W.H. and Gaspar, A.R.M. (2010) Savicalin, a lipocalin from hemocytes of the soft tick, *Ornithodoros savignyi*. *Experimental & Applied Acarology* 52, 313–326. DOI: 10.1007/s10493-010-9368-6.

Chmelař, J., Calvo, E. and Kotsyfakis, M. (2012) Tick salivary secretion as a source of antihemostatics. *Journal of Proteomics* 75/13, 3842–3854. DOI: 10.1016/j.jprot.2012.04.026.

Chmelař, J., Kotál, J., Karim, S., Kopacek, P., Francischetti, I.M. *et al.* (2016) Sialomes and mialomes: A systems-biology view of tick tissues and tick-host interactions. *Trends in Parasitology* 32/3, 242–254. DOI: 10.1016/j.pt.2015.10.002.

Chmelař, J., Kotál, J., Langhansová, H. and Kotsyfakis, M. (2017) Protease inhibitors in tick saliva: The role of serpins and cystatins in tick-host-pathogen interaction. *Frontiers in Cellular Infection and Microbiology* 7, 216. DOI: 10.3389/fcimb.2017.00216.

Constantinoiu, C.C., Jackson, L.A., Jorgensen, W.K., Lew-Tabor, A.E., Piper, E.K. *et al.* (2010) Local immune response against larvae of *Rhipicephalus* (*Boophilus*) *microplus* in *Bos taurus indicus* and *Bos taurus taurus* cattle. *International Journal for Parasitology* 40, 865–875. DOI: 10.1016/j.ijpara.2010.01.004.

Corral-Rodríguez, M.A., Macedo-Ribeiro, S., Pereira, P.J.B. and Fuentes-Prior, P. (2009) Tick-derived Kunitz-type inhibitors as antihemostatic factors. *Insect Biochemistry and Molecular Biology* 39/9, 579–595. DOI: 10.1016/j.ibmb.2009.07.003.

Costa, G.C.A., Ribeiro, I.C.T., Melo-Junior, O., Gontijo, N.F., Sant'Anna, M.R. *et al.* (2021) *Amblyomma sculptum* salivary protease inhibitors as potential anti-tick vaccines. *Frontiers in Immunology* 11, 611104. DOI: 10.3389/fimmu.2020.611104.

Crooks, S.W. and Stockley, R.A. (1998) Molecules in focus. Leukotriene B4. *International Journal of Biochemistry & Cell Biology* 30, 173–178.

Cuffari, B. (2022) What are ligands? *News Medical Life Sciences*. Available at: https://www.news-medical.net/life-sciences/Ligands-An-Overview.aspx (accessed 5 May 2024).

Dahlén, S.-E., Björk, J., Hedqvist, P., Arfors, K.-E., Hammarström, S. *et al.* (1981) Leukotrienes promote plasma leakage and leukocyte adhesion in postcapillary venules: *In vivo* effects with relevance to the acute inflammatory response. *Proceedings of the National Academy of Sciences of the USA* 78/6, 3887–3891.

Denisov, S.S. and Dijkgraaf, I. (2021) Immunomodulatory proteins in tick saliva from a structural perspective. *Frontiers in Cellular and Infection Microbiology* 11, 769574. DOI: 10.3389/fcimb.2021.769574.

Denisov, S.S., Ippel, J.H., Castoldi, E., Mans, B.J., Hackeng, T.M. *et al.* (2021) Molecular basis of anticoagulant and anticomplement activity of the tick salivary protein Salp14 and its homologs. *Journal of Biological Chemistry* 297/1, 100865. DOI: 10.1016/j.jbc.2021.100865.

de Veer, M.J., Kemp, J.M. and Meeusen, E.N. (2007) The innate host defence against nematode parasites. *Parasite Immunology* 29, 1–9.

Elder, J.K., Emmerson, F.R., Kearnan, J.F., Waters, K.S., Dunwell, G.H. *et al.* (1980a) A survey concerning cattle tick control in Queensland. 3. Chemical Control. *Australian Veterinary Journal* 56/5, 212–218.

Elder, J.K., Kearnan, J.F., Waters, K.S., Dunwell, G.H., Emmerson, F.R. *et al.* (1980b) A survey concerning cattle tick control in Queensland. 4. Use of resistant cattle and pasture spelling. *Australian Veterinary Journal* 56/5, 219–223.

Elder, J.K., Waters, K.S., Dunwell, G.H., Emmerson, F.R., Kearnan, J.F. *et al.* (1980c) A survey concerning cattle tick control in Queensland. 2. Managerial aspects which indirectly affect tick control. *Australian Veterinary Journal* 56/5, 205–211.

Francis, J. and Ashton, G.C. (1967) Tick resistance in cattle: Its stability and correlation with various genetic characteristics. *Australian Journal of Experimental Biological and Medical Science* 45, 131–140. DOI: 10.1038/icb.1967.10.

Francischetti, I.M., Sá-Nunes, A., Mans, B.J., Santos, I.M. and Ribeiro, J.M.C. (2009) The role of saliva in tick feeding. *Frontiers in Bioscience* 14, 2051–2088.

Franzin, A.M., Maruyama, S.R., Garcia, G.R., Oliveira, R.P., Ribeiro, J.M.C. *et al.* (2017) Immune and biochemical responses in skin differ between bovine hosts genetically susceptible and resistant to the cattle tick *Rhipicephalus microplus*. *Parasites & Vectors* 10/1, 51. DOI: 10.1186/s13071-016-1945-z.

Fridman, W.H. (1991) Fc receptors and immunoglobulin binding factors. *FASEB Journal* 5/12, 2684–2690. DOI: 10.1096/fasebj.5.12.1916092.

Gasparin, G., Miyata, M., Coutinho, L.L., Martinez, M.L., Teodoro, R.L. *et al.* (2007) Mapping of quantitative trait loci controlling tick [*Riphicephalus* [sic] (*Boophilus*) *microplus*] resistance on bovine chromosomes 5, 7 and 14. *Animal Genetics* 38, 453–459. DOI: 10.1111/j.1365-2052.2007.01634.x.

Goto, A., Matsushita, K., Gesellchen, V., Chamy, L.E., Kuttenkeuler, D. *et al.* (2008a) Akirins are highly conserved nuclear proteins required for NF-κB-dependent gene expression in drosophila and mice. *Nature Immunology* 9, 97–104. DOI: 10.1038/ni1543.

Goto, A., Matsushita, K., Gesellchen, V., Chamy, L.E., Kuttenkeuler, D. *et al.* (2008b) Erratum: Akirins are highly conserved nuclear proteins required for NF-κB-dependent gene expression in drosophila and mice. *Nature Immunology* 9, 216. DOI: 10.1038/ni0208-216.

Guizzo, M.G., Mans, B., Pienaar, R. and Ribeiro, J.M.C. (2023) A comparison of illumina and pacbio methods to build tick salivary gland transcriptomes confirms large expression of lipocalins and other salivary protein families that are not represented in available tick genomes. *Ticks & Tick-Borne Diseases* 14/6, 102209. DOI: 10.1016/j.ttbdis.2023.102209.

Hertzog, P., Forster, S. and Samarajiwa, S. (2011a) Systems biology of interferon responses. *Journal of Interferon & Cytokine Research* 31/1, 5–11.

Hertzog, P.J., Mansell, A., Van Driel, I.R. and Hartland, E.L. (2011b) Sculpting the immune response to infection. *Nature Immunology* 12/7, 579–582.

Hewetson, R.W. (1972) The inheritance of resistance by cattle to cattle tick. *Australian Veterinary Journal* 48/5, 299–303. DOI: https://10.1111/j.1751-0813.1972.tb05161.x.

Hovius, M., Levi, M and Fikrig, E. (2008) Salivating for knowledge: Potential pharmacological agents in tick saliva. *PLoS Medicine* 5/2, e43. DOI: 10.1371/journal.pmed.0050043.

Hüe, T., Hurlin, J.-C., Teurlai, M. and Naves, M. (2014) Comparison of tick resistance of crossbred Senepol x Limousin to purebred Limousin cattle. *Tropical Animal Health and Production* 46/2, 447–453. DOI: 10.1007/s11250-013-0512-2.

Hynes, A.P., Villion, M. and Moineau, S. (2014) Adaptation in bacterial CRISPR-Cas immunity can be driven by defective phages. *Nature Communications* 5, Article number 4399. DOI: 10.1038/ncomms5399.

Janeway, C., Travers, P., Walport, M. and Shlomchik, M. (eds) (2001) The major histocompatibility complex and its functions. In: *Immunobiology: The Immune System in Health and Disease*, 5th edn. Garland Science, New York. Available at: https://www.ncbi.nlm.nih.gov/books/NBK27156/ (accessed 29 September 2024).

Janssen, Y.M.W., Barchowsky, A., Treadwell, M., Driscoll, K.E. and Mossman, B.T. (1995) Asbestos induces nuclear factor cB (NF-KcB) DNA-binding activity and NF-cB-dependent gene expression in tracheal epithelial cells. *Proceedings of the National Academy of Sciences of the USA* 92/18, 8458–8462. DOI: 10.1073/pnas.92.18.8458.

Jaworski, D.C., Simmen, F.A., Lamoreaux, W., Coons, L.B., Muller, M.T. *et al.* (1995) A secreted calreticulin protein in ixodid tick (*A americanum*) saliva. *Journal of Insect Physiology* 41/4, 369–375.

Jonsson, N.N., Piper, E.K. and Constantinoiu, C.C. (2014) Host resistance in cattle to infestation with the cattle tick *Rhipicephalus microplus*. *Parasite Immunology* 36/11, 553–559. DOI: 10.1111/pim.12140.

Karasuyama, H., Miyake, K. and Yoshikawa, S. (2020) Immunobiology of acquired resistance to ticks. *Frontiers in Immunology* 11, 601504. DOI: 10.3389/fimmu.2020.601504.

Kelley, R.B. (1932) *Zebu (Brahman) Cross Cattle and Their Possibilities in North Australia*. Pamphlet no. 27, Council for Scientific and Industrial Research, Rockhampton, Australia.

Kim, T.K., Ibelli, A.M.G. and Mulenga, A. (2015a) *Amblyomma americanum* tick calreticulin binds C1q but does not inhibit activation of the classical complement cascade. *Ticks & Tick-Borne Diseases* 6/1, 91–101. DOI: 10.1016/j.ttbdis.2014.10.002.

Kim, T.K., Tirloni, L., Radulovic, Z., Lewis, L., Bakshi, M. *et al.* (2015b) Conserved *Amblyomma americanum* tick Serpin19, an inhibitor of blood clotting factors Xa and XIa, trypsin and plasmin, has anti-haemostatic functions. *International Journal for Parasitology* 45/9-12, 613–627. DOI: 10.1016/j.ijpara.2015.03.009.

Kim, T.K., Radulovic, Z. and Mulenga, A. (2016a) Target validation of highly conserved *Amblyomma americanum* tick saliva serine protease inhibitor 19. *Ticks & Tick-Borne Diseases* 7, 405–414. DOI: 10.1016/j.ttbdis.2015.12.017.

Kim, T.K., Tirloni, L., Pinto, A.F., Moresco, J., Yates III, J.R. *et al.* (2016b) *Ixodes scapularis* tick saliva proteins sequentially secreted every 24 h during blood feeding. *PLoS Neglected Tropical Diseases* 10/1, e0004323. DOI: 10.1371/journal.pntd.0004323.

Konnai, S., Nishikado, H., Yamada, S., Imamura, S., Ito, T. *et al.* (2011) Molecular identification and expression analysis of lipocalins from blood feeding taiga tick, *Ixodes persulcatus* Schulze. *Experimental Parasitology* 127/2, 467–474. DOI: 10.1016/j.exppara.2010.10.002.

Lander, F. and Russell, T. (2018) The archaeological evidence for the appearance of pastoralism and farming in southern Africa. *PLoS One* 13/6, e0198941. DOI: 10.1371/journal.pone.0198941.

Letinic, B.D., Contreras, M., Dahan-Moss, Y., Linnekugel, I., de la Fuente, J. *et al.* (2021) Additional evidence on the efficacy of different Akirin vaccines assessed on *Anopheles arabiensis* (Diptera: Culicidae). *Parasites & Vectors* 14/1, 209. DOI: 10.1186/s13071-021-04711-8.

Liu, M., Guo, S., Hibbert, J.M., Jain, V., Singh, N. *et al.* (2011) CXCL10/IP-10 in infectious diseases pathogenesis and potential therapeutic implications. *Cytokine & Growth Factor Reviews* 22/3, 121–130. DOI: 10.1016/j.cytogfr.2011.06.001.

Loick, H.M. and Theissen, J.L. (1994) Die eicosanoide als mediatoren beim ARDS [The eicosanoids as mediators in ARDS]. *Anästhesiologie Intensivmedizin Notfallmedizin Schmerztherapie* 29/01, 3–9. DOI: 10.1055/s-2007-996677.

Macedo-Ribeiro, S., Almeida, C., Calisto, B.M., Friedrich, T., Mentele, R. *et al.* (2008) Isolation, cloning and structural characterisation of boophilin, a multifunctional kunitz-type proteinase inhibitor from the cattle tick. *PLoS One* 3/2, e1624. DOI: 10.1371/journal.pone.0001624.

Maity, A. and Wollman, R. (2020) Information transmission from NFkB signaling dynamics to gene expression. *PLoS Computational Biology* 16(8), e1008011. DOI: 10.1371/journal.pcbi.1008011.

Mans, B.J. (2005) Tick histamine-binding proteins and related lipocalins: Potential as therapeutic agents. *Current Opinion in Investigational Drugs* 6/11, 1131–1135.

Mans, B.J. and Ribeiro, J.M.C. (2008) Function, mechanism and evolution of the moubatin-clade of soft tick lipocalins. *Insect Biochemistry and Molecular Biology* 38/9, 841–852. DOI: 10.1016/j.ibmb.2008.06.007.

Mans, B.J., Steinmann, C.M.L., Venter, J.D., Louw, A.I. and Neitz, A.W.H. (2002) Pathogenic mechanisms of sand tampan toxicoses induced by the tick, *Ornithodoros savignyi*. *Toxicon* 40/7, 1007–1016. DOI: 10.1016/50041-0101(02)00098-3.

Mans, B.J., Louw, A.I. and Neitz, A.W. (2003a) The influence of tick behavior, biotope and host specificity on concerted evolution of the platelet aggregation inhibitor savignygrin, from the soft tick *Ornithodoros savignyi*. *Insect Biochemistry and Molecular Biology* 33/6, 623–629.

Mans, B.J., Louw, A.I. and Neitz, A.W. (2003b) The major tick salivary gland proteins and toxins from the soft tick, *Ornithodoros savignyi*, are part of the tick Lipocalin family: Implications for the origins of tick toxicoses. *Molecular Biology and Evolution* 20/7, 1158–1167. DOI: 10.1093/molbev/msg126.

Mans, B.J., Venter, J.D., Coons, L.B., Louw, A.I. and Neitz, W.H. (2004) A reassessment of argasid tick salivary gland ultrastructure from an immuno-cytochemical perspective. *Experimental & Applied Acarology* 33, 119–129.

Mans, B.J., Andersen, J.F., Francischetti, I.M., Valenzuela, J.G., Schwan, T.G. *et al.* (2008) Comparative sialomics between hard and soft ticks: implications for the evolution of blood-feeding behavior. *Insect Biochemistry and Molecular Biology* 38/1, 42–58.

Mapholi, N.O. (2015) Exploring genetic architecture of tick resistance in south African Nguni cattle. PhD thesis, Stellenbosch University, Stellenbosch, South Africa.

Mapholi, N.O., Marufu, M.C., Maiwashe, A., Banga, C.B., Muchenje, V. *et al.* (2014) Towards a genomics approach to tick (Acari: Ixodidae) control in cattle: A review. *Ticks & Tick-Borne Diseases* 5, 475–483. DOI: 10.1016/j.ttbdis.2014.04.006.

Martins, K.R., Garcia, M.V., Bonatte-Junior, P., Duarte, P.O., Csordas, B.G. *et al.* (2022) Seasonal fluctuations of *Babesia bigemina* and *Rhipicephalus microplus* in Brangus and Nellore cattle reared in the Cerrado biome, Brazil. *Parasites & Vectors* 15(1), 395. DOI: 10.1186/s13071-022-05513-2.

Meeusen, E.N., de Veer, M., Hertzog, P.J., Stear, M.J., Mallard, B.A. *et al.* (2013) New approaches to innate immunity in livestock and the potential for manipulation - review. MLA final report B.BSC.0321 180pp. Available at: https://www.mla.com.au/research-and-development/search-rd-reports/?q=b.bsc.0321&sort=1 (accessed 15 October 2023).

Mejri, N. and Brossard, M. (2007) Splenic dendritic cells pulsed with *Ixodes ricinus* tick saliva prime naive CD4+T to induce th2 cell differentiation *in vitro* and *in vivo*. *International Immunology* 19/4, 535–543. DOI: 10.1093/intimm/dxm019.

Narasimhan, S., Koski, R.A., Beaulieu, B., Anderson, J.F., Ramamoorthi, N. *et al.* (2002) A novel family of anticoagulants from the saliva of *Ixodes scapularis*. *Insect Molecular Biology* 11/6, 641–650. DOI: 10.1046/j.1365-2583.2002.00375.x.

Narasimhan, S., Montgomery, R.R., DePonte, K., Tschudi, C., Marcantonio, N. *et al.* (2004) Disruption of *Ixodes scapularis* anticoagulation by using RNA interference. *Proceedings of the National Academy of Sciences of the USA* 101/5, 1141–1146.

Neelakanta, G. and Sultana, H. (2022) Tick saliva and salivary glands: What do we know so far on their role in arthropod blood feeding and pathogen transmission? *Frontiers in Cellular and Infection Microbiology* 11, 816547. DOI: 10.3389/fcimb.2021.816547.

Paesen, G.C., Adams, P.L., Nuttall, P.A. and Stuart, D.L. (2000) Review. Tick histamine-binding proteins: Lipocalins with a second binding cavity. *Biochimica et Biophysica Acta* 1482, 92–101.

Palucka, K. and Banchereau, J. (1999) Dendritic cells: A link between innate and adaptive immunity. *Journal of Clinical Immunology* 19/1, 12–25.

Peperzak, V., Veraar, E.A., Xiao, Y., Bąbała, N., Thiadens, K. *et al.* (2013) CD8+ T cells produce the chemokine CXCL10 in response to CD27/CD70 costimulation to promote generation of the CD8+ effector T cell pool. *Journal of Immunology* 191/6, 3025–3036. DOI: 10.4049/jimmunol.1202222.

Pham, M., Underwood, J. and Oliva Chávez, A.S. (2021) Changing the recipe: Pathogen directed changes in tick saliva components. *International Journal of Environmental Research and Public Health* 18, 1806. DOI: 10.3390/ijerph18041806.

Piper, E.K. (2010) Bovine immune responses to cattle tick infestation. PhD thesis, University of Queensland, Brisbane, Australia.

Piper, E.K., Jonsson, N.N., Gondro, C., Lew-Tabor, A.E., Moolhuijzen, P. *et al.* (2009) Immunological profiles of *Bos taurus* and *Bos indicus* cattle infested with the cattle tick, *Rhipicephalus* (*Boophilus*) *microplus*. *Clinical and Vaccine Immunology* 16/7, 1071–1086.

Proell, M., Riedl, S.J., Fritz, J.H., Rojas, A.M. and Schwarzenbacher, R. (2008) The nod-like receptor (NLR) family: A tale of similarities and differences. *PLoS One* 3/4, e2119. DOI: 10.1371/journal.pone.0002119.

Ramesh, G., MacLean, A.G. and Philipp, M.T. (2013) Cytokines and chemokines at the crossroads of neuroinflammation, neurodegeneration, and neuropathic pain. *Mediators of Inflammation* 480739. DOI: 10.1155/2013/480739.

Ranasinghe, S. and McManus, D.P. (2013) Structure and function of invertebrate Kunitz serine protease inhibitors. *Developmental and Comparative Immunology* 39/3, 219–227. DOI: 10.1016/j.dci.2012.10.005.

Raza, A., Schulz, B.L., Nouwens, A., Jackson, L.A., Piper, E.K. *et al.* (2021) Serum proteomes of Santa Gertrudis cattle before and after infestation with *Rhipicephalus australis* ticks. *Parasite Immunology* 43/7, e12836. DOI: 10.1111/pim.12836.

Raza, A., Schulz, B.L., Nouwens, A., Naseem, M.N., Kamran, M. *et al.* (2023) Application of quantitative proteomics to discover biomarkers for tick resistance in cattle. *Frontiers in Immunology* 14, 1091066. DOI: 10.3389/fimmu.2023.1091066.

Robbertse, L., Richards, S.A. and Maritz-Olivier, C. (2017) Bovine immune factors underlying tick resistance: Integration and future directions. *Frontiers in Cellular and Infection Microbiology* 7, 522. DOI: 10.3389/fcimb.2017.00522.

Rodriguez-Valle, M., Xu, T., Kurscheid, S. and Lew-Tabor, A.E. (2015) *Rhipicephalus microplus* serine protease inhibitor family: Annotation, expression and functional characterisation assessment. *Parasites & Vectors* 8, 7. DOI: 10.1186/s13071-014-0605-4.

Sajiki, Y., Konnai, S., Ochi, A., Okagawa, T., Githaka, N. *et al.* (2020) Immunosuppressive effects of sialostatin L1 and L2 isolated from the taiga tick *Ixodes persulcatus* Schulze. *Ticks & Tick-Borne Diseases* 11/2, 101332. DOI: 10.1016/j.ttbdis.2019.101332.

Salmon, J.A. and Higgs, G.A. (1987) Prostaglandins and leukotrienes as inflammatory mediators. *British Medical Bulletin* 43/2, 285–296. DOI: 10.1093/oxfordjournals.bmb.a072183.

Samuelson, L.C., Phillips, R.S. and Swanberg, L.J. (1996) Amylase gene structures in primates: Retroposon insertions and promoter evolution. *Molecular Biology and Evolution* 13/6, 767–779.

Sarma, J.V. and Ward, P.A. (2011) The complement system. *Cell and Tissue Research* 343/1, 227–235. DOI: 10.1007/s00441-010-1034-0.

Söderbom, G. and Zeng, B.-Y. (2020) The NLRP3 inflammasome as a bridge between neuroinflammation in metabolic and neurodegenerative diseases. *International Review of Neurobiology* 154, 345–391. DOI: 10.1016/bs.irn.2020.03.023.

Spickett, A.M., De Klerk, D., Enslin, C.B. and Scholtz, M.M. (1989) Resistance of Nguni, Bonsmara and Hereford cattle to ticks in a bushveld region of South Africa. *Onderstepoort Journal of Veterinary Research* 56, 245–250.

St Charles, R., Padmanabhan, K., Arni, R.V., Padmanabhan, K.P. and Tulinsky, A. (2000) Structure of tick anticoagulant peptide at 1.6 Å resolution complexed with bovine pancreatic trypsin inhibitor. *Protein Science* 9, 265–272.

Steen, N.A., Barker, S.C. and Alewood, P.F. (2006) Proteins in the saliva of the Ixodida (ticks): Pharmacological features and biological significance. *Toxicon* 47/1, 1–20. DOI: 10.1016/j.toxicon.2005.09.010.

Stutzer, C., Mans, B.J., Gaspar, A.R.M., Neitz, A.W.H. and Maritz-Olivier, C. (2009) *Ornithodoros savignyi*: Soft tick apyrase belongs to the 5'-nucleotidase family. *Experimental Parasitology* 122, 318–327. DOI: 10.1016/j.exppara.2009.04.007.

Sutherst, R.W., Wagland, J.A. and Roberts, J.A. (1978) The effect of density on the survival of *Boophilus microplus* on previously unexposed cattle. *International Journal for Parasitology* 8/4, 321–324. DOI: 10.1016/0020-7519(78)90097-8.

Sutherst, R.W., Roberts, J.A. and Wagland, B.M. (1979) Resistance in cattle to *Haemaphysalis* (*Kaiseriana*) *longicornis*. *International Journal for Parasitology* 9, 183–188.

Swain, S.L., McKinstry, K.K. and Strutt, T.M. (2012) Expanding roles for CD4+ T cells in immunity to viruses. *Nature Reviews Immunology* 12, 136–148. DOI: 10.1038/nri3152.

Swanson, K.V., Deng, M. and Ting, J.P.-Y. (2019) The NLRP3 inflammasome: Molecular activation and regulation to therapeutics. *Nature Reviews Immunology* 19, 477–489.

Tirloni, L., Kim, T.K., Coutinho, M.L., Ali, A., Seixas, A. *et al.* (2016) The putative role of *Rhipicephalus microplus* salivary serpins in the tick–host relationship. *Insect Biochemistry and Molecular Biology* 71, 12–28. DOI: 10.1016/j.ibmb.2016.01.004.

Toyomane, K., Konnai, S., Niwa, A., Githaka, N., Isezaki, M. *et al.* (2016) Identification and the preliminary *in vitro* characterization of IRIS homologue from salivary glands of *Ixodes persulcatus* schulze. *Ticks & Tick-Borne Diseases* 7/1, 119–125. DOI: 10.1016/j.ttbdis.2015.09.006.

Valdes, J.J., Schwarz, A., Vaca, I., Calvo, E., Pedra, J.H. *et al.* (2013) Tryptogalinin is a tick Kunitz serine protease inhibitor with a unique intrinsic disorder. *PLoS One* 8/5, e62562. DOI: 10.1371/journal.pone.0062562.

Van Asbeck, E.C., Hoepelman, A.I., Scharringa, J., Herpers, B.L. and Verhoef, J. (2008) Mannose binding lectin plays a crucial role in innate immunity against yeast by enhanced complement activation and enhanced uptake of polymorphonuclear cells. *BMC Microbiology* 8, 229. DOI: 10.1186/1471-2180-8-229.

Vasselon, T. and Detmers, P.A. (2002) Toll receptors: A central element in innate immune responses. *Infection and Immunity* 70/3, 1003–1041. DOI: 10.1128/IAI.70.3.1033-1041.2002.

Wagland, B.M. (1978) Host resistance to cattle tick (*Boophilus microplus*) in Brahman (*Bos indicus*) cattle. III. Growth on previously unexposed animals. *Australian Journal of Agricultural Research* 29/2, 401–409. DOI: 10.1071/AR9780401.

White, M. (1999) Mediators of inflammation and the inflammatory process. *Journal of Allergy and Clinical Immunology* 103/3, Part 2, S378–S381.

Wikel, S.K. (1996) Host immunity to ticks. *Annual Review of Entomology* 41/1, 1–22. DOI: 10.1146/annurev.en.41.010196.000245.

Wikel, S.K. (1999) Tick modulation of host immunity: An important factor in pathogen transmission. *International Journal for Parasitology* 29/6, 851–859. DOI: 10.1016/S0020-7519(99)00042-9.

Wikel, S.K., Ramachandra, R.N. and Bergman, D.K. (1994) Tick induced modulation of the host immune response. *International Journal for Parasitology* 24/1, 59–66.

Willadsen, P. and McKenna, R.V. (1983) Binding of antigens to tissues: The example of *Boophilus microplus* and bovine skin. *International Journal for Parasitology* 13/6, 593–598.

Willadsen, P., Williams, P.G., Roberts, J.A. and Kerr, J.D. (1978) Responses of cattle to allergens from *Boophilus microplus*. *International Journal for Parasitology* 8, 89–95.

Xu, T., Lew-Tabor, A. and Rodriguez-Valle, M. (2016) Effective inhibition of thrombin by *Rhipicephalus microplus* serpin-15 (RmS-15) obtained in the yeast *Pichia pastoris*. *Ticks & Tick-Borne Diseases* 7/1, 180–187. DOI: 10.1016/j.ttbdis.2015.09.007.

Xu, Z., Yan, Y., Zhang, H., Cao, J., Zhou, Y. *et al.* (2020) A serpin from the tick *Rhipicephalus haemaphysaloides*: Involvement in vitellogenesis. *Veterinary Parasitology* 279, 109064. DOI: 10.1016/j.vetpar.2020.109064.

Yu, Y., Wan, Y. and Huang, C. (2009) The biological functions of NF-kB1 (p50) and its potential as an anti-cancer target. *Current Cancer Drug Targets* 9/4, 566–571. DOI: 10.2174/156800909788486759.

Zheng, W., Hu, H., Jiang, J., Sun, X., Fu, R. *et al.* (2022) *Haemaphysalis longicornis* calreticulin is not an effective molecular tool for tick bite diagnosis and disruption of tick infestations. *Veterinary Parasitology* 309, 109775. DOI: 10.1016/j.vetpar.2022.109775.

4 Naturally Acquired Adaptive Immunity

Abstract

Adaptive immunity is a seamless continuation from the innate response to an initial pathogen incursion. It relies on the successful collaboration of a complex system of humoral and cellular components and signalling networks. Tick infestation presents the host with a dynamic 'cocktail' of antigens. The cellular and humoral host immune response is mostly aimed at preventing the tick from successfully completing its engorgement. Fewer ticks complete their bloodmeals on immune hosts and those that do are reproductively less successful. Serological and molecular evidence provides further proof of an adaptive immune response to ticks. Ticks counter the inflammatory and immune responses and prevent blood coagulation interfering with their feeding. In a balanced system, ticks and hosts coexist successfully, each allowing the other to survive, thrive and reproduce, with neither causing the demise of the other, but many factors can affect this equilibrium.

The main driver of the adaptive immune response in vertebrates is the innate immune system, with which it works in close collaboration (Luckheeram *et al.*, 2012). The first contact of a pathogen with the innate immune system, the interaction of a PAMP (pathogen-associated molecular pattern) with its PRR (pathogen recognition receptor), determines the strength and direction of the ensuing adaptive immunity and the ultimate effector response. This additional level of immune protection is characterized by specific receptors. It needs to be activated by an antigen (acquired, for example, by infection or vaccination), of which it will retain a memory to allow quicker and stronger reactions to subsequent exposure to the same antigen. The adaptive immune response can be of type 1, characterized by production of interferon (IFN)-γ and cell-mediated immunity (CMI) against bacteria and viruses. A type 2 immune response promotes eosinophil and mast cell-mediated immunity against multicellular pathogens, e.g. helminths (Meeusen *et al.*, 2013) and ticks (Brossard and Fivaz, 1982).

Whereas the pattern recognition pathways of innate immunity are non-clonal, B- and T-lymphocytes of the adaptive immune system are able to create large numbers of clones expressing distinct antigen receptors, by rearrangement of their immunoglobulin or T-cell receptor (TCR) genes. They need prior instruction from the cells of the innate immune system (Palucka and Banchereau, 1999).

4.1 Components of the Adaptive Immune System

The term immunoglobulin (Ig) superfamily (IgSF) was initially used when it was found that immunoglobulins and other proteins involved in the immune response shared a common three-dimensional structure called the Ig fold, which is a sandwich of two β sheets held together by disulfide bonds. Subsequent discovery of the Ig fold in proteins not functionally related to the immunoglobulins led to the definition of new functional families within the IgSF, such as cytokine receptors and MHC antigens (Williams and Barclay, 1988; Halaby and Mornon, 1998).

The components of the adaptive immune system are graphically represented in Fig. 4.1.

4.1.1 Major histocompatibility complex (MHC)

The MHC is a collection of polymorphic genes which encode proteins, called MHC molecules, involved in antigen processing and presentation. They are located on more than one chromosome

DOI: 10.1079/9781800625761.0004

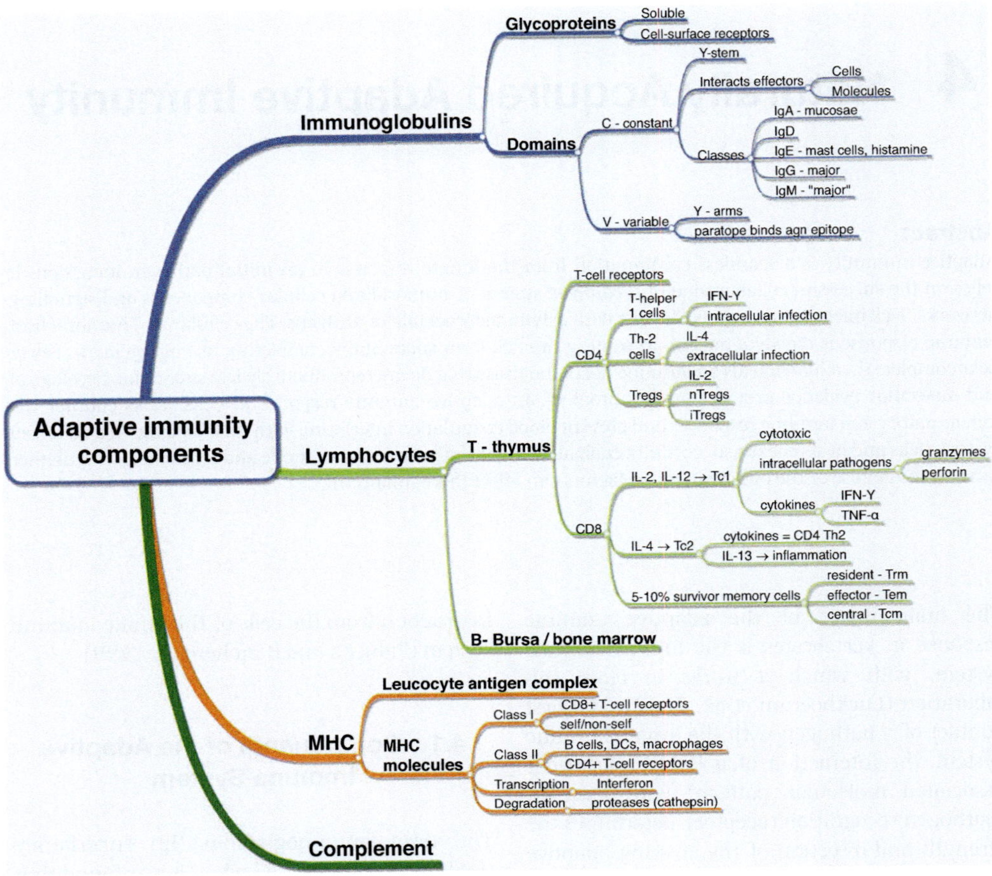

Fig. 4.1. Graphic representation of the components of the adaptive immune system, drawn from cited references, using MindMapper 21 Pro© software. Abbreviations in the illustration are explained in the text. Courtesy of Johann Schröder.

in the genome and are grouped into three classes. Polymorphism in MHC class I and II genes can affect resistance or susceptibility to disease. The human MHC is also referred to as the human leucocyte antigen (HLA) complex, while for livestock there are the SLA (swine) and BoLA (bovines) complexes (Anon., 2024).

The presentation of antigen peptides by MHC cell surface glycoproteins for recognition by the receptors at the surface of T-cells (TCRs) is one of the key elements of the adaptive immune response (Kaas and Lefranc, 2005). The MHC distinguishes auto- from alloantigens, preventing the immune system from targeting the organism's own cells (Janeway Jr *et al.*, 2001a). The desetope is the domain of the MHC molecule that binds to the antigen (Matsunaga *et al.*, 1993). The same TCR can distinguish between a 'healthy self' cell and an allogenic cell, e.g. that same type of cell infected with a virus (Zinkernagel and Doherty, 1977). MHC class I molecules are expressed by most host cells and their peptides recognized by TCRs on CD8$^+$ T-cells. MHC class II molecules are constitutively expressed by B-cells, dendritic cells (DC) and macrophages, and their peptides recognized by TCRs on CD4$^+$ T-cells (see below). MHC molecules alert the host to an infection by displaying pathogen peptides on the surfaces of host cells (Riese *et al.*, 1998; Tubo and Jenkins, 2014).

Because the MHC genes are polymorphic, there is polymorphism in the expressed MHC molecules, enabling the individual's immune system to recognize a diversity of antigens. In rare cases, protein processing will not generate any peptides suitable for binding to the MHC molecules and the individual fails to respond to the antigen. Such immune response gene defects were first reported in inbred animals. This was the first indication of the antigen-presenting function of the MHC molecules, and that MHC genotype controlled the ability of the immune system to respond to antigens (Janeway Jr *et al.*, 2001a).

After presentation, the MHC class II molecule–antigen complex is degraded by proteolysis to allow subsequent binding of peptides, regeneration of antigenic peptides and removal of the non-polymorphic invariant chain chaperone of the MHC II molecule. This process is facilitated by lysosomal/endosomal cysteine, aspartyl and serine proteases, of which the cathepsins form an important group (Matsunaga *et al.*, 1993; Riese *et al.*, 1998; Riese and Chapman, 2000; Burster *et al.*, 2010). Cathepsins are classified as endo- or exopeptidases and they are involved in many cellular processes, such as activation of the NLRP3 inflammasome (Campden and Zhang, 2019) and MHC class II molecule binding to antigens.

The activity of the lysosomal cathepsins is in turn regulated by numerous protease inhibitors, of which the cystatins form one large group (Riese and Chapman, 2000; Turk *et al.*, 2002, 2012). Inhibition of cathepsin S has been proposed as a possible method for increasing $CD8^+$ T-cell immunity, by decreasing apoptosis of $CD8^+$ T-cells (Yan *et al.*, 2017).

Interferons (see section 3.1.2, this volume), produced early in viral infections in an innate immune response, cause an increase in transcription of MHC genes. This increases the ability of cells to process foreign proteins and present their peptides to the appropriate T-cells and initiate the adaptive immune response.

Other MHC genes are under different regulatory control and are induced by cellular stress, e.g. heat shock. Some MHC genes are expressed in fibroblasts and epithelial cells, playing a part in innate immunity in circumstances where interferons are not produced. Some MHC molecules are recognized by receptors on NK, gamma:delta (γ:δ) T-cells and some CD8 T-cells, prompting these cells to kill cells presenting these molecules (Janeway Jr *et al.*, 2001a).

The MHC, cattle, and ticks

Cattle typed for 30 (MHC class I) BoLAs were found to be more susceptible to induced infestation with [*B. microplus*] *R. australis* when they were positive for antigens W6 and CA31. Tick burdens on the experimental cattle were recorded by more than one observer, in May, July and October in northern Queensland, and tick resistance assessed not on actual tick numbers but on each animal's ranking within the group, to account for seasonal variation in tick challenge and infestation. Genotypically, the cattle were three-quarter Brahman and one-quarter Shorthorn. Previous research had hinted at tick resistance associated with two, and tick susceptibility associated with one, of 11 detected antigens (Stear *et al.*, 1989). Follow-up investigations revealed that Belmont Red cattle with bovine MHC antigens W6.1 and W7 carried significantly fewer ticks than those without (Stear *et al.*, 1990). W6 antigens can either be of wide tissue distribution (W6/32, /34, /45 and /46) or mainly found on erythrocytes (W6/1 and W6/28). In humans, antierythrocyte W6/1 antibodies reacted with A erythrocytes but not B nor O (Barnstable *et al.*, 1978). Substitution of W6.1 for other antigens increased heifer weight at first calving and protein yield, but also the treatment cost for disease in Canadian Holstein cattle. It was unclear whether W6.1 was itself associated with disease susceptibility or in linkage disequilibrium with a disease susceptibility allele (Batra *et al.*, 1989).

4.1.2 T- and B-lymphocytes and their regulating chemicals

The adaptive immune system depends on three main classes of lymphocytes: B-cells, $CD8^+$ T-cells and $CD4^+$ T-cells. Each developing lymphocyte produces an antigen receptor, resulting in millions of single copies of different antigen receptors, with each newly formed lymphocyte able to express many copies of a single antigen receptor. Each antigen receptor has a unique binding pocket that accommodates an antigen with a defined shape. Antigen receptor-binding pockets have random shapes, so that the set of lymphocytes in an individual is likely to contain only a few cells that express antigen receptors with shapes that match the molecular shapes of antigens produced by a given pathogen. The adaptive immune response to that antigen depends on the expansion and differentiation of these few lymphocytes (Tubo and Jenkins, 2014).

T-lymphocytes

T-cell (thymus-derived lymphocyte) precursors originate from a common lymphoid stem cell and leave the bone marrow to mature in the thymus, considered to be a primary lymphoid organ, indispensable for T-lymphocyte development. This process prepares the T-cells for antigen recognition, using TCRs, and the expression of surface molecules, such as the glycoproteins CD4 and CD8. Mature naïve T-cells are deployed to secondary lymphoid tissue in the spleen, lymph nodes and mucosae, to perform their surveillance and antigen recognition (Luckheeram *et al.*, 2012).

Antigen-specific $CD4^+$ and $CD8^+$ T-cells exist at very low frequencies in naïve hosts. Transient exposure to antigen, whether by infection or immunization, activates naïve $CD4^+$ and $CD8^+$ T-cells to multiply and develop, culminating in a higher frequency of antigen-specific cells with a more rapid effector function and long-lived immune memory (Seder and Ahmed, 2003).

Having recognized a pathogen-encoded antigen, T-cells undergo multiple rounds of replication, generating enormous numbers of cytotoxic T-cell effector progeny that can be regarded as the foot soldiers of the adaptive immune response (Zhang and Bevan, 2011). $CD4^+$ TCRs recognize peptides from extracellular proteins that are taken up into endosomes or phagosomes, and $CD8^+$ TCRs recognize short peptides from cytosolic proteins (Tubo and Jenkins, 2014). They are a principal component of immunity against intracellular pathogens such as viruses (Laidlaw *et al.*, 2016). The multiple functions of γδ T-cells are not fully known but they are thought to play a role in integrating innate and adaptive immune responses (Constantinoiu *et al.*, 2010).

Antigen-presenting cells (APCs, e.g. dendritic cells; see section 3.5, this volume) take up foreign antigens in their PRRs and are stimulated to upregulate their expression of MHC class II molecules, costimulatory molecules (e.g. CD80 and CD86) and proinflammatory cytokines, e.g. type I IFNs, TNF, IL-1, IL-6 and IL-12. They migrate to the draining lymph nodes, inducing naïve $CD4^+$ T-cells to differentiate into different effector T-lymphocytes (Swain *et al.*, 2012). $CD4^+$ T-cells differentiate into type 1 T helper (Th1) cells, characterized by IFN-γ production, or Th2 cells, characterized by production of IL-4. Th1 cells are essential for protection against a variety of intracellular infections, whereas Th2 responses can be protective against certain extracellular infections (Seder and Ahmed, 2003). The balance between Th1 and Th2 ensures an integrated immune system (Kuo *et al.*, 2024).

Interleukin 2 is a pleiotropic cytokine and a key regulator of T-cell metabolic programmes. IL-2-responsive T-cell subsets have diverse characteristics and both pro- and anti-inflammatory biological roles. IL-2 receptors are expressed by $CD4^+$ regulatory T-cells (Tregs), which can be thymically derived ('natural', nTregs) or antigen-activated ('induced', iTregs) (Ross and Cantrell, 2018), and are essential for the balance between pro- and anti-inflammatory responses (Schmidt and Williams, 2013).

Other subsets of $CD4^+$ T helper lymphocytes have been identified, each with a characteristic effector cytokine profile, such as Th9, Th17 and follicular helper T (T_{FH}) cells (Luckheeram *et al.*, 2012). $CD4^+$ effector functions which have been described include inflammation (Th17 cells – IL-17, IL-22), regulation of inflammation (T_{Reg} cells – IL-10), allergic and helminth responses (Th2 cells – IL-4, IL-5, IL-13), germinal centre help (T_{FH} cells – IL-4, IL-21), macrophage activation and inflammation (Th1 cells – IFN-γ, TNF) and killing of infected cells (cytolytic $CD4^+$ T-cells – granzyme B, perforin) (Swain *et al.*, 2012).

Naïve $CD8^+$ T-cells are similarly primed by APCs in secondary lymphoid organs to differentiate into effector cells. A single naïve $CD8^+$ T-cell can differentiate into a diverse population of short-lived effector and memory precursor effector cells (Zhang and Bevan, 2011). $CD8^+$ T-cells need less antigen exposure time than $CD4^+$ cells, divide sooner and have a faster rate of cell division, developing into effector cells (Seder and Ahmed, 2003; Laidlaw *et al.*, 2016). The dramatic rate of multiplication of

$CD8^+$ T-cells in response to a pathogen-encoded antigen depends on signals from multiple receptors impinging upon cell division and survival. Proinflammatory cytokines such as IL-2, predominantly produced by activated $CD4^+$ T-cells, play a key role in the terminal differentiation of $CD8^+$ effector cells, also promoted by IL-12 (Zhang and Bevan, 2011). $CD4^+$ T-cells regulate memory $CD8^+$ T-cell maturation and function. $CD4^+$ T-cells also support $CD8^+$ T-cells by facilitating their interaction with DC. Whereas antibodies (see section 4.1.3) recognize proteins expressed on pathogen surfaces, $CD8^+$ T-cells respond to peptide sequences on the surface of APCs (Laidlaw *et al.*, 2016).

Effector $CD8^+$ T-cells have diverse functions. Differentiation into cytotoxic T-lymphocytes (Tc1 cells) is enhanced by IL-2 and IL-12. Tc1 cells eliminate intracellular pathogens by killing the host cells with cytotoxic molecules (e.g. granzymes and perforin) and secreting cytokines to accelerate the adaptive immune response, such as IFN-γ and TNF-α (Mittrücker *et al.*, 2014; Laidlaw *et al.*, 2016). Differentiation into Tc2 cells can be induced *in vitro* with IL-4, and their cytokine profile overlaps with that of Th2 $CD4^+$ T-cells. They have a low level of cytotoxicity and enhance inflammation by producing IL-13. Tc9, producing IL-9, Tc17, producing IL-17, and $CD8^+$ T_{reg} lymphocytes have also been described (Mittrücker *et al.*, 2014).

In addition to the killing of infected cells and releasing cytokines at the site of infection, effector $CD8^+$ T-cells prevent excessive tissue injury by secreting the immunosuppressive cytokine IL-10. IL-10 is also secreted by Th2, B and NK cells, and macrophages, DC and monocytes (Zhang and Bevan, 2011).

Following viral clearance, the majority of $CD8^+$ T-cells die. The surviving 5–10% are maintained by IL-7 and IL-15 signals, and are divided into resident (T_{RM}), effector (T_{EM}) and central (T_{CM}) memory cells. They provide overlapping layers of protection against potential reinfection and can respond rapidly to re-exposure to the antigen (Mittrücker *et al.*, 2014; Laidlaw *et al.*, 2016), forming the basis for protective immunity against infection and disease in concert with antibody responses (Seder and Ahmed, 2003).

Natural killer (NK) T-cells are also thymus-derived lymphocytes (Luckheeram *et al.*, 2012) and are considered as part of the innate immune system (see section 3.1.1, this volume).

The various forms and functions of thymus-derived lymphocytes are represented graphically in the form of a mind map in Fig. 4.2.

B-lymphocytes

B- (bursa-derived) lymphocytes are named for the bursa of Fabricius in poultry, described in anatomical terms by Hieronymus Fabricius (or Girolamo Fabrizio) at Padua in 1621 (Cullen, 1982; Ribatti, 2015). The role of the bursa was discovered serendipitously when bursectomized chickens failed to raise antibodies in response to an induced *Salmonella pullorum* infection (Glick *et al.*, 1956). Subsequent research revealed how the role of antibody production in chickens was transferred, prior to regression of the bursa (Glick, 1994), to secondary lymphoid tissue such as the aggregations in Peyer's patches (Jung *et al.*, 2010; Reboldi and Cyster, 2016). The search for the mammalian equivalent of the bursa included a demonstration of antigenic specificities between thymus- and bursa-derived lymphocytes (Forget *et al.*, 1970). In mammals, B-cells arise from haemopoietic stem cells in the bone marrow (Fischer *et al.*, 2020).

B-cells use antibodies to recognize extracellular macromolecules (Tubo and Jenkins, 2014). The expression of antibody as an antigen receptor on the surface of B-cells is important for their development and survival (Küppers *et al.*, 1999). A diversity of antibody specificities is generated during antigen-independent B-cell maturation in the bone marrow (Mix *et al.*, 2006). Naïve mature B-cells leave the bone marrow and can recirculate in the spleen or bone marrow, and migrate to B-cell areas of lymph nodes, Peyer's patches and the spleen (Allman and Pillai, 2008). Antigen-dependent B-cell maturation occurs in peripheral lymphatic tissue (Mix *et al.*, 2006). Transcriptomic analysis revealed the transition from naïve to memory B-cells in germinal centres in secondary lymphoid tissue, following activation by T-cell-dependent antigen receptor stimulation, with costimulatory signals from immune helper cells (Klein *et al.*, 2003). These memory B-cells and plasma cells egress from the germinal centres into the circulation, thus conferring long-lived humoral immunity (Reboldi and Cyster, 2016; Suan *et al.*, 2017).

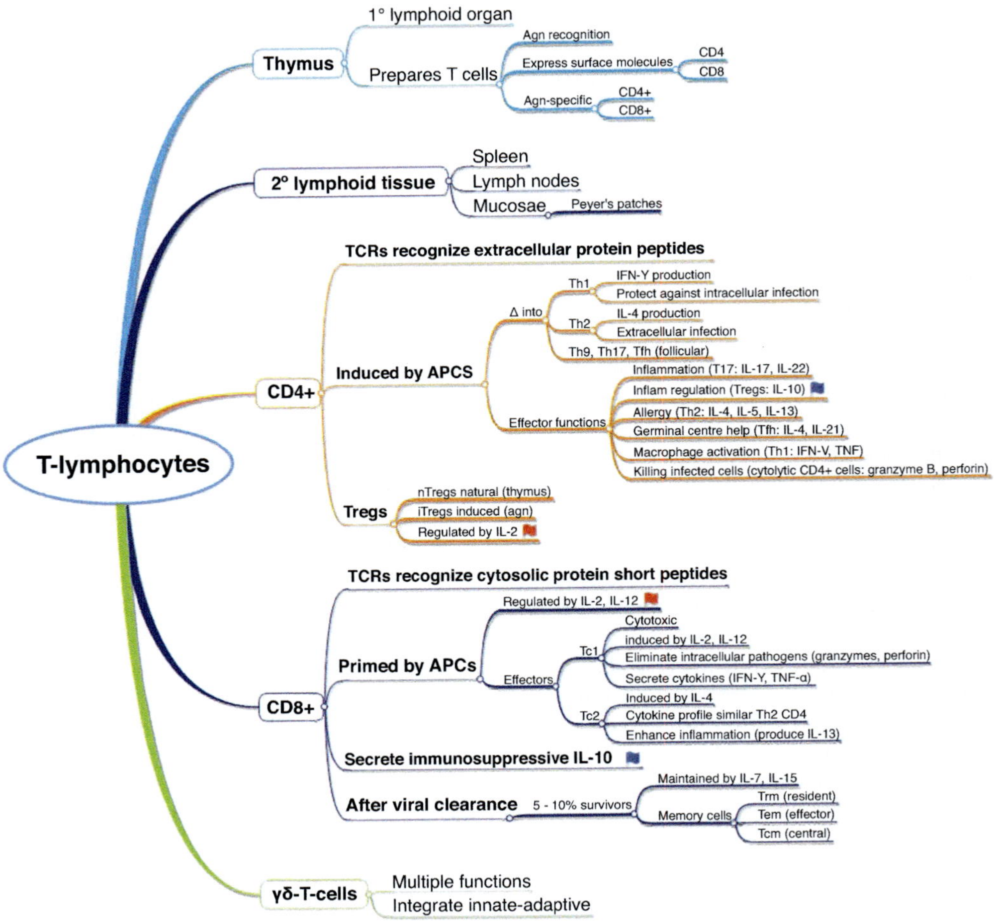

Fig. 4.2. The origins, forms and functions of T lymphocytes, drawn from references cited in the text, using MindMapper 21 Pro© software. Abbreviations in the illustration are explained in the text. Courtesy of Johann Schröder.

The longevity of mature B-cells expressing surface IgM and IgD (see below) depends on antigen selection. After leaving the bone marrow, unstimulated cells live only days or weeks. B-cells are rescued from apoptosis by their response to a cognate antigen. T-cell-independent stimulation induces differentiation of B-cells into short-lived plasma cells, whereas T-cell-dependent stimulation leads to differentiation into the long-lived pools of plasma cells or memory B-cells (Schroeder and Cavacini, 2010). Unstimulated apoptotic B-cells in the lymph node germinal centres are cleared by phagocytic histiocytes known as tingible body macrophages (TBMs). These are large cells containing condensed apoptotic nuclei, referred to as 'tingible bodies' (Gurwicz *et al.*, 2023).

4.1.3 Antibodies

The existence of an agent in the blood that could neutralize a bacterial toxin was reported in 1890. The term 'antibody' was coined the following year, and the substance inducing its production was referred to as the 'antigen' (Schroeder and Cavacini, 2010). Immunoglobulins (Ig) or antibodies (Abs) are produced by B-cells and plasma cells and are the principal operators of the adaptive humoral response (Mix *et al.*, 2006). They serve as cell surface receptors for antigens that permit cell signalling and activation, and as soluble effector molecules that can individually bind and neutralize antigens. They are glycoproteins and their glycosylation affects their antibody function, such as coating antigens to activate effector cells, e.g. NK cells or monocytes. They can bind to a virtually unlimited array of antigens sharing little or no similarity, owing their variability to a complex array of mechanisms that break and recombine the DNA sequence of individual B-cells (Schroeder and Cavacini, 2010).

Every Ig molecule is made up of one pair each of heavy and light polypeptide chains, held together by disulfide bonds. Their complex structure includes a constant (C) domain which determines the effector function and a variable (V) domain that confers antigenic specificity (Schroeder and Cavacini, 2010). X-ray crystallography determined the roughly Y-shaped structure of Ab molecules. The two arms of the Y contain the V regions involved in antigen binding. The stem of the Y contains the C region that interacts with effector cells and molecules (Janeway Jr *et al.*, 2001b). The stem of the Y is known as the Fc (fragment, crystallizable) and the arms of the Y as the Fab (fragment, antigen binding) region of the antibody.

There are five classes of the C domain which define the IgM, IgG, IgA, IgD and IgE isotypes (Schroeder and Cavacini, 2010). IgG is the major component, and they neutralize bacterial toxins, enhance phagocytosis of microorganisms and may activate the complement sequence, leading to cell lysis. IgA appears in seromucous secretions of tears, saliva, nasal and gastrointestinal mucus. IgM ('macroglobulins' due to their size) appear early in immune responses, probably to deal with bacterial invasions with their agglutinating and cytolytic properties. IgE can fix mast cells and provoke the release of histamine (Bradley, 1974). IgD is found at low levels in serum, with a short half-life. It is expressed on the membranes of B-cells when they leave the bone marrow and populate secondary lymphoid organs but its function is poorly understood. It is not known to participate in major antibody effector mechanisms (Bradley, 1974; Schroeder and Cavacini, 2010).

Ig–antigen interactions consist of the *paratope* on the Ig binding to the *epitope* on the antigen. The epitope is a conformational structure and makes it possible for B-cells to discriminate between closely related antigens. Divergent antigens that share equivalent or similar epitopes will be recognized by the same antibody, known as cross-reactivity (Schroeder and Cavacini, 2010).

4.1.4 Complement

The complement system plays a receptor role in innate immunity (see section 3.1.3, this volume). It links the host innate and adaptive immune responses, being activated via its three pathways. Its role in adaptive immunity is to maintain immunological memory, helping T- and B-cells in the elimination of pathogens (Sarma and Ward, 2011; Aounallah *et al.*, 2020).

4.2 Cell-mediated and Humoral Adaptive Immunity

The 1908 Nobel Prize in Medicine was shared by the two proponents of cellular and humoral immunity. A century later, these two views of immunology had become unified in the paradigm of type 1/type 2 immunity. Types 1 and 2 immunity are not strictly synonymous with cell-mediated (CMI) and humoral immunity. Th1 cells also stimulate moderate levels of antibody production, whereas Th2 cells actively suppress phagocytosis.

Type 1 immunity is protective against most infections, other than those caused by large eukaryotic pathogens. Type 2 immune responses assist with resolving cell-mediated inflammation (Spellberg and Edwards, 2001). The cytokines IL-4 and IL-13 orchestrate type 2 immunity, dominated by basophils, eosinophils, mast cells, B-cell IgE production, Th2 and T_{FH} cells, to helminth infections (identified in some insects, but not [yet] in other arthropods). It is a response aimed at expulsion and decreased fecundity, rather than killing, of macroparasites (Heeb *et al.*, 2020).

4.3 Adaptive Immunity to Ticks

In vitro and live animal experiments using serology and molecular methods have demonstrated that there are both humoral and cellular, and both innate and adaptive, components to the host's immune response to repeated or sustained tick infestation. The nature of the immunity differs between host species with differing host–parasite relationships, and between breeds within the same host species. Manifestation of this immunity is recognizable by various indicators.

4.3.1 Lower tick burdens

Observation of progressively diminishing numbers of engorging larvae of *D. variabilis* reared on guinea pigs and rabbits led to the conclusion that the hosts were acquiring an immunity to repeated infestation. Prior exposure to larvae did not have any noticeable effect on the numbers of nymphs engorging successfully but the engorged nymphs were substantially lighter in weight, indicating that they had ingested less blood (Trager, 1939a). Subsequent experiments confirmed the humoral response by complement fixation (Trager, 1939b). These results could not be replicated with argasid ticks. Neither chickens infested with *A. persicus* nor guinea pigs infested with *Ornithodoros venezuelensis* developed any demonstrable immunity, presumably because their feeding time is much shorter than that of ixodid ticks (Trager, 1940).

Ixodes rubicundus feeding on previously infested and presumably immunized sheep were seen to fail to fully engorge and to have a different colouring from ticks engorging fully on susceptible sheep (Stampa and Du Toit, 1958). The nature of this immune response, in the case of *Rhipicephalus e. evertsi* infestation of sheep, was thought to rely not on lymphocyte transformation but on histamine release by basophils, suggesting a hypersensitivity reaction which did not interfere with tick feeding (Neitz *et al.*, 1993).

Cattle are probably the best studied host that demonstrates adaptive immunity, manifest as fewer, smaller and less fecund ticks. Prolonged exposure to [*B. microplus*] *R. australis* leads to some degree of immunologically mediated resistance in cattle but stabilizes at a level at which economical losses still occur. Brahman cattle with high levels of resistance to [*B. microplus*] *R. australis* reject up to 80% of larvae from induced infestations within the first 24 hours and newly moulted nymphs are fewer in number and slower to engorge (Wagland, 1979). Naturally-acquired immunity is largely directed at tick larvae, reducing the number of ticks reaching engorged adulthood but with little or no effect on engorgement or reproduction of surviving ticks (Willadsen *et al.*, 1988). A strong T-cell-mediated response directed against larval stages, as mounted by indicine cattle, seems to be protective (Jonsson *et al.*, 2014).

4.3.2 Immune indicators

Early research on the immune reaction to tick infestation in cattle skin seemed to yield conflicting results. Some cattle displayed a strong hypersensitivity reaction, with a greater increase in numbers of eosinophils and histamine concentration accumulating at tick attachment sites than others (Piper *et al.*, 2010). Likewise, some studies indicated that strong IgG responses to tick antigens are not protective (Jonsson *et al.*, 2014). This variability was attributable to genetic breed differences (see section 4.4).

Humoral immunity to ticks was proven to be passively transferrable when plasma from adult cattle immunized by repeat daily exposure to larvae of [*B. microplus*] *R. australis* was injected into calves raised tick free. The calves were infested with tick larvae 24 hours after the plasma transfusion and allowed the engorgement of significantly fewer ticks, based on the collection of engorged adult females (Roberts and Kerr, 1976).

In the quest to clarify the bovine immune response to ticks, purified extract of [*B. microplus*] *R. australis* larvae was found to contain a component responsible for an immediate hypersensitivity reaction in previously exposed European cattle. It was found to be an esterase that retained its antigenic property, even if its enzymatic activity had been inhibited with di-isopropyl phosphorofluoridate (DFP), which causes little alteration to the enzyme's tertiary structure (Willadsen and Williams, 1976). Identifying an antigenic protein with a biochemical function was a significant discovery (Willadsen, 1976). The larval extract contained a second component that caused an immediate hypersensitivity reaction in naïve cattle that was more pronounced in previously exposed animals (Willadsen *et al.*, 1978).

The nature and components of the immune response to tick infestation have been studied extensively, and from different points of view, revealing a complex array of elements, some of which appear sequentially and some which seem to act in concert. Basophil, eosinophil and mast cell infiltration and degranulation at the site of attachment is one of the earliest observed events. A changing assortment of tick salivary proteins induces a corresponding array of antibodies. The mediators released by the granulocytes include histamine, leukotrienes, prostaglandins and other cytokines. Antigens are collected by dermal DC (Langerhans cells) and presented to lymphocytes in the draining lymph nodes. Activated antigen-specific $CD4^+$ T-lymphocytes outnumber $CD8^+$ cells and express their cytokines (Brossard and Wikel, 1997).

The role of T-lymphocytes in the response to ticks needed further elucidation, but the tick-mediated polarization of the immune response away from Th1 (IFN-γ production) towards a Th2 (IL-4) cytokine profile (see section 4.1.2) (Brossard and Wikel, 2004) made it tempting to surmise that it is the Th1 response which is aimed at ticks and which they try to modulate, as was confirmed by subsequent research.

Rabbits displayed more pronounced immediate type hypersensitivity reactions to a second induced infestation with *I. ricinus*, as evidenced by greater numbers of eosinophils and degranulated basophils. Mast cells were seen in low numbers and showed a modest increase in the early stages of reinfestation (Brossard and Fivaz, 1982). Subsequent work demonstrated a progressive sensitization of basophils and an increase in specific anti-*I. ricinus* IgG titres, but a partial decline in basophil degranulation with four sequential tick infestations (Brossard *et al.*, 1982). Female *I. ricinus* ingested less blood on immunized rabbits and could no longer digest ingested haemoglobin effectively (Brossard and Papatheodorou, 1990).

Ixodid tick infestation stimulates APCs, T- and B-lymphocytes, basophils, mast cells and eosinophils in the immune response, and bioactive molecules like cytokines, immunoglobulins and complement (Brossard and Wikel, 1997).

Serum samples from guinea pigs immunized by repeated induced infestation with adult *R. appendiculatus* were analysed by SDS-PAGE against tick salivary gland, cement and gut antigens. At least five of these were strongly recognized. The amount and number of specific antigens changed during the course of tick feeding and differed between males and females. Most of the antigens from adult salivary glands were not detectable in larvae or nymphs (Shapiro *et al.*, 1986).

Dendritic cells incubated *in vitro* with *I. ricinus* saliva initiated Th2 differentiation of $CD4^+$ T-cells. Fluorescence-activated cell sorting demonstrated enhanced expression of costimulatory molecules by DC, thus stimulating $CD4^+$ T-cell proliferation. The *in vitro* results were confirmed *in vivo* by injecting tick saliva pulsed DC into mice and eliciting a Th2 immune response (Mejri and Brossard, 2007).

Lymph node transcriptome analysis revealed differential gene expression in cattle infested with *R. microplus*. This was more intense upon larval attachment than during adult feeding. Comparisons of different tick life stages provide insights into the underlying dynamics of the development of an immune response in bovines. Leucocytes were recruited to the lymph node via upregulated chemokines, chemokine receptors and chemotaxis. Galectins are carbohydrate-binding proteins expressed in vascular and lymphatic endothelial cells, where they regulate leucocyte tissue entry during inflammation. They also mediate DC activation. Two galectins were differentially expressed, which may offer a rapid way of suppressing the activation of cellular immunity in the lymph nodes (Robbertse, 2018).

The interferon regulatory factor, IRF4, was also found to be upregulated in lymph node tissues following tick infestation and then diminished during adult tick feeding stages. It is involved in differentiation of multiple lineages of $CD4^+$ T-helper cells, in the development of cytotoxic T-cell responses and differentiation of $CD4^+$ follicular helper cells in secondary lymphoid germinal centres for production of high-affinity neutralizing antibodies. Due to the additional role of IRF4 in $CD8^+$ T-lymphocyte responses, this transcription factor has functions in both humoral and cellular immunity (Robbertse, 2018).

4.4 Breed and Individual Differences in Adaptive Immunity

It is not only cattle that display breed diversity in tick susceptibility. Based on the assertion that calves of all breeds are born equally susceptible to ticks (Hewetson, 1972), differences in susceptibility to three successive induced infestations of unfed adult *R. appendiculatus* between Nguni and Saanen goats were ascribed to differing adaptive immune responses. Based on higher γ-globulin levels, lower engorged female tick weights and fewer replete female ticks, South African indigenous Nguni were deemed to acquire a better immunity than Saanen goats (Gopalraj *et al.*, 2013).

Cattle breeds differ not only in their innate immune response to ticks (see section 3.3.2, this volume). Various breeds of beef and dairy cattle with experience of previous exposure to ticks were challenged with induced infestations of ca. 20,000 larvae of [*B. microplus*] *R. australis*. Their resistance levels were determined as the percentage of tick larvae that failed to survive to maturity. Zebu and Zebu-cross were most resistant among the beef breeds, while Jersey cattle were more resistant than Guernsey, Illawarra Shorthorn or Friesians (Utech *et al.*, 1978b).

Illawarra Shorthorn cattle previously exposed to tick infestation were ranked on their tick counts after induced infestation with [*B. microplus*] *R. australis* larvae. Parent cows consistently carrying fewer ticks were selected for breeding and their progeny were significantly more resistant than calves from low-resistance cows (Utech *et al.*, 1978a).

4.4.1 Immunological differences

Variations between breeds in titres of IgG reacting with salivary Ig-binding proteins offer one possible explanation for the higher loads of reproductively successful ticks carried by some breeds compared to others. Hereford and Simmental cattle exposed to natural infestations of *A. hebraeum*, *R. appendiculatus* and *R. e. evertsi* carried more ticks and had higher serum Ig levels than cograzing Brahmans (Rechav, 1987; Rechav *et al.*, 1990). Susceptible tick-naïve Holsteins reacted to repeated induced infestations of *R. microplus* with significantly higher increases in IgG levels than Nelore cattle in the same experiment. Antibodies from the Nelores recognized twice as many salivary proteins as those from Holsteins. Based on serum productivity profiles, extracts of salivary glands indicated that ticks modify their salivary protein repertoire according to the host they feed on. IgE levels did not vary between breeds, increasing during successive initial infestations but subsiding by the end of the third infestation, 7 months after the first (Garcia *et al.*, 2017). What these results seem to indicate is the futility of an IgG response against tick salivary proteins, because it does not reduce the tick burden.

Within-breed individual variation in tick susceptibility offers the possibility of selection for resistance. After 13 weeks of induced infestation with [*R. microplus*] *R. australis*, a group of previously tick-naïve Santa Gertrudis (a composite breed with a high Zebu genetic component) heifers displayed divergent phenotypes in their tick resistance. Susceptible cattle (based on regular tick counts) developed significantly higher tick-specific IgG_1 titres than tick-resistant animals, again indicating that a heightened antibody response does not impart protection against infestation (Piper *et al.*, 2017). A different interpretation might be that the susceptible cattle had higher Ig titres because they carried more ticks and had therefore received a bigger dose of antigen, or that they were anaemic, thus increasing the Ig concentration (Rechav, 1987). Based on flow cytometry of the peripheral blood mononuclear cell (PBMC) population prior to infestation, there was no difference in the percentages of $CD14^+$, $CD25^+$, $CD3^+$, $CD8^+$, $MHC\text{-}II^+$, $WC1^+$ γδ T or $WC3^+$ cells, but resistant animals had 4.9% more $CD4^+$ cells. After infestation, $CD4^+$ increased in susceptible and decreased in resistant animals. IgG_1 levels were significantly higher in susceptible animals (Piper *et al.*, 2017).

Other marked differences in the adaptive immune responses have also been described. Previously repeatedly infested Brahman cattle yielded fewer engorged female ticks than did Shorthorn cattle, when challenged with an induced infestation with [*B. microplus*] *R. australis* (Wagland, 1975). Brahman cattle acquired their adaptive immunity quicker than Shorthorn cattle, based on tick counts following repeated induced infestations of previously unexposed cattle (Wagland, 1978). The immunological basis for this phenotypic difference based on visible tick numbers was explained in a series of publications (Piper *et al.*, 2008, 2009, 2010; Constantinoiu *et al.*, 2010).

The higher expression of many gene transcripts involved in innate immunity at attachment sites of [*R. microplus*] *R. australis* in European breed cattle was deemed as evidence of a non-directed pathological response to tick infestation. Many of the upregulated transcripts in the taurine cattle form part of TLR pathway, playing a role in triggering cell-mediated inflammation and recognizing molecules produced by damaged tissue, e.g. at tick attachment sites. No gene transcripts were expressed more abundantly in Zebu cattle, by comparison. It was assumed that Zebu cattle acquire high levels of resistance to tick infestation differently from the cell-mediated hypersensitivity-type reaction in European cattle (Piper *et al.*, 2008).

Based on the composition of the PBMC population, cytokine expression by circulating leucocytes and tick-specific IgG1 titres, Zebu cattle were shown to mount a stabilized T-cell-mediated response, whereas European cattle demonstrated a sustained inflammatory response to infestation. High tick-specific antibody levels suggest that there is also a T-cell component to their immune reaction (Piper *et al.*, 2009). In European cattle, upregulated genes are involved in the cellular inflammatory response to tick infestation whereas in Zebu cattle, upregulated genes encode the constituents of the extracellular matrix (Piper *et al.*, 2010).

At tick attachment sites, fewer basophils were present in susceptible cattle (*R. appendiculatus* nymphs), there was a greater influx of eosinophils in susceptible cattle (*R. microplus* but not *H. longicornis*), and there is a greater increase in mast cell numbers in tick-resistant cattle (*R. microplus*). Using induced infestations with *R. microplus* as a model shows that cell infiltrations and histamine release fluctuate during the tick's life cycle (Robbertse *et al.*, 2017), but this is likely to be of little consequence under conditions of natural infestations, where all life cycle stages can be present at the same time.

Skin and lymph node samples were collected from Brahman, Bonsmara and Holstein-Friesian cattle before and after infestation with *R. microplus* larvae. Compared to the baseline before induced tick infestation, 183 DEG were found in Bonsmara whereas few transcripts were identified as differentially expressed within the Holstein-Friesian and Brahman breeds during larval and adult tick feeding. Bonsmara animals at the larval life stage (compared to uninfested animals) represented the majority of DEG, with 68 being downregulated and 90 upregulated (Robbertse, 2018). The animals represented highly resistant, resistant and susceptible breeds. The samples were subject to histology, immunohistochemistry and flow cytometry to elucidate the cellular dynamics of the immune response. All cattle displayed a significant influx of $CD20^+$ B-lymphocytes in the dermis, while $CD3^+$ T-lymphocytes were significantly increased in the more tick-resistant breeds. In the lymph node germinal centres, all cattle breeds had an eosinophil influx but TBM were significantly increased in the Brahmans. More resistant cattle showed negligible fluctuation in $CD20^+$ and CD79α B-lymphocytes in the lymph nodes, but susceptible cattle displayed an initial decrease in B-cells, followed by an increase as the ticks progressed to adulthood. Tick susceptibility seemed to be associated with differential B-lymphocyte regulation, increased variability in $WC1^+$ $\gamma\delta$ T-lymphocytes and a decrease in T-helper lymphocytes in lymph nodes. In Brahman cattle, the lymph node T-helper lymphocyte population was stable. The impression was that animals of a susceptible breed develop a more gradual, slower cutaneous response to tick bites than resistant breeds (Robbertse *et al.*, 2018).

Nguni and Bonsmara heifers exposed to natural infestation by several tick species for at least 1 month received intradermal injections of unfed larval extracts of *R. decoloratus* and *R. microplus* in different ears. Bonsmara cattle showed a more intense immediate reaction than did Nguni, judged by ear thickness at the injection site 1 hour after injection. Only the Nguni displayed a delayed hypersensitivity reaction 72 hours after injection. *R. decoloratus* elicited a more intense skin response than did *R. microplus*. The study indicated the need for further investigation of the cellular responses to tick infestation in Nguni cattle (Marufu *et al.*, 2013).

Skin punch biopsies were taken from Zebu and European breed cattle after they had been repeatedly infested with *R. microplus* larvae. Infiltrations with T-cell subsets ($CD3^+$, $CD4^+$, $CD8^+$ and γδ) followed the same pattern in both breeds, substantially increasing 7 weeks after the first infestation. T-cells and MHC class II-expressing cells were seen in greater numbers in Zebu cattle, but the difference was only significant for γδ T-cells. More granulocytes infiltrated more rapidly and in higher numbers in European cattle. Granulocytes and MHC class II-expressing cells infiltrated closest to the mouthparts of the larvae, and a large volume of granulocyte antigen was seen in the gut of attached feeding larvae. It was speculated that granulocytes might be a nutrient source for tick larvae, with lower granulocyte numbers reducing their feeding success on Zebu cattle. Zebu cattle seemed to be better able to recruit T-cells and monocytes to the skin around tick bite sites. Although the final number of challenge larvae was the same for both cattle breeds, only the European cattle suffered from tick-sore lesions. It was suggested that the greater numbers of γδ T-cells limited the inflammatory process in the Zebu cattle (Constantinoiu *et al.*, 2010).

4.4.2 Genomic/proteomic indicators

Once the immunological basis for differences in susceptibility to ticks is known, it would be useful if this could be selected for by genomic means or by way of biomarkers.

Efforts to relate genomic differences identified by microsatellites and SNPs to phenotypic differences in tick burdens have yielded inconsistent results. Gene expression studies found increased expression of TLRs, MHC class II molecules, Ca-binding proteins and complement proteins, with an increase in the number of neutrophils in the skin of susceptible cattle after tick feeding. There were higher numbers of T-cells, eosinophils, mast cells and basophils, with upregulated proteases, cathepsins, keratins, collagens and extracellular matrix proteins in the skin of resistant cattle (Tabor *et al.*, 2017).

Proteomic analysis of serum samples from the Santa Gertrudis cattle in which variation in their immune responses had been demonstrated (Piper *et al.*, 2017) revealed differential abundance of several proteins between tick-resistant and susceptible animals. The differential abundance of 28 proteins seen between resistant and susceptible naïve Santa Gertrudis cattle (see section 3.3.2, this volume) persisted after tick infestation, when an additional eight proteins differed highly in their abundance. The differentially abundant proteins in resistant cattle were associated with complement activation, enabling a better protective cellular response, chemotaxis for immune cells and acute-phase elements of the immune response. Tick-resistant cattle seemed to develop a more controlled inflammatory response, which is protective instead of facilitating tick feeding. Tick-susceptible cattle developed significantly higher IgG1 titres than resistant cattle, suggesting that the antibody response plays no role in resistance or might contribute to increased susceptibility to infestation. This discovery could be used to define a proteomics profile of tick resistance (Raza *et al.*, 2021, 2023).

The CD45 leucocyte antigen receptor (see section3.1.3, this volume) is encoded by the protein tyrosine phosphatase receptor type-C gene (PTPRC), of which there are four variants/families, distributed unevenly between Zebu and European breeds of cattle. Although the PTPRC genotype affects leucocyte count, $CD8^+$ cells, haematocrit, haemoglobin concentration, erythrocyte count and IgG1 titre differently in the different cattle breeds, there was no significant association between PTPRC genotype and tick count (Jonsson *et al.*, 2021).

4.5 Adaptive Cross-immunity to Ticks

Cattle that become resistant to one species of tick are likely to also become resistant to other species after they have been infested (Rechav and Kostrzewski, 1991). Cattle ranked for resistance based on the numbers of one species were ranked similarly based on the numbers of another in the case of Zebu cattle in Uganda, infested with *R. appendiculatus, A. variegatum, [B.] R. decoloratus, R. e. evertsi, R. simus, R. compositus* and *H. m. rufipes* (Kaiser *et al.*, 1982). The same was true for European cattle in Australia, but the adaptive immunity seems to be species specific. Cattle previously exposed to *H. longicornis* were as susceptible as naïve cattle upon first exposure to [*B. microplus*] *R. australis* (Wagland *et al.*, 1985), and cattle with acquired resistance to [*B.*] *R. microplus* were as susceptible as naïve cattle to *H. a. anatolicum* (Miranpuri, 1989).

4.6 Modulation of Adaptive Immunity

Ticks are confronted with the host's immediate defensive haemostatic, inflammatory and immune responses of the innate immune system (see section 3.4, this volume) every time they penetrate a host's skin with their mouthparts (Steen *et al.*, 2006; Van Oosterwijk and Wikel, 2021). It is a cascade of components composed of antigen-presenting cells, B- and T-lymphocytes, antibodies, granulocytes and an array of cytokines and other biologically active molecules. But this immunity is only partially effective. During their secondary and subsequent infestations, ticks have to also withstand the adaptive immune response.

There are distinct advantages for ticks in modulating the host cytokine and T-cell proliferation aimed at reducing their ability to obtain a bloodmeal (Brossard and Wikel, 2004). Ticks defend themselves against microbial insult and injury with their innate immune system. This includes interaction with host immune molecules acquired during the bloodmeal (Boulanger and Wikel, 2021).

4.6.1 Defensive molecules in tick saliva

Due to considerable gene duplication, ticks possess a diverse arsenal of closely related proteins from several classes to modulate the host's adaptive immune response. They include chemokine-binding proteins, complement pathway inhibitors and ion channel modulators (Denisov and Dijkgraaf, 2021).

The immunosuppressive countermeasures mounted by ticks inhibit antibody responses, complement activation (in both the innate and adaptive phases), B- and T-cell proliferation and elicitation of cytokines (macrophages: IL-1, TNF-α; Th1 lymphocytes: IFN-γ; Th2 cells: IL-4, IL-5, IL-10). Secreted tick saliva components include enzymes, enzyme inhibitors, amine-binding proteins and cytokine homologues that act as anti-inflammatory or immune-modulatory antihaemostatic agents, to allow extended feeding (Neitz and Vermeulen, 1987; Brossard and Wikel, 1997; Wikel, 1999; Steen *et al.*, 2006; Hovius *et al.*, 2008; Zavašnik-Bergant *et al.*, 2017).

Figure 4.3 provides a schematic presentation of some tick salivary proteins acting on various aspects of the host's adaptive immunity. The immunomodulatory components in tick saliva are predominantly made up of proteinaceous salivary compounds, but also non-peptide molecules, lipid derivatives and non-coding RNA (ncRNA), that target both the innate and adaptive immune systems (Chmelař *et al.*, 2016; Aounallah *et al.*, 2020). These proteins have different expression patterns in each developmental stage, and between salivary gland and midgut expression. They have been shown to belong to different protein families such as metalloproteases, serpins, cysteine protease, histamine-binding proteins, lipoglycoproteins and esterases (Rodriguez-Valle *et al.*, 2013).

Whereas some of the salivary components remain in the immediate vicinity of the attachment site (see section 3.4, this volume) (Willadsen and McKenna, 1983) to inhibit blood coagulation, inflammation and local immune reactions, others, such as venom and toxins, probably enter the general circulation (Steen *et al.*, 2006).

Some of the immunomodulatory components of tick saliva have been identified as candidates for targeted immunotherapy (Aounallah *et al.*, 2020).

4.6.2 Cytokine interference

Some tick salivary compounds interfere with dendritic cells and change their capacity to present antigens, or prevent lymphocyte proliferation, or T-cell cytokine production (Aounallah *et al.*, 2020). Saliva of *I. scapularis* contains an IL-2-binding protein which can affect activated T-cells, B-cells, NK cells, cytotoxic T-cells, monocytes and macrophages, all known to express IL-2 receptors (Brossard and Wikel, 2004).

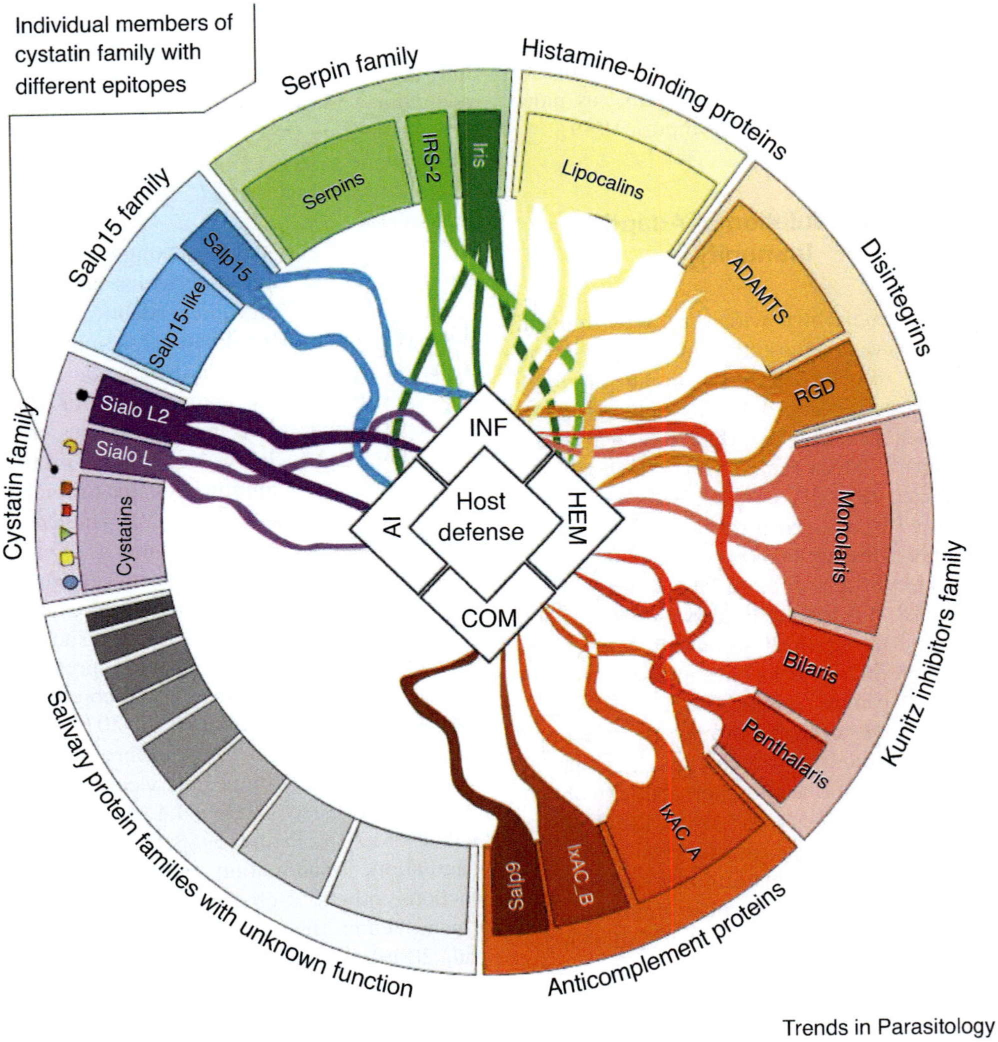

Fig. 4.3. Schematic representation of some tick salivary components acting on host adaptive immunity. From Chmelař et al. (2016) with permission of Elsevier.

4.6.3 Complement inhibition

Several molecules with anticomplement activity have been identified in the salivary glands of *I. scapularis* and *I. ricinus*, inhibiting formation of complement C3 convertase. Soft ticks have been reported to inhibit the classical complement pathway (see section 3.1.3, this volume), with lipocalins from *O. moubata* and *O. savignyi* (Aounallah *et al.*, 2020). One of the diverse biological functions of calreticulin (CRT) is binding of the first complement component C1q (Brossard and Wikel, 2004; Kim *et al.*, 2015). CRT is secreted in the saliva of *A. americanum*, *D. variabilis* and [*B.*] *R. microplus* (Brossard and Wikel, 2004). Modulation of the proteolytic activity of cysteine proteases (such as cathepsin) may be another mechanism to interfere with the immune response. Cystatin OmC2 is naturally present in the saliva, salivary glands and gut of *O. moubata* (Zavašnik-Bergant *et al.*, 2017).

4.6.4 Antibody neutralization

The suppression of antibody production by tick infestation was demonstrated in guinea pigs infested with *D. andersoni* larvae and in rabbits infested with adult *R. appendiculatus* (Brossard and Wikel, 1997). IgG-binding proteins have been found in *A. variegatum*, *I. hexagonus* and *R. appendiculatus*. They could be important in eliminating antibody molecules crossing the gut into the haemocoele (Brossard and Wikel, 2004). Salivary components from *I. ricinus* and *H. asiaticum* were also shown to disarm humoral immunity by inhibiting B-cell responses, such as the production of specific anti-tick antibodies (Aounallah *et al*., 2020).

Host anti-tick immunoglobulin has been found in the haemolymph, salivary glands and saliva of feeding ticks of more than one species (Ackerman *et al*., 1981; Wang and Nuttall, 1994; Boulanger and Wikel, 2021). The reason for this is not yet clear. It could be a part of the tick's removal of large proteins from the bloodmeal. But there is the possibility that host antibodies recycled back into the tick bite site could downregulate the host's immune defences (Boulanger and Wikel, 2021).

4.6.5 MHC interference and T-lymphocyte impediment

Numerous inhibitors of T-cell functions have been identified in tick saliva and salivary glands. T-lymphocyte proliferation was suppressed by salivary proteins from *R. appendiculatus* (Fivaz *et al*., 1984; Fivaz, 1989), *D. andersoni* (Brossard and Wikel, 2004), [*B. microplus*] *R. australis* (Turni *et al*., 2004), *H. longicornis* and *R. haemaphysaloides* (Aounallah *et al*., 2020). Recombinant versions of these proteins inhibited the expression of cytokines such as IL-2, IL-12 and TNF-α. *R. haemaphysaloides* serpin 2 can prevent the activation of CD4 and CD8 T-cells, inhibiting the Th1 immune response. Sialostatins from *I. scapularis* suppressed proliferation of CD4 and CD8 T-cells, neutrophil migration in severe inflammation, the secretion of cytokines by mast cells, dendritic cells and lymphocytes, and reduced the release of IL-9 by Th9 cells (Aounallah *et al*., 2020). The host's immune response influences the composition of salivary gland extract from [*B. microplus*] *R. australis* and the level of inhibition of lymphocyte proliferation (Turni *et al*., 2004).

Different mitogens have been used *in vitro* to study the inhibitory effect of tick salivary gland extract (SGE) on T-cell proliferation. Concanavalin A and phytohaemagglutinin were more stimulatory than pokeweed mitogen. Reduction of lymphocyte proliferative responses by the addition of SGE was not significantly different for the three mitogens. In an adjunct experiment, it was shown that SGE did not inhibit the stimulation of B-cell proliferation by lipopolysaccharide (Turni *et al*., 2007).

In addition to being a membrane-bound early marker of lymphocyte activation, CD69 also regulates the differentiation of T_{reg} cells and the secretion of IFN-γ, IL-17 and Il-22 (Cibrián and Sánchez-Madrid, 2017). Salivary gland extract from *I. ricinus* inhibits expression of CD69 on both B- and T-cells (Brossard and Wikel, 2004).

Several tick salivary compounds are pleiotropic and target haemostatic and immune system components. One such multifunctional protein is Salp15, which binds to dendritic cells, inhibits CD4 and T-cell activation and proliferation, and blocks the liberation of IL-2 (Chmelař *et al*., 2016; Aounallah *et al*., 2020).

Iris (*I. ricinus* immunosuppressor) was the first tick serpin described to inhibit T-cell and splenocyte proliferation, alter PBMC-derived cytokine levels, bind macrophages and suppress the secretion of TNF (Chmelař *et al*., 2017).

A serpin cloned from dissected *R. microplus* salivary gland, gut and ovary was predicted to have B- and T-cell epitopes, using bioinformatics. The serpin and its B-cell epitope were recognized immunologically by ELISA, using sera from tick-resistant Santa Gertrudis cattle previously exposed to induced and natural tick infestation, and shown to have IgG titres against the recombined serpin. The T-cell epitopes were not well exposed and did not stimulate lymphocyte proliferation *in vitro*. *In vitro* feeding on sheep sera with antibodies against a synthesized B-cell epitope conjugated to keyhole limpet hemocyanin (KLH) reduced ticks' reproductive capacity by 81.16% (Rodriguez-Valle *et al*., 2012).

The differentiation of $CD8^+$ T-lymphocytes into NK T-cells or cytotoxic T-cells is downregulated during the immature feeding stages of *R. microplus* on Bonsmara cattle. Such activity was also reported from salivary gland extracts of *D. reticulatus*, *A. variegatum*, *Haemaphysalis inermis* and *I. ricinus*. NK cells can differentiate and mature in the lymph nodes and can also regulate T-cell interactions of endothelial, dendritic and macrophage cell lineages. This suggests that in response to tick infestation, there is a suppression of cytotoxic T-cell immunity in the host (Robbertse, 2018).

The sialostatins (C1-type cysteine protease inhibitors; cystatins) suppress cathepsins, which play an important role in MHC II antigen processing and presentation. They also play a role in suppressing chemokines such as IP-10 and cytokines such as TNF-α, IL-1β, IL-9 and IL-12. Sialostatin L decreases activation of signalling in mast cells and dendritic cells and dampens antigen-mediated $CD4^+$ proliferation (Zavašnik-Bergant *et al.*, 2017; Pham *et al.*, 2021).

4.6.6 Enhanced pathogen transmission

Altering the host immune defences also provides an environment favourable to the establishment of tick-transmitted pathogens, which is already evident during the innate immune phase (Brossard and Wikel, 2004). Tick-transmitted pathogens take advantage of this privileged environment and are suspected of manipulating the composition of tick saliva to enhance their own survival, transmission and evasion of immune defences (Pham *et al.*, 2021).

Tick salivary gland molecules potentiate infection with tick-borne pathogens, such as Thogoto virus and TBEV, demonstrated for *I. ricinus*, *D. reticulatus* and *R. appendiculatus*. *R. appendiculatus* enhanced the susceptibility of bovine lymphocytes to infection with *Theileria parva*, the causative agent of East Coast fever (Brossard and Wikel, 2004).

Using the available information from the *R. microplus* genome in a bioinformatics approach, the three-dimensional structure of the lipocalin family, known as histamine-binding proteins, was discovered to be conserved, despite high sequence variability. B- and T-cell epitopes in these lipocalins were predicted and used to examine host immune interactions with sera and PBMC collected from tick-susceptible (Holstein-Friesian) and tick-resistant (Brahman) cattle challenged with [*R. microplus*] *R. australis*. Antilipocalin titres were higher in resistant than in susceptible cattle 28–60 days after tick infestation, but then declined in both groups. PBMCs from tick-susceptible cattle, challenged with T-cell epitopes in a cell proliferation assay, displayed a higher number of IFN-γ-secreting Th1 cells than those from resistant cattle. This relationship was reversed in the expression of the Th2 IL-4 cytokine, which was higher in PBMCs from Brahman cattle (Rodriguez-Valle *et al.*, 2013).

Needle injection of pathogens with tick SGE was used to demonstrate enhanced infection. Only a small number of salivary components have been described. Sialostatin L and L2 enhance the transmission of *A. phagocytophilum*, TBEV and *B. burgdorferi*. Increased numbers of infected neutrophils at tick bite sites may explain transfer of infection to uninfected ticks, also in the case of *B. burgdorferi* (Pham *et al.*, 2021).

4.6.7 Extraneous interference

Described in 1966 as having anthelmintic activity, levamisole (l-tetramisole), the laevo-rotating isomer of tetramisole (O'Neil *et al.*, 2013), was later discovered to also have immunomodulatory characteristics, such as macrophage stimulation, neutrophil chemotaxis, lymphocyte proliferation, T-cell differentiation and an effect on IL-1 production (Renoux, 1978, 1980). It seems this 'adjuvant' effect has mostly been investigated in the context of vaccines against bacteria and viruses (Sajid *et al.*, 2006). Whether it might be useful in a future tick vaccine remains to be seen.

A recent discovery is the disturbance of immune responses by an acaricide. Fipronil (FPN) is an N-phenylpyrazole that induces hyperexcitation neuronal toxicity by antagonizing insect γ-aminobutyric acid (GABA)-gated chloride channels. When administered orally to mice sensitized to ovalbumin (OVA), FPN was found not to cause any clinical signs of intoxication but to increase OVA-specific IgG titres (but not IgM). FPN caused splenocytes to significantly increase production of the antigen-specific cytokines IL-2, IL-4 and IFN-γ. Dysregulated Th1/Th2 cytokine production has the potential to contribute to the development of autoimmune disorders and allergic conditions. Because mRNA expression of Th1/Th2 cytokines and their respective upstream transcription factors remained unchanged or slightly decreased, the immunomodulatory effects of FPN on antigen-specific T-cell responses is possibly not through the regulation of Th1/Th2 differentiation and cytokine gene expression.

Immunostimulatory effects of FPN have also been reported in human nasal epithelial cells. FPN induced both protein levels and mRNA expression *in vitro* of proinflammatory cytokines, including IL-1β, IL-6 and IL-8 through activation of ERK1/2 MAPK, p38 MAPK and the NF-κB pathway.

GABA is an inhibitory neurotransmitter which can also be synthesized and released by immune cells. GABAergic signalling genes and functional proteins are also expressed in mononuclear phagocytes and lymphocytes. GABA has diverse roles in the immune system, acting as an intercellular signalling molecule to modulate monocyte migration and suppress T-cell activation, proliferation and cytokine production. GABA participates in T-cell-mediated immunity via GABA transporters and receptors. GABA treatment can inhibit antigen-specific T-cell proliferation and the T-cell responses to foreign and self-antigens *in vitro*. Antigen-specific T-cell response can be directly inhibited by the GABAergic agents. Dysregulation of GABAergic genes in immune cells might be a potential mechanism of FPN-induced immunotoxicity (Kuo *et al.*, 2024).

4.6.8 Therapeutic uses for tick-secreted proteins

The hundreds of proteins secreted in tick saliva with antihaemostatic, anticomplement, anti-inflammatory and immunomodulatory effects lend themselves to exploitation in the treatment of a number of human diseases. Listed possibilities include conjunctivitis, allergic rhinitis, pancreatitis, rheumatoid arthritis, muscular dystrophy, osteoporosis, neurodegeneration, psoriasis, atherosclerosis, emphysema, chronic obstructive pulmonary disease and cystic fibrosis. The functional specificity of tick serpins and cystatins is regarded as an advantage in developing bespoke immunotherapeutic strategies (Mans, 2005; Chmelař *et al.*, 2017).

References

Ackerman, S., Clare, F.B., McGill, T.W. and Sonenshine, D.E. (1981) Passage of host serum components, including antibody, across the digestive tract of *Dermacentor variabilis* (Say). *Journal of Parasitology* 76/5, 737–740.

Allman, D. and Pillai, S. (2008) Peripheral B cell subsets. *Current Opinion in Immunology* 20/2, 149–157. DOI: 10.1016/j.coi.2008.03.014.

Anon. (2024) Major histocompatibility complex. Available at: https://en.wikipedia.org/w/index.php?title=Major_histocompatibility_complex&oldid=1192764972 (accessed 29 September 2024).

Aounallah, H., Bensaoud, C., M'ghirbi, Y., Faria, F., Chmelař, J. *et al.* (2020) Tick salivary compounds for targeted immunomodulatory therapy. *Frontiers in Immunology* 11, 583845. DOI: 10.3389/fimmu.2020.583845.

Barnstable, C.J., Bodmer, W.F., Brown, G., Galfre, G., Milstein, C. *et al.* (1978) Production of monoclonal antibodies to Group A erythrocytes, HLA and other human cell surface antigens – new tools for genetic analysis. *Cell* 14, 9–20. DOI: 10.1016/0092-8674(78)90296-9.

Batra, T.R., Lee, A.J., Gavora, J.S. and Stear, M.J. (1989) Class I alleles of the bovine major histocompatibility system and their association with economic traits. *Journal of Dairy Science* 72/8, 2115–2124. DOI: 10.3168/jds.S0022-0302(89)79336-X.

Boulanger, N. and Wikel, S. (2021) Induced transient immune tolerance in ticks and vertebrate host: A keystone of tick-borne diseases? *Frontiers in Immunology* 12, 625993. DOI: 10.3389/fimmu.2021.625993.

Bradley, J. (1974) Immunoglobulins. *Journal of Medical Genetics* 11, 80–90.
Brossard, M. and Fivaz, V. (1982) *Ixodes ricinus* L.: Mast cells, basophils and eosinophils in the sequence of cellular events in the skin of infested or re-infested rabbits. *Parasitology* 85/3, 583–592. DOI: 10.1017/S0031182000056365.
Brossard, M. and Papatheodorou, V. (1990) Immunity against female *Ixodes ricinus* L.: Effect on feeding and haemoglobin digestion. *Annales de Parasitologie Humaine et Comparée* 65/1, 32–36. DOI: 10.1051/parasite/1990651032.
Brossard, M.L. and Wikel, S.K. (1997) Immunology of interactions between ticks and hosts. *Medical and Veterinary Entomology* 11/3, 270–276. DOI: 10.1111/j.1365-2915.1997.tb00406.x.
Brossard, M.L. and Wikel, S.K. (2004) Tick immunobiology. *Parasitology* 129, S161–S176. DOI: 10.1017/S0031182004004834.
Brossard, M., Monneron, J.P. and Papatheodorou, V. (1982) Progressive sensitization of circulating basophils against *Ixodes ricinus* L. antigens during repeated infestations of rabbits. *Parasite Immunology* 4/5, 355–361. DOI: 10.1111/j.1365-3024.1982.tb00447.x.
Burster, T., Macmillan, H., Hou, T., Boehm, B.O. and Mellins, E.D. (2010) Cathepsin G: Roles in antigen presentation and beyond. *Molecular Immunology* 47/4, 658–665. DOI: 10.1016/j.molimm.2009.10.003.
Campden, R.I. and Zhang, Y. (2019) The role of lysosomal cysteine cathepsins in NLRP3 inflammasome activation. *Archives of Biochemistry and Biophysics* 670, 32–42. DOI: 10.1016/j.abb.2019.02.015.
Chmelař, J., Kotál, J., Kopecký, J., Pedra, J.H.F. and Kotsyfakis, M. (2016) All for one and one for all on the tick–host battlefield. *Trends in Parasitology* 32/5, 368–377. DOI: 10.1016/j.pt.2016.01.004.
Chmelař, J., Kotál, J., Langhansová, H. and Kotsyfakis, M. (2017) Protease inhibitors in tick saliva: The role of serpins and cystatins in tick–host–pathogen interaction. *Frontiers in Cellular Infection and Microbiology* 7, 216. DOI: 10.3389/fcimb.2017.00216.
Cibrián, D. and Sánchez-Madrid, F. (2017) CD69: From activation marker to metabolic gatekeeper. *European Journal of Immunology* 47/6, 946–953. DOI: 10.1002/eji.201646837.
Constantinoiu, C.C., Jackson, L.A., Jorgensen, W.K., Lew-Tabor, A.E., Piper, E.K. *et al*. (2010) Local immune response against larvae of *Rhipicephalus (Boophilus) microplus* in *Bos taurus indicus* and *Bos taurus taurus* cattle. *International Journal for Parasitology* 40, 865–875. DOI: 10.1016/j.ijpara.2010.01.004.
Cullen, G.A. (1982) The bursa: Fabricius to Delaware. *Journal of the Royal Society of Medicine* 75/7, 507–512.
Denisov, S.S. and Dijkgraaf, I. (2021) Immunomodulatory proteins in tick saliva from a structural perspective. *Frontiers in Cellular and Infection Microbiology* 11, 769574. DOI: 10.3389/fcimb.2021.769574.
Fischer, U., Yang, J.J., Ikawa, T., Hein, D., Vicente-Dueñas, C. *et al*. (2020) Cell fate decisions: The role of transcription factors in early B-cell development and leukemia. *Blood Cancer Discovery* 1/3, 224–233. DOI: 10.1158/2643-3230.BCD-20-0011.
Fivaz, B.H. (1989) Immune suppression induced by the brown ear tick *Rhipicephalus appendiculatus* Neuman, 1901. *Journal of Parasitology* 75/6, 946–952.
Fivaz, B.H., Norval, R.A.I. and Brown, A. (1984) Immunity of the ox to the brown ear tick *Rhipicephalus appendiculatus*. *Proceedings of the 13th World Congress on Diseases of Cattle, Durban, South Africa* 1, 455–460.
Forget, A., Potworowski, E.F., Richer, G. and Borduas, A.G. (1970) Antigenic specificities of bursal and thymic lymphocytes in the chicken. *Immunology* 19/3, 465–468.
Garcia, G.R., Maruyama, S.R., Nelson, K.T., Ribeiro, J.M.C., Gardinassi, L.G. *et al*. (2017) Immune recognition of salivary proteins from the cattle tick *Rhipicephalus microplus* differs according to the genotype of the bovine host. *Parasites & Vectors* 10/1, 144. DOI: 10.1186/s13071-017-2077-9.
Glick, B. (1994) The bursa of fabricius: The evolution of a discovery. *Poultry Science* 73/7, 979–983. DOI: 10.3382/ps.0730979.
Glick, B., Chang, T.S. and Jaap, R.G. (1956) The Bursa of Fabricius and antibody production. *Poultry Science* 35/1, 224–225.
Gopalraj, J.B.P., Clarke, F.C. and Donkin, E.F. (2013) Assessment of acquired immune response to *Rhipicephalus appendiculatus* tick infestation in different goat breeds. *Onderstepoort Journal of Veterinary Research* 80/1, 614. DOI: 10.4102/ojvr.v80i1.614.
Gurwicz, N., Stoler-Barak, L., Schwan, N., Bandyopadhyay, A., Meyer-Hermann, M. *et al*. (2023) Tingible body macrophages arise from lymph node-resident precursors and uptake B cells by dendrites. *Journal of Experimental Medicine* 220/4, e20222173. DOI: 10.1084/jem.20222173.

Halaby, D.M. and Mornon, J.P.E. (1998) The immunoglobulin superfamily: an insight on its tissular, species, and functional diversity. *Journal of Molecular Evolution* 46, 389–400.

Heeb, L.E.M., Egholm, C. and Boyman, O. (2020) Evolution and function of interleukin-4 receptor signaling in adaptive immunity and neutrophils. *Genes & Immunity* 21/3, 143–149. DOI: 10.1038/s41435-020-0095-7.

Hewetson, R.W. (1972) The inheritance of resistance by cattle to cattle tick. *Australian Veterinary Journal* 48/5, 299–303. DOI: 10.1111/j.1751-0813.1972.tb05161.x.

Hovius, J.W.R., Levi, M. and Fikrig, E. (2008) Salivating for knowledge: Potential pharmacological agents in tick saliva. *PLoS Medicine* 5/2, e43. DOI: 10.1371/journal.pmed.0050043.

Janeway Jr, C.A., Travers, P., Walport, M. and Shlomchik, M.J. (eds) (2001a) The major histocompatibility complex and its functions. In: *Immunobiology: The Immune System in Health and Disease*, 5th edn. Garland Science, New York. Available at: https://www.ncbi.nlm.nih.gov/books/NBK27156/ (accessed 02 January 2025).

Janeway Jr, C.A., Travers, P., Walport, M. and Shlomchik, M.J. (eds) (2001b) The structure of a typical antibody molecule. In: *Immunobiology: The Immune System in Health and Disease*, 5th edn. Garland Science, New York. Available at: https://www.ncbi.nlm.nih.gov/books/NBK27144/ (accessed 02 January 2025).

Jonsson, N.N., Piper, E.K. and Constantinoiu, C.C. (2014) Host resistance in cattle to infestation with the cattle tick *Rhipicephalus microplus*. *Parasite Immunology* 36/11, 553–559. DOI: 10.1111/pim.12140.

Jonsson, N.N., Cox, D.K., Piper, E.K., Valdivieso, E.F.M., Constantinoiu, C. *et al*. (2021) Allelic variation in protein tyrosine phosphatase receptor type-C in cattle influences erythrocyte, leukocyte and humoral responses to infestation with the cattle tick *Rhipicephalus australis*. *Frontiers in Immunology* 12, 675979. DOI: 10.3389/fimmu.2021.675979.

Jung, C., Hugot, J.P. and Barreau, F. (2010) Peyer's patches: The immune sensors of the intestine. *International Journal of Inflammation*. DOI: 10.4061/2010/823710.

Kaas, Q. and Lefranc, M.-P. (2005) T cell receptor/peptide/MHC molecular characterization and standardized pMHC contact sites in IMGT/3dstructure-DB. *In Silico Biology* 5, 505–528.

Kaiser, M.N., Sutherst, R.W. and Bourne, A.S. (1982) Relationship between ticks and Zebu cattle in southern Uganda. *Tropical Animal Health and Production* 14/2, 63–74. DOI: 10.1007/bf02282583.

Kim, T.K., Ibelli, A.M.G. and Mulenga, A. (2015) *Amblyomma americanum* tick calreticulin binds C1q but does not inhibit activation of the classical complement cascade. *Ticks & Tick-Borne Diseases* 6/1, 91–101. DOI: 10.1016/j.ttbdis.2014.10.002.

Klein, U., Tu, Y., Stolovitzky, G.A., Keller, J.L., Haddad Jr, J. *et al*. (2003) Transcriptional analysis of the B cell germinal center reaction. *Proceedings of the National Academy of Sciences* 100/5, 2639–2644. DOI: 10.1073_pnas.0437996100.

Kuo, J.-F., Cheng, A.H., Tung, C.-W. and Wang, C.-C. (2024) Fipronil disturbs the antigen-specific immune responses and GABAergic gene expression in the ovalbumin-immunized BALB/c mice. *BMC Veterinary Research* 20, 30. DOI: 10.1186/s12917-024-03878-3.

Küppers, R., Klein, U.L., Hansmann, M.L. and Rajewsky, K. (1999) Cellular origin of human B-cell lymphomas. *New England Journal of Medicine* 341/20, 1520–1529.

Laidlaw, B.J., Craft, J. and Kaech, S.M. (2016) The multifaceted role of CD4+ T cells in the regulation of CD8+ T cell memory maturation. *Nature Reviews Immunology* 16/2, 102–111. DOI: 10.1038/nri.2015.10.

Luckheeram, R.V., Zhou, R., Verma, A.D. and Xia, B. (2012) CD4+T cells: Differentiation and functions. *Clinical and Developmental Immunology* 2012, 925135. DOI: 10.1155/2012/925135.

Mans, B.J. (2005) Tick histamine-binding proteins and related lipocalins: Potential as therapeutic agents. *Current Opinion in Investigational Drugs* 6/11, 1131–1135.

Marufu, M.C., Chimonyo, M., Mans, B.J. and Dzama, K. (2013) Cutaneous hypersensitivity responses to *Rhipicephalus* tick larval antigens in pre-sensitized cattle. *Ticks & Tick-Borne Diseases* 4/4, 311–316. DOI: 10.1016/j.ttbdis.2012.12.001.

Matsunaga, Y., Saibara, T., Kido, H. and Katunuma, N. (1993) Participation of cathepsin B in processing of antigen presentation to MHC class II. *FEBS Letters* 324/3, 325–330. DOI: 10.1016/0014-5793(93)80144-j.

Meeusen, E.N., de Veer, M., Hertzog, P.J., Stear, M.J., Mallard, B.A. *et al*. (2013) New approaches to innate immunity in livestock and the potential for manipulation – review. MLA final report B.BSC.0321.

Available at: https://www.mla.com.au/research-and-development/search-rd-reports/?q=b.bsc.0321 &sort=1 (accessed 15 October 2023).

Mejri, N. and Brossard, M. (2007) Splenic dendritic cells pulsed with *Ixodes ricinus* tick saliva prime naive CD4$^+$T to induce Th2 cell differentiation *in vitro* and *in vivo*. *International Immunology* 19/4, 535–543. DOI: 10.1093/intimm/dxm019.

Miranpuri, G.S. (1989) Relationship between the resistance of crossbred cattle to ticks, *Boophilus microplus* (Canestrini, 1887) and *Hyalomma anatolicum anatolicum* (Koch, 1844). *Veterinary Parasitology* 31, 289–301.

Mittrücker, H.-W., Visekruna, A. and Huber, M. (2014) Heterogeneity in the differentiation and function of CD8$^+$ T cells. *Archivum Immunologiae et Therapiae Experimentalis* 62, 449–458. DOI: 10.1007/s00005-014-0293-y.

Mix, E., Goertsches, R. and Zettl, U.K. (2006) Immunoglobulins – basic considerations. *Journal of Neurology* 253/Suppl 5, V9–V17. DOI: 10.1007/s00415-006-5002-2.

Neitz, A.W.H. and Vermeulen, N.M.J. (1987) Biochemical studies on the salivary glands and haemolymph of *Amblyomma hebraeum*. *Onderstepoort Journal of Veterinary Research* 54, 443–450.

Neitz, A.W.H., Gothe, R., Pawlas, S. and Groeneveld, H.T. (1993) Investigations into lymphocyte transformation and histamine release by basophils in sheep repeatedly infested with R*hipicephalus evertsi evertsi* ticks. *Experimental & Applied Acarology* 17, 551–559.

O'Neil, M.J., Heckelman, P.E., Dobbelaar, P.H. and Roman, K.J. (eds) (2013) *The Merck Index*, 15th edn. Royal Society of Chemistry, Cambridge.

Palucka, K. and Banchereau, J. (1999) Dendritic cells: A link between innate and adaptive immunity. *Journal of Clinical Immunology* 19/1, 12–25.

Pham, M., Underwood, J. and Oliva Chávez, A.S. (2021) Changing the recipe: Pathogen directed changes in tick saliva components. *International Journal of Environmental Research and Public Health* 18, 1806. DOI: 10.3390/ijerph18041806.

Piper, E.K., Jackson, L.A., Bagnall, N.H., Kongsuwan, K.K., Lew, A.E. *et al*. (2008) Gene expression in the skin of *Bos taurus* and *Bos indicus* cattle infested with the cattle tick, *Rhipicephalus (Boophilus) microplus*. *Veterinary Immunology and Immunopathology* 126/1-2, 110–119. DOI: 10.1016/j.vetimm.2008.06.011.

Piper, E.K., Jonsson, N.N., Gondro, C., Lew-Tabor, A.E., Moolhuijzen, P. *et al*. (2009) Immunological profiles of *Bos taurus* and *Bos indicus* cattle infested with the cattle tick, *Rhipicephalus (boophilus) microplus*. *Clinical and Vaccine Immunology* 16/7, 1071–1086.

Piper, E.K., Jackson, L.A., Bielefeldt-Ohmann, H., Gondro, C., Lew-Tabor, A.E. *et al*. (2010) Tick-susceptible *Bos taurus* cattle display an increased cellular response at the site of larval *Rhipicephalus (Boophilus) microplus* attachment, compared with tick-resistant *Bos indicus* cattle. *International Journal for Parasitology* 40/4, 431–441. DOI: 10.1016/j.ijpara.2009.09.009.

Piper, E.K., Jonsson, N.N., Gondro, C., Vance, M.E., Lew-Tabor, A.E. *et al*. (2017) Peripheral cellular and humoral responses to infestation with the cattle tick *Rhipicephalus microplus* in Santa Gertrudis cattle. *Parasite Immunology* 39, e12402. DOI: 10.1111/pim.12402.

Raza, A., Schulz, B.L., Nouwens, A., Jackson, L.A., Piper, E.K. *et al*. (2021) Serum proteomes of Santa Gertrudis cattle before and after infestation with *Rhipicephalus australis* ticks. *Parasite Immunology* 43/7, e12836. DOI: 10.1111/pim.12836.

Raza, A., Schulz, B.L., Nouwens, A., Naseem, M.N., Kamran, M. *et al*. (2023) Application of quantitative proteomics to discover biomarkers for tick resistance in cattle. *Frontiers in Immunology* 14, 1091066. DOI: 10.3389/fimmu.2023.1091066.

Reboldi, A. and Cyster, J.G. (2016) Peyer's patches: Organizing B-cell responses at the intestinal frontier. *Immunological Reviews* 271/1, 230–245. DOI: 10.1111/imr.12400.

Rechav, Y. (1987) Resistance of Brahman and Hereford cattle to African ticks with reference to serum gamma globulin levels and blood composition. *Experimental & Applied Acarology* 3, 219. DOI: 10.1007/BF01270458.

Rechav, Y. and Kostrzewski, M.W. (1991) Relative resistance of six cattle breeds to the tick *Boophilus decoloratus* in South Africa. *Onderstepoort Journal of Veterinary Research* 58, 181–186.

Rechav, Y., Dauth, J. and Els, D.A. (1990) Resistance of Brahman and Simmentaler cattle to southern African ticks. *Onderstepoort Journal of Veterinary Research* 57, 7–12.

Renoux, G. (1978) Modulation of immunity by levamisole. *Pharmacology & Therapeutics. Part A: Chemotherapy, Toxicology and Metabolic Inhibitors* 2/2, 397–423. DOI: 10.1016/0362-5478(78)90024-4.

Renoux, G. (1980) The general immunopharmacology of levamisole. *Drugs* 20, 89–99. DOI: 10.2165/00003495-198020020-00001.

Ribatti, D. (2015) The Bursa of Fabricius. In: *The Development of Immunologic Competence*. Springer, Cham, pp. 13–23.

Riese, R.J. and Chapman, H.A. (2000) Cathepsins and compartmentalization in antigen presentation. *Current Opinion in Immunology* 12, 107–113.

Riese, R.J., Mitchell, R.N., Villadangos, J.A., Shi, G.P., Palmer, J.T. *et al.* (1998) Cathepsin S activity regulates antigen presentation and immunity. *Journal of Clinical Investigation* 101/1, 2351–2363.

Robbertse, L. (2018) Comparative immune-profiling of three cattle breeds infested with *Rhipicephalus microplus* and *Ixodes ricinus*-infested BALB/c mice. PhD thesis, University of Pretoria, Pretoria, South Africa.

Robbertse, L., Richards, S.A. and Maritz-Olivier, C. (2017) Bovine immune factors underlying tick resistance: Integration and future directions. *Frontiers in Cellular and Infection Microbiology* 7, 522. DOI: 10.3389/fcimb.2017.00522.

Robbertse, L., Richards, S.A., Clift, S.J., Barnard, A.C., Leisewitz, A. *et al.* (2018) Comparison of the differential regulation of T and B-lymphocyte subsets in the skin and lymph nodes amongst three cattle breeds as potential mediators of immune-resistance to *Rhipicephalus microplus*. *Ticks & Tick-Borne Diseases* 9/4, 976–987. DOI: 10.1016/j.ttbdis.2018.03.034.

Roberts, J.A. and Kerr, J.D. (1976) *Boophilus microplus*: Passive transfer of resistance in cattle. *Journal of Parasitology* 62/3, 485–489.

Rodriguez-Valle, M., Vance, M., Moolhuijzen, P., Tao, X. and Lew-Tabor, A.E. (2012) Differential recognition by tick-resistant cattle of the recombinantly expressed *Rhipicephalus microplus* serine protease inhibitor-3 (RMS-3). *Ticks & Tick-Borne Diseases* 3/3, 159–169. DOI: 10.1016/j.ttbdis.2012.03.002.

Rodriguez-Valle, M., Moolhuijzen, P., Piper, E.K., Weiss, O., Vance, M. *et al.* (2013) *Rhipicephalus microplus* lipocalins (LRMs): Genomic identification and analysis of the bovine immune response using in silico predicted B and T cell epitopes. *International Journal for Parasitology* 43/9, 739–752. DOI: 10.1016/j.ijpara.2013.04.005.

Ross, S.H. and Cantrell, D.A. (2018) Signaling and function of interleukin-2 in T lymphocytes. *Annual Review of Immunology* 36, 411–433. DOI: 10.1146/annurev-immunol-042617-053352.

Sajid, M.S., Iqbal, Z., Muhammad, G. and Iqbal, M.U. (2006) Immunomodulatory effect of various anti-parasitics: A review. *Parasitology* 132/3, 301–313. DOI: 10.1017/S0031182005009108.

Sarma, J.V. and Ward, P.A. (2011) The complement system. *Cell and Tissue Research* 343/1, 227–235. DOI: 10.1007/s00441-010-1034-0.

Schmidt, E.G. and Williams, C.B. (2013) Generation and function of induced regulatory T cells. *Frontiers in Immunology* 4, Article 152. DOI: 10.3389/fimmu.2013.00152.

Schroeder, H.W. and Cavacini, L. (2010) Structure and function of immunoglobulins. *Journal of Allergy and Clinical Immunology* 125/2 Suppl 2, S41–S52. DOI: 10.1016/j.jaci.2009.09.046.

Seder, R.A. and Ahmed, R. (2003) Similarities and differences in $CD4^+$ and $CD8^+$ effector and memory T cell generation. *Nature Immunology* 4/9, 835–842. DOI: 10.1038/ni969.

Shapiro, S.Z., Voigt, W.P. and Fujisaki, K. (1986) Tick antigens recognized by serum from a guinea pig resistant to infestation with the tick *Rhipicephalus appendiculatus*. *Journal of Parasitology* 72/1, 454–463.

Spellberg, B. and Edwards, J.E. (2001) Type 1/Type 2 immunity in infectious diseases. *Clinical Infectious Diseases* 32, 76–102.

Stampa, S. and Du Toit, R. (1958) Paralysis of stock due to the Karoo paralysis tick (*Ixodes rubicundus* Neu.). *South African Journal of Science* 241–246.

Stear, M.J., Nicholas, F.W., Brown, S.C. and Holroyd, R.G. (1989) Class I antigens of the bovine major histocompatibility system and resistance to the cattle tick (*Boophilus microplus*) assessed in 3 different seasons. *Veterinary Parasitology* 31, 303–315.

Stear, M.J., Hetzel, D.J.S., Brown, S.C., Gershwin, L.J., Mackinnon, M.J. *et al.* (1990) The relationships among ecto- and endoparasite levels, class I antigens of the bovine major histocompatibility system, immunoglobulin E levels and weight gain. *Veterinary Parasitology* 34, 303–321.

Steen, N.A., Barker, S.C. and Alewood, P.F. (2006) Proteins in the saliva of the Ixodida (ticks): Pharmacological features and biological significance. *Toxicon* 47/1, 1–20. DOI: 10.1016/j.toxicon.2005.09.010.

Suan, D., Sundling, C. and Brink, R. (2017) Plasma cell and memory B cell differentiation from the germinal center. *Current Opinion in Immunology* 45, 97–102.

Swain, S.L., McKinstry, K.K. and Strutt, T.M. (2012) Expanding roles for CD4+ T cells in immunity to viruses. *Nature Reviews Immunology* 12, 136–148. DOI: 10.1038/nri3152.

Tabor, A.E., Ali, A., Rehman, G., Rocha Garcia, G., Zangirolamo, A.F. *et al.* (2017) Cattle tick *Rhipicephalus microplus*–host interface: A review of resistant and susceptible host responses. *Frontiers in Cellular and Infection Microbiology* 7, 506. DOI: 10.3389/fcimb.2017.00506.

Trager, W. (1939a) Acquired immunity to ticks. *Journal of Parasitology* 25/1, 57–81.

Trager, W. (1939b) Further observations on acquired immunity to the tick *Dermacentor variabilis* Say. *Journal of Parasitology* 25/2, 137–139.

Trager, W. (1940) A note on the problem of acquired immunity to argasid ticks. *Journal of Parasitology* 26/1, 71–74.

Tubo, N.J. and Jenkins, M.K. (2014) CD4+ T-cells: Guardians of the phagosome. *Clinical Microbiology Reviews* 27/2, 200–213. DOI: 10.1128/CMR.00097-13.

Turk, V., Turk, B., Gunčar, G., Turk, D. and Kos, J. (2002) Lysosomal cathepsins: Structure, role in antigen processing and presentation, and cancer. *Advances in Enzyme Regulation* 42, 285–303.

Turk, V., Stoka, V., Vasiljeva, O., Renko, M., Sun, T. *et al.* (2012) Cysteine cathepsins: From structure, function and regulation to new frontiers. *Biochimica et Biophysica Acta* 1824/1, 68–88. DOI: 10.1016/j.bbapap.2011.10.002.

Turni, C., Lee, R.P. and Jackson, L.A. (2004) A comparison of the immunosuppressive effects of salivary gland extracts from two laboratory strains of *Boophilus microplus*. *International Journal for Parasitology* 34, 833–838. DOI: 10.1016/j.ijpara.2004.03.002.

Turni, C., Lee, R.P. and Jackson, L.A. (2007) The effects of salivary gland extracts from *Boophilus microplus* ticks on mitogen-stimulated bovine lymphocytes. *Veterinary Research Communications* 31, 545–552. DOI: 10.1007/s11259-007-3461-2.

Utech, K.B.W., Seifert, G.W. and Wharton, R.H. (1978a) Breeding Australian Illawarra Shorthorn cattle for resistance to *Boophilus microplus*, I. Factors affecting resistance. *Australian Journal of Agricultural Research* 29/2, 411–422. DOI: 10.1071/AR9780411.

Utech, K.B.W., Wharton, R.H. and Kerr, J.D. (1978b) Resistance to *Boophilus microplus* (Canestrini) in different breeds of cattle. *Australian Journal of Agricultural Research* 29, 885–895.

Van Oosterwijk, J.G. and Wikel, S.K. (2021) Resistance to ticks and the path to anti-tick and transmission blocking vaccines. *Vaccines* 9, 725. DOI: 10.3390/vaccines9070725.

Wagland, B.M. (1975) Host resistance to cattle tick (*Boophilus microplus*) in Brahman (*Bos indicus*) cattle. I. Responses of previously exposed cattle to four infestations with 20,000 larvae. *Australian Journal of Agricultural Research* 26/6, 1073–1080. DOI: 10.1071/AR9751073.

Wagland, B.M. (1978) Host resistance to cattle tick (*Boophilus microplus*) in Brahman (*Bos indicus*) cattle. II. The dynamics of resistance in previously unexposed and exposed cattle. *Australian Journal of Agricultural Research* 29, 395–400. DOI: 10.1071/AR9780395.

Wagland, B.M. (1979) Host resistance to cattle tick (*Boophilus microplus*) in Brahman (*Bos indicus*) cattle. IV. Ages of ticks rejected. *Australian Journal of Agricultural Research* 30, 211–218. DOI: 10.1071/AR9790211.

Wagland, B.M., Sutherst, R.W. and Roberts, J.A. (1985) Relationship between the resistance of cattle to *Haemaphysalis longicornis* and to *Boophilus microplus*. *Australian Veterinary Journal* 62/9, 308–310.

Wang, H. and Nuttall, P.A. (1994) Excretion of host immunoglobulin in tick saliva and detection of IgG-binding proteins in tick haemolymph and salivary glands. *Parasitology* 109/4, 525–530. DOI: 10.1017/S0031182000080781.

Wikel, S.K. (1999) Tick modulation of host immunity: An important factor in pathogen transmission. *International Journal for Parasitology* 29/6, 851–859. DOI: 10.1016/S0020-7519(99)00042-9.

Willadsen, P. (1976) Allergenic activity of an esterase from *Boophilus microplus*. *FEBS Letters* 72/2, 346–349.

Willadsen, P. and McKenna, R.V. (1983) Binding of antigens to tissues: The example of *Boophilus microplus* and bovine skin. *International Journal for Parasitology* 13/6, 593–598.

Willadsen, P. and Williams, P.G. (1976) Isolation and partial characterization of an antigen from the cattle tick, *Boophilus microplus*. *Immunochemistry* 13, 591–597. DOI: 10.1016/0019-2791(76)90171-3.

Willadsen, P., Williams, P.G., Roberts, J.A. and Kerr, J.D. (1978) Responses of cattle to allergens from *Boophilus microplus*. *International Journal for Parasitology* 8, 89–95.

Willadsen, P., McKenna, R.V. and Riding, G.A. (1988) Isolation from the cattle tick, *Boophilus microplus*, of antigenic material capable of eliciting a protective immunological response in the bovine host. *International Journal for Parasitology* 18/2, 183–189. DOI: 10.1016/0020-7519(88)90059-8.

Williams, A.F. and Barclay, A.N. (1988) The immunoglobulin superfamily-domains for cell surface recognition. *Annual Review of Immunology* 6, 381–405.

Yan, X., Wu, C., Chen, T., Santos, M.M., Liu, C.L. *et al.* (2017) Cathepsin S inhibition changes regulatory T-cell activity in regulating bladder cancer and immune cell proliferation and apoptosis. *Molecular Immunology* 82, 66–74. DOI: 10.1016/j.molimm.2016.12.018.

Zavašnik-Bergant, T., Vidmar, R., Sekirnik, A., Fonović, M., Salát, J. *et al.* (2017) Salivary tick cystatin OmC2 targets lysosomal cathepsins S and C in human dendritic cells. *Frontiers in Cellular and Infection Microbiology* 7, 288. DOI: 10.3389/fcimb.2017.00288.

Zhang, N. and Bevan, M.J. (2011) $CD8^+$ T cells: Foot soldiers of the immune system. *Immunity* 35, 161–168. DOI: 10.1016/j.immuni.2011.07.010.

Zinkernagel, R.M. and Doherty, P.C. (1977) The concept that surveillance of self is mediated via the same set of genes that determines recognition of allogenic cells. *Cold Spring Harbor Symposia on Quantitative Biology* 41, 505–510. DOI: 10.1101/SQB.1977.041.01.058.

5 Adaptive Immunity Elicited by Vaccination

Abstract

Vaccination can induce an adaptive immunity to ticks. Depending on the chosen antigen or antigen combination, this immunity can interfere with tick feeding, survival, reproduction and/or pathogen transmission. Various techniques have been used to select from a rich source of candidate subunit antigens in tick secretions, and in structural and functional proteins. Coevolution of ticks and their hosts means that ticks can avoid or neutralize many of the natural immune mechanisms they encounter. Having to empirically test the protective immunogenic efficacy of candidate vaccines, and comparing antigens with each other, has uncovered a new field of scientific endeavour. Formulating the antigen(s) in a vaccine that will optimize the degree and duration of protection presents additional challenges.

Vaccination is a cornerstone of health management, due to its low cost, proven efficacy, duration of effect, safety profile and ease of delivery (Meeusen *et al.*, 2013). Research into immunological control of ticks follows two main approaches – investigating the antigens eliciting the complex physiological and immunological reactions to tick infestation, and the effects of immune reactions that do not occur as a result of natural infestation (Willadsen and Jongejan, 1999). Tick bites elicit both innate (cutaneous basophil hypersensitivity, leucocyte infiltration) and adaptive (T- and B-lymphocytes, plasma cell, macrophage and DC involvement) immune responses, with an important role ascribed to cell-mediated immunity. It is desirable to develop vaccines with the broadest possible application (Trimnell *et al.*, 2005).

Translational biotechnology over the past three decades has uncovered many tick–host–pathogen interactions at the molecular level and offers the promise of several avenues towards better tick control, with engagement of the immune system a major player (de la Fuente, 2021).

The objective of vaccinating against ticks is worth considering. The reviewed literature investigates many antigens that will elicit a protective immune response which interferes with tick physiology, ultimately leading to the demise of the tick. It requires ticks to ingest host antibodies raised against internal antigenic epitopes (hidden or concealed antigens: shifting the 'battlefield' into the tick). There is the alternative paradigm of immunizing the host against the harmful secreted components of tick saliva, including the pathogens they may transmit (waging the 'battle' inside the host). In the latter case, interfering with the tick's vector competence will most probably again require an ingested immunoglobulin (Merino *et al.*, 2013a). A vaccine containing a mixture of antigens seems to offer the promise of achieving both these goals and against multiple tick species, to broaden its global appeal (Parthasarathi *et al.*, 2021).

It is also vitally important not to forget that resistance to ticks has many effector mechanisms, of which the innate and adaptive immune response is one (Jonsson *et al.*, 2014). In addition to using a vaccine to reduce reliance on chemical acaricides, integrated tick management will include efforts to select for and breed tick-resistant cattle, using additional resources such as genomic and proteomic profiling (see sections 2.3 and 4.4.2, this volume).

DOI: 10.1079/9781800625761.0005

5.1 Early Successes

5.1.1 Protozoa and helminths

The concept of eliciting adaptive immunity to parasites is not new. Immunizing livestock against parasites was first achieved in the case of *Eimeria* spp. in chickens (Chapman, 2014). Irradiated third-stage larvae of lungworm (*Dictyocaulus* spp.) have been used for a long time to immunize cattle and sheep against husk (Cornwell, 1961; Benitez-Usher, 1975; Benitez-Usher *et al.*, 1976). Protozoa of the genus *Babesia* are still being attenuated by serial passage before being used to immunize cattle, with or without chemical intervention against any possible adverse vaccine reaction (de Vos and Jorgensen, 1992). The infect-and-treat method (ITM) achieves immunity in cattle against East Coast fever and tropical theileriosis, without attempting to attenuate the parasites (Irvin, 1985). A live attenuated isolate of *Toxoplasma gondii* is available as a commercial vaccine in New Zealand (Kelly, 2018). Although a protective immunogenic replica could not be expressed by recombinant technology, a gut antigen of the gastrointestinal helminth *Haemonchus contortus* was isolated and a vaccine successfully commercialized (Smith, 1993; Smith and Smith, 1993; Smith *et al.*, 1994, 2001).

Technological advances enabling the recombinant expression of gene products and precision fermentation have led to rapid advances in the development of vaccines with subunit antigens against infectious disease, but less so in the case of helminth, protozoal and arthropod parasites.

5.1.2 Ticks

Immunizing guinea pigs and cattle in Canada with antigens extracted from the gut and other internal organs of partially fed ticks, collected before they had completed their bloodmeal (Allen and Humphreys, 1979), followed soon after by reports of immunizing rats against *D. variabilis* with tick midgut extracts (Ackerman *et al.*, 1980), opened the door to a revolution in tick control of livestock.

In preparation for further work, a sequential histological examination traced the development and function of gut cells in pharate (unmoulted) and feeding nymphs and adult female [*B. microplus*] *R. australis*. Stem cells develop into secretory and digest cells, the former containing glycoprotein granules and the latter packed with endosomes filled with ingested host cells and fluid (Agbede and Kemp, 1985). This was followed by an ultrastructural study to confirm the identity of the secretory cell types identified earlier, their origin and the formation of their granules (Agbede and Kemp, 1987).

Engorged female ticks were collected 18–20 days after larval infestation, suspended in buffered saline and disrupted in a blender before the suspension was filtered to remove the tick cuticles and centrifuged. In a series of three experiments, centrifuge supernatant and pellet material were used singly or combined, with Freund's complete adjuvant, to vaccinate Hereford (European) and Droughtmaster (composite Zebu) cattle by various regimes. Vaccinated cattle were exposed to induced infestations with varying numbers of [*B. microplus*] *R. australis* larvae. The effect of vaccination was evaluated by indirect radioimmunoassay and gel diffusion of antibody levels, histopathology of tick gut mucosae, numbers of ticks engorging and laying eggs, and visible signs of damage (Fig. 5.1). The histological lesions had not previously been seen in ticks from cattle with naturally acquired resistance. Antibody titres in individual cattle were not correlated with their immunity. Tick survival, engorgement and ovipositioning were compromised to varying degrees. Larvae feeding on vaccinated cattle were largely unaffected (Agbede and Kemp, 1986; Johnston *et al.*, 1986; Kemp *et al.*, 1986).

A different approach was taken with the dissection of synganglia and midguts from semi-engorged [*B. microplus*] *R. australis* removed from cattle and processing these to yield three fractions. Vaccines were prepared by emulsifying soluble gut antigens in Freund's incomplete adjuvant, suspending particulate gut antigens in saponin or suspending disrupted synganglion cells in Freund's incomplete adjuvant. Hereford cattle were vaccinated three times in 6 weeks and challenged with larval infestations 8, 9 and 10 weeks later. Vaccinated cattle dropped fewer engorged ticks that weighed less and laid fewer eggs than those from unvaccinated animals. The

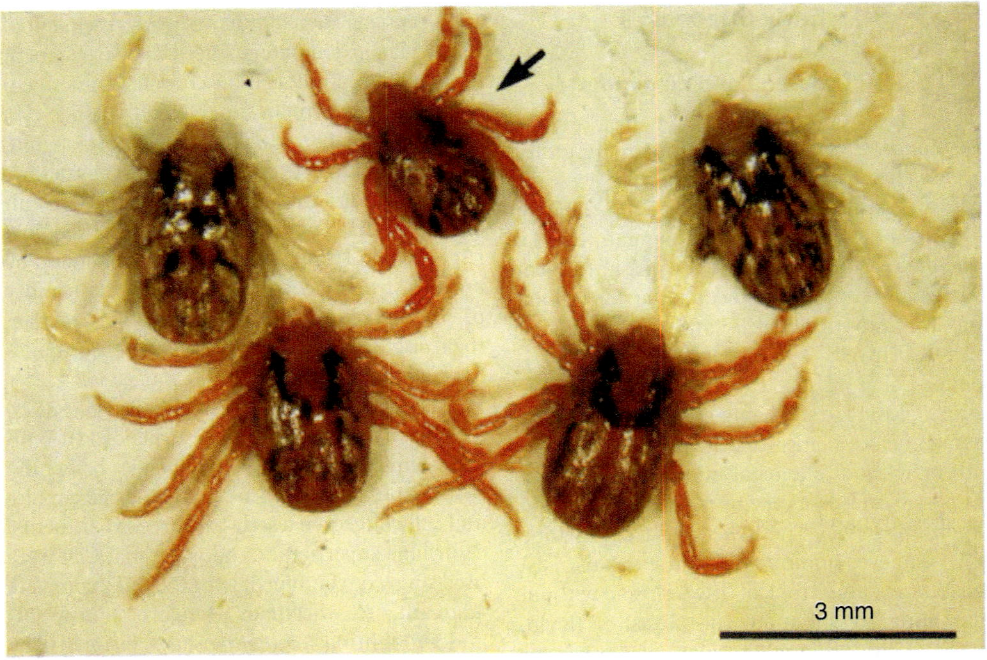

Fig. 5.1. Evidence of damage to gut epithelium in *R. microplus* adults feeding on vaccinated cattle, with host erythrocytes leaking into haemolymph causing red leg discolouration. From Kemp *et al.* (1986) with permission of Elsevier.

'gut vaccine' gave 87% protection, compared with 80% when a gut–synganglion combination was given. A synganglion-alone vaccination did not provide protection. Antibody titres were demonstrated by ELISA (Opdebeeck *et al.*, 1988).

Differing from naturally acquired immunity directed largely at tick larvae, vaccination with antigens extracted from adult [*B. microplus*] *R. australis* results in direct damage to the adult tick, decreasing replete weight and affecting egg laying. Numerous purification steps were required for final identification of the antigen(s) responsible for inducing the immunity (Willadsen *et al.*, 1988).

Salivary gland extracts of *H. a. anatolicum* were used to vaccinate European/Zebu cross-bred cattle twice, 2 weeks apart, prior to challenging them with unfed adult ticks. Whole extract (as opposed to centrifugal sediment or supernatant) administered with Freund's complete adjuvant was most effective in reducing weight and egg production (Banerjee *et al.*, 1990), but no distinction was made between antigen(s) that may have been secreted or constitutional.

5.1.3 Bm86

The successful cloning in *E. coli* of a cDNA encoding for a tick gut epithelium surface glycoprotein was a landmark achievement. The responsible tick gut antigen was designated Bm86. It is present in very low abundance in extracts of partially engorged adult female ticks and has an affinity for wheat germ lectin. Microgram amounts of this antigen were shown to induce effective protection in cattle against [*B. microplus*] *R. australis*, as shown by the decreased survival of ticks on vaccinated cattle and a reduction in engorgement weight and severely impaired reproductive capability of the survivors. Antisera to the antigen react with the surface of digest cells in the tick gut, strongly and rapidly inhibiting their endocytotic activity, which is a critical step in bloodmeal digestion. A number of peptides from this antigen were sequenced and one was found to have homology with the epidermal growth factor (EGF) precursor and a second to be homologous with a putative protective antigen from *Plasmodium falciparum* (Willadsen and Kemp, 1988; Rand *et al.*, 1989; Willadsen *et al.*, 1989, 1992). Improvements and refinements followed, such as high yield expression by *Pichia pastoris* with improved immunogenicity (Rodríguez *et al.*, 1994).

Glycosylation is common in cell surface proteins such as on the surface of tick gut cells and protects against proteolysis. It would also be expected for some salivary proteins secreted at the tick attachment site. This explains why antibodies from animals infested with ticks will react with tick-derived Bm86 (through the carbohydrate epitopes) but not with recombinant Bm86 which only has the polypeptide epitope. The damage to the gut of [*B. microplus*] *R. australis* and the decrease in engorgement weight and egg production are much less in cattle with naturally acquired immunity than in vaccinated cattle (Willadsen and McKenna, 1991; Willadsen *et al.*, 1993a).

The recombinant Bm86 vaccine Gavac™ ('garapatas de vacca' – tick of the cow) was tested in dairy and beef cattle exposed to natural tick (this is assumed to be *R. microplus*, although it is not explicitly stated in the publication) infestations in Brazil. In a field study in Cuba, tick-naïve calves were vaccinated with Gavac, kept on natural pasture and challenged with an induced *R. microplus* larval infestation. In both cases, the antibody response was monitored by ELISA and efficacy by the numbers of engorged ticks, which were substantially reduced (Rodriguez *et al.*, 1995a, b).

Gavac was initially commercialized in Cuba, Colombia, Dominican Republic, Brazil and Mexico. In field trials, it was 55–100% effective in controlling infestations of [*B.*] *R. microplus* for 12–36 weeks (de La Fuente *et al.*, 1998, 1999). It led to an 82% reduction in the use of chemical acaricides in Cuba within 8 years, and a dramatic drop in the numbers of clinical cases of babesiosis (Valle *et al.*, 2004; de la Fuente *et al.*, 2007a). A similar reduction (83.7% within 2 years) in acaricide use was seen in Venezuela (Suarez *et al.*, 2016) but Gavac has been less successful commercially in Mexico, where cattle are concurrently infested with *Amblyomma cajennense* which is not affected by the vaccine (de la Fuente *et al.*, 2007a).

Marketed as TickGARD® (with the antigen expressed by *E. coli*) and later TickGARD®PLUS (expression by *Pichia pastoris*) (Tabor, 2021), Bm86 was not a commercial success in Australia for several reasons. Having to inject cattle more than once a year to maintain an effective antibody titre is impractical in northern Australia, where cattle face the greatest challenge from [*R. microplus*] *R. australis* but are routinely mustered only once a year.

Australian dairy cattle vaccinated with TickGARDPLUS in southern Queensland carried fewer ticks, with lower tick reproductive efficiency. The cows gained more weight than unvaccinated controls and had lower milk somatic cell counts (Jonsson *et al.*, 2000). On Friesian cattle immunized with two TickGARD injections and challenged with [*B.*] *Rhipicephalus annulatus* larvae in Israel, the ticks did not develop to nymphs and adults. Larvae derived from *Babesia bovis*-infected female ticks transmitted the infection to vaccinated cattle but nymphs from females infected with *Babesia bigemina* did not, supporting the observation that Bm86 does affect the larval stage of *R. annulatus* (Pipano *et al.*, 2003).

More than 30 years after its registration (de la Fuente, 2021), the commercial success of the Bm86 recombinant antigen against infestations of *R. microplus* has not yet been equalled, but its success is hampered by a narrow efficacy spectrum, genomic variation and limited duration of immunity (de la Fuente *et al.*, 2017).

Cattle vaccinated with Bm86 were exposed to induced infestations of [*B.*] *R. microplus* and *R. decoloratus* simultaneously and displayed 74 and 70% reduction in reproductive capacity, respectively. Induced infestations with *H. a. anatolicum*, *H. dromedarii*, *R. appendiculatus* and *A. variegatum* were affected in varying to non-significant extent (de Vos *et al.*, 2001). Bm86 confers partial protection against *Hyalomma* and *Rhipicephalus* spp. that are phylogenetically closely related but fails to protect against the phylogenetically more distant *Amblyomma* spp. (Almazán *et al.*, 2003). Camels and cattle were vaccinated with Bm86 and challenged with induced infestations of *H. dromedarii* and *A. cajennense*. The effect on the various assessment criteria for *H. dromedarii* nymphs and adults was variable, but no effect against *A. cajennense* was seen (Rodríguez-Valle *et al.*, 2012a).

This limited success has evidently not hampered the search for an improved solution, and a host of alternative antigens have been investigated (de la Fuente *et al.*, 2017). More is said below (see section 5.2.5) about Bm86 orthologues in other tick species. Table 5.1 lists some examples of subunit antigens investigated in vaccines against ticks.

5.2 Finding the Right Antigen

Ectoparasitic arthropods are large and complex, with genome sizes not unlike those of their hosts, and spend most of their lives outside or on the surface of their hosts. This poses a considerable challenge to vaccine development (Meeusen *et al.*, 2007). The tick genome is large (Jongejan *et al.*, 2007), with the genome of *R. microplus* estimated to be 7.1 gigabase pairs, more than twice the size of the human genome (Fogaça *et al.*, 2021), but it also contains significant amounts of repetitive DNA, potentially problematic for genome assembly. Whole-genome sequencing (WGS) relies on inbred colonies with minimal polymorphism, which is not available for many Acari. Evolutionary distance between ticks and insects may limit homology-based gene predictions (Van Zee *et al.*, 2007). Having access to an annotated tick genome has been valuable in the discovery of potential antigens (Bellgard *et al.*, 2012) but hampered by the fact that 60% of the (in this case, *R. microplus*) genome lacks similarity with sequences from other organisms, making transcriptomic analysis difficult. Cross-species microarray technology was used to identify genes shared by *R. microplus* and *R. decoloratus* (van Zyl *et al.*, 2015), both of which infest cattle in southern Africa and should ideally be controlled by the same vaccine.

Whether by chemical or immunogenic means, when tick management interventions are devised, the chosen gene function(s) target must be sufficiently conserved to ensure an acceptable species spectrum of susceptibility, but not so well conserved that anti-tick measures will have an unintended adverse effect on the host. Subolesin (see section 5.2.5) is an example of a gene conserved in arthropod parasites and vertebrate hosts, raising the potential for inducing autoimmune reactions. The expectation that the antibody response will be directed at non-self epitopes, thus reducing the risk to the vaccinated host, seems to have been validated (de la Fuente *et al.*, 2011).

The sources of identified antigen candidates for an anti-tick vaccine can be grouped as egg, salivary gland, midgut, Malpighian and cement associated (Abbas *et al.*, 2023).

Messenger RNA (mRNA) purified from salivary glands dissected from feeding female *A. variegatum* was used to make random cDNA clones, whose nucleotide sequences were analysed. Sequences that encode for protein components of tick cement, proteins that contribute to anticoagulant and anti-inflammatory responses, and potential immunosuppressive molecules were found. It was surmised that interference with the function of these proteins might disrupt the life cycle of *A. variegatum*, helping to control it and reduce its disease transmission capability (Nene *et al.*, 2002). Genes transcribed in the salivary glands of female *R. appendiculatus* infected with *Theileria parva* did not differ greatly from those expressed in uninfected ticks. The recognized genes coded for previously characterized tick salivary proteins, including an immunosuppressive protein (Nene *et al.*, 2004).

Because T-cell responses are important in immunity to parasites, T-cell epitope identification is an important first step in developing T-cell-directed vaccines. Mapping T-cell epitopes for BoLA MHC peptide ligands has been done with mathematical algorithms, offering an advantage in the development of T-cell-directed vaccines. T-cell epitopes can be used as vaccine components or can help with the selection of antigens for inclusion in a vaccine (De Groot *et al.*, 2003).

Twenty-two or more antigenic molecules have already been tested in trials for vaccinating cattle against *R. microplus*. Despite considerable interest in antigenic proteins in tick cement and saliva (Zhou *et al.*, 2006), concealed and dual antigens seem to predominate in vaccination experiments (Leal and Ferreira, 2021).

Characterizing the haemolymph proteome of *Hyalomma asiaticum* by liquid chromatography tandem mass spectrometry yielded 311 proteins. Thirteen of these were immunity related and included PRRs, signalling proteins and effectors. Serpins and other proteins that may participate in coagulation were also identified. These discoveries could facilitate the

Table 5.1. Examples of subunit tick antigens.

Protein	Function	Species	Author	Hidden?
Akirins; subolesin; Q38, Q41 chimeras	NF-κB gene expression, innate tick immunity	Conserved	de la Fuente *et al.*, 2011, 2013; Merino *et al.*, 2011; Carreón *et al.*, 2012; Naranjo *et al.*, 2013; Trentelman *et al.*, 2019; Contreras *et al.*, 2020; Lee *et al.*, 2020; Mendoza-Martinez *et al.*, 2021	Y
Aquaporin	Water channelling	*I. ricinus*	Campbell *et al.*, 2010	Y
ATAQ proteins?	Bloodmeal digestion	*R. microplus* *R. appendiculatus* *H. longicornis*	Nijhof *et al.*, 2010 Kiper, 2013 Adjou Moumouni *et al.*, 2023	Y
Bm86	Bloodmeal digestion	*R. microplus* *R. australis* *R. decoloratus*	Willadsen and McKenna, 1991; Willadsen *et al.*, 1993a; Rodriguez *et al.*, 1995a, b; de Vos *et al.*, 2001	Y
Bm86 orthologues		*R. annulatus* *H. a. anatolicum* *H. m. marginatum* *H. excavatum* *H. dromedarii* *I. scapularis*	Canales *et al.*, 2008; Azhahianambi *et al.*, 2009; Canales *et al.*, 2009a; Ben Said *et al.*, 2012a; Kočí *et al.*, 2021	Y
Bm91		*R. australis*	Jarmey *et al.*, 1995; Nijhof *et al.*, 2007	Y
Bm95		*R. microplus*	García-García *et al.*, 2000	Y
BmVDAC	Mitochondrial porin	*R. microplus*	Ortega-Sánchez *et al.*, 2020	Y
Calreticulin	Ca-binding, anticoagulant	*H. longicornis*	Zheng *et al.*, 2022; Parizi *et al.*, 2023	N
Cathepsin	Proteolytic processes	*R. microplus*	Leal *et al.*, 2006a	Y
Cement protein RH50	Attachment, feeding	*R. haemaphysaloides*	Zhou *et al.*, 2006	N
Cement protein 64P	Attachment, feeding	*R. appendiculatus*	Havlíková *et al.*, 2009; Saimo *et al.*, 2011	N
Cystatin	Blood digestion Immune modulation	*R. appendiculatus* *R. microplus* *I. scapularis* *O. moubata*	Rangel *et al.*, 2017; Lu *et al.*, 2020; Parizi *et al.*, 2020	
Ferritin 2	Fe metabolism	*I. ricinus* *R. microplus* *R. annulatus*	Hajdusek *et al.*, 2010	Y

Continued

Table 5.1. Continued

Protein	Function	Species	Author	Hidden?
GPCRs	Signal transduction	*R. microplus*	Brock *et al.*, 2019	Y
Lipocalin	Histamine binding	*I. persulcatus* *H. longicornis*	Mans *et al.*, 2003; Konnai *et al.*, 2011; Wang *et al.*, 2021; Pérez-Sánchez *et al.*, 2022	N
Metalloproteases	Anticoagulant	*R. microplus*	Ali *et al.*, 2015	N
Paramyosin	Immune modulation	*R. microplus* *H. longicornis*	Leal *et al.*, 2013; Wu *et al.*, 2021	Y
Ribosomal phosphoproteins	Protein synthesis	*R. microplus* *A. mixtum* *R. haemaphysaloides* *H. longicornis*	Rodríguez-Mallón *et al.*, 2012, 2015, 2020a, b	Y
Serpins	Anticoagulant	*A. americanum* *R. australis* *R. haemaphysaloides*	Rodriguez-Valle *et al.*, 2012b; Kim *et al.*, 2016a; Xu *et al.*, 2020	Y
Silk	Cement component	*R. microplus*	Zivkovic *et al.*, 2010a; Antunes *et al.*, 2014	N
TIM	Glycolysis	*H. longicornis*	Liang *et al.*, 2022	Y
TROSPA	Pathogen transmission	*R. microplus*	Merino *et al.*, 2013b	Y
Ubiquitin	Protein turnover	*I. scapularis* *A. americanum* *D. variabilis* *H. longicornis*	de la Fuente *et al.*, 2007b; Choy *et al.*, 2013; Bullard *et al.*, 2016b; McClure Carroll *et al.*, 2019; Wang *et al.*, 2020	Y

identification of new targets for control of tick-borne pathogens (Yuan *et al.*, 2022).

5.2.1 Immuno-screening

A cDNA library constructed from mRNA extracted from partially fed female *H. longicornis* was immuno-screened in rabbits. The cDNAs of two genes encoding salivary gland proteins were cloned and their expression sites determined by RT-PCR on dissected tick salivary glands and midguts. The recombinant version of one of the genes was expressed *in vitro* in *E. coli*. The feeding of immature and adult ticks feeding on rabbits vaccinated with the recombinant protein was impaired (Tsuda *et al.*, 2001).

Another cDNA expression library was constructed from an *I. scapularis* cell line initially derived from tick embryos. Mice were immunized with pools of the cDNA clones and challenged with *I. scapularis* larvae, in a process labelled expression library immunization (ELI). Clones in pools that induced immunity were sequenced and individual antigens identified. Interpreting the results of this work can be complicated. Failure to demonstrate an effect of immunization could be due to a cellular rather than a humoral effect (i.e. no antibodies transferred from bloodmeal to haemolymph). Or immunization could have unintended consequences, such as promotion of tick feeding because the expressed antigens encode for tick immunosuppressants or anticoagulants, for example. A protective antigen (4D8) from one of the cDNA subpools was later designated subolesin (see section 5.2.5) (Almazán *et al.*, 2003).

5.2.2 Reverse vaccinology (RV)

This process, aimed at producing an immunogenic recombinant subunit antigen, starts with an annotated map of the organism's genome sequence, working backwards to find proteins essential for the organism's function and survival, determining their molecular structure and site(s) of expression *in silico*, cloning these genes and expressing them in a suitable system, testing the immunity they elicit, and its utility as a protective mechanism (Goodswen *et al.*, 2012). The *in silico* process of selection can be refined by using machine learning algorithms to reduce the number of false candidates (Goodswen *et al.*, 2013) and by using predicted scores for peptide-MHC molecule binding to T-cell receptors (Goodswen *et al.*, 2014a) and can be accelerated by automation (Goodswen *et al.*, 2014b). The probability of failure is high because protective immunity will clearly only be elicited by antigenic proteins which are accessible to the vaccinated animal's immune response.

Reverse vaccinology cannot replace experimental work, but computationally helps to narrow down the candidates by attempting to predict, from a sequence of letters, whether the three-dimensional (3D) protein they encode for will induce the memory helper T- and B-cells needed in a protective immune response. RV has become a reality thanks to an exponential increase in the amount of publicly available molecular biological data, and an exponential increase in computer processing, data storage and communication, among others (Goodswen *et al.*, 2023).

Effective vaccines have been produced by the RV approach against a number of infectious diseases, but multicellular parasites such as ticks present the obstacles of genome size and complexity, antigenic variability and probably the need for more than just a humoral immune response (Meeusen *et al.*, 2007; Lew-Tabor and Rodriguez-Valle, 2016; Bhakta *et al.*, 2022).

The tick vaccine project in the adaptation and cattle welfare programme of the Australian Cooperative Research Centre for Beef Genetic Technologies (Beef CRC3) ran from 2005 to 2012. By means of RV, it identified approximately 20 vaccine candidates (short peptides representing 'non-concealed' B-cell epitopes). Twelve of these were tested in a series of efficacy trials against induced tick infestations in Australia (*R. australis*) and Brazil (*R. microplus*). To compensate for the low immunogenicity of the short peptides, initial vaccine booster doses were formulated with Freund's complete adjuvant, and the second booster with Freund's incomplete adjuvant. Three antigens achieved efficacies of 63–66% when administered singly, but mixing of the peptides resulted in lower efficacy rather than the anticipated additive/cumulative, or possibly synergistic, effect (Tabor *et al.*, 2017).

5.2.3 Gene silencing and editing

In the absence of an annotated tick genome, an alternative approach to RV for establishing the importance of a gene or its expression product for tick survival, and thus its potential as a vaccine antigen, was to either silence the gene by a process called RNA interference (RNAi) (Lew-Tabor *et al.*, 2011; de la Fuente and Kocan, 2022) or to remove the gene from the tick's genome by so-called gene editing, or CRISPR/Cas-9.

Clustered regularly interspersed short palindromic repeats (CRISPR) and their associated protein genes serve as a prokaryotic adaptive immune system providing protection against foreign DNA, such as from bacteriophages. They function by incorporating short DNA spacers, homologous to the invading DNA sequences, into a CRISPR array that is then transcribed to interfere with the phage replication. Genetic manipulation of CRISPR arrays has enabled their use as targeted genome editing tools (Hynes *et al.*, 2014).

First described for use in ticks in 2002, RNAi involves the introduction of double-stranded RNA (dsRNA) into the organism by various means. Tick salivary glands have been incubated with dsRNA to demonstrate disruption of gene transcription *in vitro* or dsRNA injected into whole female *A. americanum* to affect their feeding pattern *in vivo* (Aljamali *et al.*, 2002). The first report of RNAi in the single host [*B.*] *R. microplus* described the injection of dsRNA into engorged females and the consequent silencing of Bm86, Bm91 and subolesin genes in eggs and larvae (Nijhof *et al.*, 2007). Unless care is taken with the size of the dsRNA, off-target effects may occur. Smaller dsRNA fragments reduce the risk of off-target effects (Lew-Tabor *et al.*, 2011).

Recombinant dsRNA was injected into ticks to investigate their feeding mechanism and the importance of tick cement (Hollmann *et al.*, 2018). Ubiquitin and Bm86 dsRNA were fed to individual ticks in various combinations of whole blood and serum and the knockdown confirmed by the quantitative reverse transcription polymerase chain reaction (qRT-PCR) (Lew-Tabor *et al.*, 2014).

5.2.4 Secreted and excreted antigens

Immunological control of ticks requires a vaccine antigen not normally involved in host responses to infestation. Salivary gland-derived molecules introduced to the host during tick engorgement are not the ideal antigens for an optimal immunization strategy. The induction of an intense host skin reaction to tick feeding is to be avoided (Wikel, 1988). Coevolution over millennia has led to ticks developing various mechanisms for avoiding and modulating the host immune response (see sections 3.4 and 4.6, this volume).

Despite this intuitively logical argument, the development of a vaccine targeting tick saliva components became the focus of much tick vaccine development research (Zhou *et al.*, 2006). Perceived benefits of exposed over concealed antigens lay in their expected greater spectrum of efficacy (species and stages, due to greater conservation), longer lasting immunity (repeated boosting from natural infestation) and deterrent action against tick attachment (thus also reducing pathogen transmission) (Nuttall *et al.*, 2006). The express objective of the Beef CRC3 was to identify antigens that were not concealed (Tabor *et al.*, 2017). Many attempts at immunizing against ticks using secreted and excreted tick antigens have been described and have met with varying degrees of success.

Tick saliva contains hundreds of proteins, depending on tick species, developmental stage, feeding stage and host. Because these proteins facilitate successful tick attachment and engorgement, potentially disabling them with a host immune reaction makes them an attractive port of call in the search for novel antigens. Some of them have been shown to be immunologically more antigenic, inducing a robust protective tick immunity (Černý *et al.*, 2020). Salivary glands in adult ticks have three (females) or four (males) types of acini to secrete this variety of molecules (Havlíková *et al.*, 2009). A vaccine against tick salivary proteins can interfere with tick attachment or pathogen transmission (Bhowmick and Han, 2020).

The composition of tick saliva has been investigated through analysis of salivary gland transcriptomes which revealed more than 1000 polypeptides for hard ticks. But there is a discrepancy between this number of coding sequences and the number that can be inferred from the genome sequences of *R. zambeziensis* and *I. scapularis* for lipocalins and metalloproteases. These discrepancies can be blamed on different technologies and analytical methods, differences in expression rates between strains of the same species or elevated mutation rates in highly expressed protein families (Guizzo *et al.*, 2023). Soft ticks may secrete up to 200 different proteins, belonging to different protein families, during the feeding process (Cheng, 2010). Using urea and sodium dodecyl sulfate extraction, 654 proteins were found just in the attachment cement of *R. microplus*, a metastriate hard tick of the Brevirostrata (short mouthparts) (Villar *et al.*, 2020).

Choosing the right protein(s) in tick saliva to incorporate into a vaccine is further complicated by the fact that the composition of tick saliva changes in the course of the tick's sojourn on the host (Bullard *et al.*, 2016b; Kim *et al.*, 2016b; Abbas *et al.*, 2023). The immune response to an individual salivary antigen probably has a limited window of opportunity within which to exert its effect and a high degree of redundancy probably means that the effect on the secreting tick might be minimal (Antunes and Domingos, 2023).

Comparing the salivary gland transcriptomes of *R. microplus* fed on tick-susceptible (Holstein) and -resistant (Nelore) hosts revealed

137 differentially expressed genes. Proteins expressed by upregulated genes in ticks from susceptible cattle were involved in the stress response mechanism during feeding. Ticks fed on susceptible cattle expressed a molecule with a sequence similar to that of a small heat shock protein (HSP) cloned from the salivary glands of *R. annulatus* and shown to have a strong immunogenic effect in rabbits. Increased expression of HSPs during feeding indicates that they may be required to stabilize tick proteins during ingestion of warm blood. They have also been found to play a role in fibrinogenolysis during feeding. This study was expected to shed new light on possible vaccine targets (Giachetto *et al.*, 2020).

Proteomic characterization demonstrated that the composition of tick saliva differs from that of tick cement in *Ixodes scapularis*, with vitellogenin-like lipoproteins the most abundant proteins in cement. Partially engorged ticks were removed from rabbits and the cement material adhering to the hypostomes manually removed and cleansed prior to freezing. The material was not washed and assumed to be contaminated with some non-cement saliva. Saliva was collected from replete detached ticks by stimulation with pilocarpine (Lynn *et al.*, 2022). This may necessitate a reassessment of earlier work examining tick salivary gland secretions.

Tick cement

Because they are essential for tick attachment and feeding, the protein components of the cement from metastriate ixodid ticks, assumed to have short hypostomes, seem to be logical candidates for vaccination against tick infestation. The cDNA encoding one such protein in the *e* cell granules of type III salivary gland acini of *R. appendiculatus* was cloned. The recombinant protein, expressed by *E. coli*, reacted with sera from cattle infested with *R. appendiculatus*. This work stopped short of attempting to demonstrate protective immunity in vaccinated host animals (Bishop *et al.*, 2002).

Even though *Ixodes* spp. are prostriate ticks with long hypostomes, considered not to need cement for attachment (Francischetti *et al.*, 2009; Hall-Mendelin *et al.*, 2011), guinea pigs were immunized with cement extract from *I. scapularis*, causing premature tick detachment and up to 41% reduction in engorged tick weights (Lynn *et al.*, 2022). This might be similar to the decline in tick infestation seen in response to naturally acquired adaptive immunity (see Chapter 4, this volume).

Cement consists of many carbohydrate components and interacting proteins. Purified extracts of cement proteins are immunogenic and immunoprotective. Cement protein 64P was identified on its amino acid composition and shown to have close compositional similarity to mammalian skin keratin and collagen, most likely to avoid rejection by the host's immune system during tick feeding. Sera from guinea pigs with naturally acquired adaptive immunity to *R. appendiculatus* did not react with the protein. It was shown by *in situ* hybridization to be expressed in the salivary gland of *R. appendiculatus* females at the beginning of feeding, but not in unfed females, and waned as feeding progressed to engorgement. Female ticks expressed 64P mRNA in type II and III acini (Havlíková *et al.*, 2009). As many as 160 proteins were identified in tick cement cones recovered from the mouthparts of manually detached *A. americanum*. These were classified as protease inhibitors (serpin, Kunitz serpins), lipocalins, storage (ferritin, vitellogenin, calmodulin), detoxification and housekeeping proteins (Hollmann *et al.*, 2018). Some proteins found in tick cement might actually not be actively secreted but contaminants from sloughed salivary gland cells (Zhou *et al.*, 2006).

Tick recombinant protein 64 (Trp64) from *R. appendiculatus* cement, expressed in *E. coli*, in vaccine form has been shown to elicit an immune response that affects both exposed and hidden tick antigens, and in more than one tick species. Antisera from vaccinated guinea pigs cross-reacted with cement cone extract, salivary glands, haemolymph and midgut of *R. sanguineus* nymphs. Gel electrophoresis results also demonstrated cross-reactivity with extracts from *I. ricinus*, *A. variegatum* and [*B.*] *R. microplus* (Trimnell *et al.*, 2005). This is in contrast with attempts to immunize rabbits with *R. appendiculatus* Trp64 expressed by baculovirus in insect cells against induced infestation with larvae, nymphs and adults. There was no effect against immature ticks and the effect on adult tick mortality and engorged weight was not statistically significant (Saimo *et al.*, 2011).

The salivary gland cDNA libraries from Brevirostrata ticks contained more sequences of glycine-rich proteins similar to silks of true spiders than those from Longirostrata ticks (Maruyama *et al.*, 2010). Very long glycine-rich proteins, similar to spider silk proteins, found in metastriate (Brevirostrata) ticks may function as cement proteins (Francischetti *et al.*, 2011). The glycine-rich protein, similar to spider silk, found in the feeding cement cone was assumed to give the cone its strength and insolubility (Bullard *et al.*, 2016a).

The gene encoding for flagelliform silk protein (100Silk) was confirmed by real-time RT-PCR to be downregulated in tick salivary glands infected with *A. marginale*. Silencing of this gene resulted in reduced *A. marginale* infection in both tick salivary glands and cultured BME26 cells, making it a candidate for development of a vaccine (Zivkovic *et al.*, 2010a). Rabbit polyclonal antibodies against silk protein added to bovine blood fed by capillary tube to engorging female *R. microplus* reduced tick weight and egg production but had no effect on infection with *A. marginale* or *B. bigemina* if these were included in the blood (Antunes *et al.*, 2014).

Tick toxins

Tick toxins potentially contain proteins that lend themselves as antigens in vaccines. Monoclonal antibodies against the paralysis-inducing toxin of *R. e. evertsi* were shown by Western blot to also recognize similar toxins from *I. rubicundus* and *A. (P.) walkerae* and were demonstrated to protect chickens from *A. (P.) walkerae* paralysis. This raised the possibility of developing a vaccine against both spring lamb and Karoo paralysis, based on a recombinant antigen (Crause *et al.*, 1994).

Masina (1999) isolated the cDNA sequence of the HT-1 neurotoxin of *I. holocyclus*, successfully expressed the toxin as a maltose-binding fusion protein (MBP) in an *E. coli* host system, and attempted expression in a baculovirus system. The recombinant fusion protein partially protected mice against the native holocyclotoxin but was not protective in dogs challenged with live ticks. At that stage, the native neurotoxins HT-2 and HT-3 had not been characterized, nor their genes isolated, which was seen as a prerequisite if a vaccine against tick paralysis were to be developed (Masina and Broady, 1999). Subsequent investigations with monoclonal antibodies indicated that the MBP had been incorrectly folded, when compared with the native toxin. It was decided to use a ubiquitin fusion protein, which was smaller than the MBP. Despite having the correct folding conformation and being recognized by commercial dog anti-tick serum, it was found not to be protective in rabbits and mice (Chung, 2001).

Recent investigation of the *I. holocyclus* salivary gland and viscera transcriptome revealed 19 holocyclotoxin moieties (Rodriguez-Valle *et al.*, 2018). Eight of these were included in an experimental cocktail vaccine. Dogs vaccinated three times over a 9-week period were monitored for holocyclotoxin-specific IgG induction and when challenged with an unfed adult female *I. holocyclus* 2 weeks after the third vaccination, were shown to be protected from toxicosis (Rodriguez-Valle *et al.*, 2021).

Calreticulin

Calreticulins are calcium-binding proteins secreted in the saliva of several tick species, potentially interfering with platelet aggregation and the classical complement pathway of the innate immune response (see sections 3.4.1 and 3.4.2, this volume). They would seem to be potential vaccine antigen candidates, but recombinant *H. longicornis* CRT expressed by *E. coli* and administered to mice and rabbits failed to elicit a humoral response (measured by ELISA) or any effect on tick engorgement, moulting (nymphs to adults) or egg production (Zheng *et al.*, 2022). There is controversy regarding the utility of CRT as a biomarker for human tick bites, with different results obtained for *A. americanum* and *H. longicornis* recombinant CRT (Kim *et al.*, 2015a; Zheng *et al.*, 2022).

Lipocalins

Lipocalins are low molecular weight proteins secreted from tick salivary glands. They are best known for their anti-inflammatory effect by binding histamine (see section 3.4.3, this volume) and play important roles in blood feeding, immune response and reproduction (Paesen *et al.*, 2000). There are at least 14 lipocalin genes in *I. ricinus*. One of them

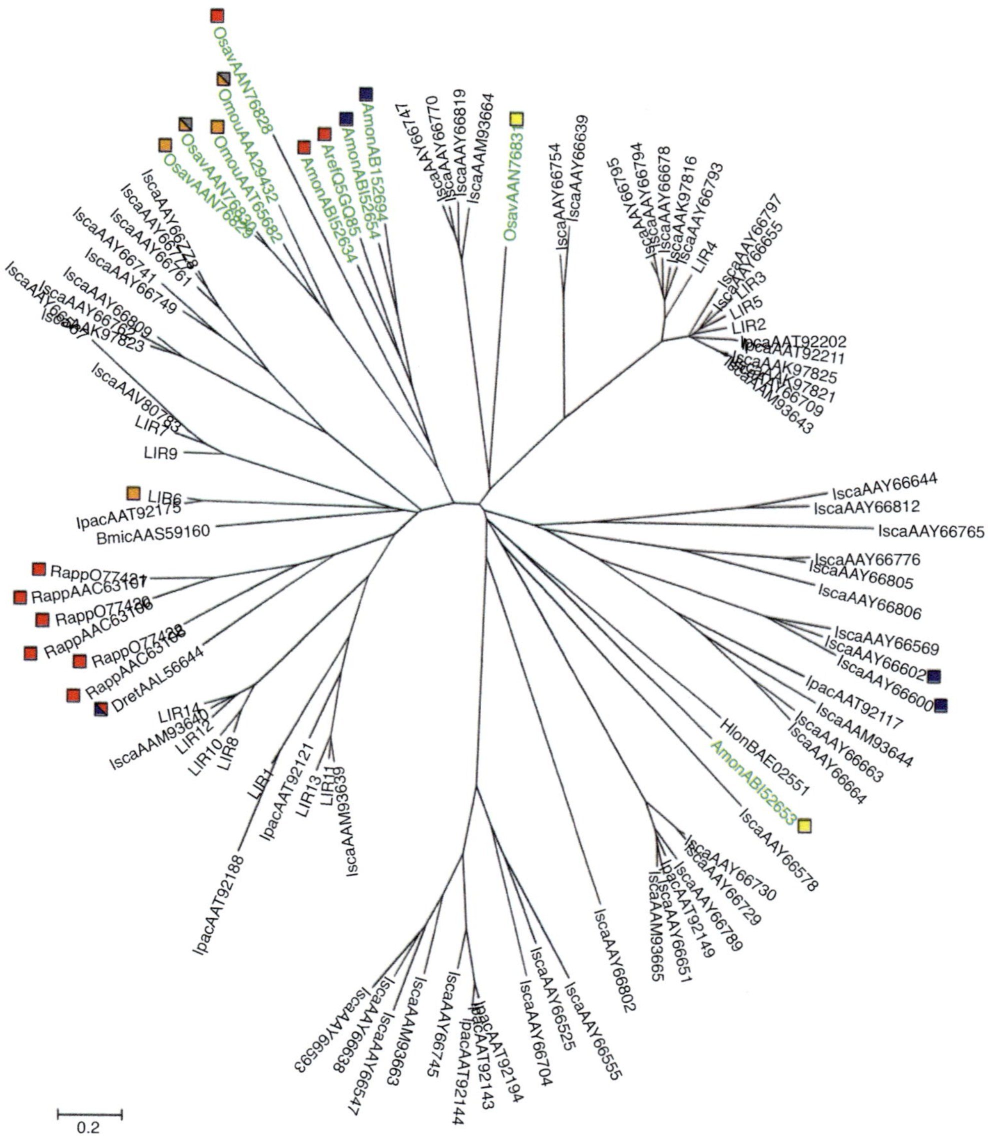

Fig. 5.2. A radial phylogenetic tree of the ixodid tick lipocalin superfamily. From Beaufays *et al.* (2008a) under the terms of the Creative Commons Attribution License.

specifically binds leukotriene B4, inhibiting neutrophil chemotaxis (Beaufays *et al.*, 2008b). Fig. 5.2 illustrates the phylogenetic relationships of tick lipocalins (Beaufays *et al.*, 2008a). They are sufficiently different from those of the rest of the lipocalin family to be considered as possible vaccine targets (Mans *et al.*, 2003).

Recombinant lipocalin from *I. persulcatus* expressed by *E. coli* was formulated with Freund's adjuvant (complete for the initial, incomplete for the booster injections) and used to vaccinate mice three times at 14-day intervals. Blood collected 7 days after the last injection contained antibodies to the recombinant lipocalin, demonstrated by Western blotting. Numbers of attaching and engorging nymphal ticks fed on immunized mice were not significantly different, but they took longer to reach engorgement and their replete weight was significantly reduced (Konnai *et al.*, 2011).

A lipocalin most abundantly expressed in the salivary gland of *H. longicornis* and with close sequence homology to *I. persulcatus* lipocalin was cloned and expressed by *E. coli* and used to immunize rabbits. This prolonged the bloodmeal and reduced replete weight, ovipositioning and egg hatchability of an induced subsequent tick infestation, amounting to 60.17% efficacy (Wang *et al.*, 2021).

Savicalin is a non-salivary lipocalin, first described in *O. savignyi* haemocytes, midgut and ovaries. Its functions are unclear but its expression relates to postfeeding events such as development, ecdysis or bacterial challenge (Cheng, 2010; Cheng *et al.*, 2010). Savicalin has since also been found in *Ornithodoros erraticus* saliva and mooted as a potential vaccine antigen (Pérez-Sánchez *et al.*, 2022).

Other tick salivary proteins

Tick saliva contains a pharmacopoeia of bioactive molecules aimed at modulating or suppressing the host's innate and adaptive immune response (see sections 3.4 and 4.6, this volume). The idea was mooted to target tick-derived immunosuppressants with an immune response, acknowledging that redundancy is probably also a feature of tick-mediated suppression of host immunity (Wikel, 1999). Analysis of the sialome of *R. pulchellus* revealed differences between the genders (Tan *et al.*, 2015), which might necessitate closer scrutiny of salivary proteins considered as vaccine antigens.

The gene encoding a glycine-rich 50 kDa protein, differentially expressed in the salivary glands of *Rhipicephalus haemaphysaloides*, was designated RH50, cloned, expressed in *E. coli* and used to immunize rabbits, which were subsequently challenged with induced infestations of nymphs and adult female ticks. The protein was also found in *R. haemaphysaloides* cement and surmised to be a membrane-bound matrix sloughing off from salivary gland cells and contaminating the tick saliva. The number of ticks attaching to immunized rabbits was markedly suppressed but mortality and feeding in those ticks that did attach were unaffected (Zhou *et al.*, 2006).

Tick-naïve calves were vaccinated four times at 15-day intervals with a recombinant *R. microplus* metalloprotease (BrRm-MP4), cloned from tick salivary glands and expressed in *E. coli*, before being challenged with an induced tick infestation. Antibodies elicited against BrRm-MP4 were confirmed by ELISA and overall protection calculated at 60% based on reductions in survival and engorgement (42.9%), fecundity (17.5%) and fertility (14.8%) (Ali *et al.*, 2015).

Proteins with α-Gal modifications (see section 1.3.4, this volume, meat allergy) may hold promise as protective antigens for prevention and treatment of anaphylactic reactions (de la Fuente *et al.*, 2017).

A vaccine cocktail of three histamine-binding proteins, two cement cone protein antigens and a subolesin homologue from *R. appendiculatus* was formulated in Montanide ISA 50 V adjuvant and used to vaccinate Friesian or Friesian/Ayrshire-cross calves. All the selected antigens had a published history of promise as potential anti-tick vaccine candidates. The calves' humoral response was monitored by indirect ELISA and the anti-tick effect evaluated by induced infestations with nymphs and adults. Despite demonstrable antibody titres to each of the antigens in the cocktail, no significant anti-tick effects were observed. A number of theories were advanced to explain the failure. Redundant salivary proteins from the challenge ticks may have circumvented the immune response. Antigenic competition was considered as unlikely, because of the natural complexity in the protein make-up of tick saliva. The wrong choice of adjuvant and protein expression system (*E. coli*) was raised as a possibility (Olds *et al.*, 2016).

Saliva collected from *I. scapularis* by pilocarpine stimulation was fractionated in an ion exchange column and each fraction separated by gel electrophoresis. The 15 fractions were grouped into five pools of three fractions each and used to immunize guinea pigs prior to induced infestation with *I. scapularis* nymphs. The fractions differed in their ability to elicit antibody production, as confirmed by ELISA, and in their effect on tick feeding, judging by nymphal tick engorgement and detachment. Antibody responses to the fractions were also different between guinea pigs vaccinated by injection and rabbits immunized by feeding ticks. Defining the subset of salivary proteins that might serve as vaccine targets will require refinement and further testing (Černý *et al.*, 2020).

Three salivary proteins from *A. sculptum*, possibly involved in haematophagy, expression of their mRNA detected in larvae, nymphs and adults, with expression levels increasing as feeding progressed, were cloned and expressed in recombinant form. All three recombinant proteins (rAsKunitz, rAs8.9kDa and rAsBasicTail) inhibited haemolysis and thrombin activity, whereas the latter two also inhibited the enzymatic activity of coagulation factor Xa and trypsin. Mice were immunized and shown to be protected against challenge by adult female ticks by 59.4% (rAsBasicTail) to more than 85% (rAsKunitz, rAs8.9 kDa). When challenged by nymphs, the efficacy was 70–100%. Thrombin inhibitors with Kunitz-like domains had previously been identified in *R. microplus*, *H. longicornis* and *I. scapularis* (Costa *et al.*, 2021).

5.2.5 Concealed ('hidden') antigens

Immunization against a hidden antigen requires a paradigm shift, because the engagement between the immune system and the pathogen no longer occurs inside the host. The product of the immune response is raised within the host but the battle is fought externally, inside the tick attached to the host's skin.

An immune response against a subunit internal ('concealed/hidden') antigen is something the tick will not have encountered before and would thus be less likely to withstand or circumvent. The tick can be damaged by the immune response if the host is first vaccinated. It might act synergistically with naturally acquired immunity (Willadsen, 1987; Willadsen *et al.*, 1993a).

Two hidden parasite antigens have thus far been commercialized – recombinant subunit Bm86 against ticks (TickGARD®, TickGARD®PLUS, Gavac; see section 5.1), and a gut antigen extracted and purified from the abomasal sheep nematode *Haemonchus contortus* (Barbervax®) (Smith, 1993; Smith and Smith, 1993; Smith *et al.*, 1994). They both require repeated administration to make up for the lack of 'boosting' by natural reinfestation.

One of the essential characteristics of a hidden antigen in a tick vaccine is its accessibility to host antibodies ingested during the bloodmeal. Immunoglobulins in ingested blood enter the tick's haemolymph and bind to internal organs, such as the ovary and salivary gland, without evidence of their degradation (Jasinskas *et al.*, 2000). The antigen also needs to be important in the tick's physiology, with limited functional redundancy or alternative pathways to achieving the same physiological outcome (Hope *et al.*, 2010). Failure of guinea pig immunization with *I. scapularis* midgut extract, the preparation of which is not described (Lynn *et al.*, 2022), may have been due to either or both these criteria not being met.

The location of the target of the vaccination plays a role in the selection of the ideal antigen for a tick vaccine. An antigen expressed closer to the tick's mouthparts will enable engagement with the host's immune response earlier in the bloodmeal, thus possibly thwarting not just tick infestation but potentially also the transmission of any tick-borne pathogen. Antigens further into the tick's digestive tract or in the internal organs will require ingestion of antibody-laden blood, by which time the tick may already have had the opportunity to secrete not only attachment cement but also saliva containing anticoagulant, anti-inflammatory and immunosuppressive molecules, toxin and possible viral, bacterial and/or protozoal pathogens.

This distinction was demonstrated by comparing the responses to tick infestation in mice immunized with either tick cement protein or midgut Bm86. The former evoked a delayed type of skin hypersensitivity response, interrupting tick feeding and preventing transmission of tick-borne encephalitis virus, whereas the latter affected tick survival but did not prevent virus transmission (Labuda *et al.*, 2006).

Two fractions of midgut protein, isolated from *A. variegatum* by detergent solubilization, were used to vaccinate rabbits and shown to reduce the reproductive capacity of a subsequently induced infestation by 48–77%. Gel electrophoresis and immunoblotting demonstrated the complexity of the antigens but more work was needed for their characterization (Kinyua *et al.*, 2002).

Different host responses to the same antigen were revealed when cattle and sheep were vaccinated with recombinant 5'-nucelotidase, a membrane-bound enzyme in the tick gut (Willadsen *et al.*, 1993b). When challenged with induced infestations of freshly moulted adult [*R. microplus*] *R. australis*, sheep with high antibody titres were protected. Cattle challenged with larvae showed no significant protection. Differences in antibody titre were found to be an unlikely reason for the discrepancy (Hope *et al.*, 2010). Despite scepticism about tick–host specificity (see section 1.2.4, this volume), sheep are not normally regarded as a preferred host for the single-host *Rhipicephalus* spp. (*R. australis*, *R. decoloratus*, *R. microplus*) (De Rose *et al.*, 1999) and may not have been the appropriate model in this instance. Inducing an infestation with freshly moulted adults of a single-host tick would involve removing them from the host on which they moulted and transferring them to a different host. This is also unconventional. Another reason for the discrepancy might be that adults (used to challenge vaccinated sheep) and larvae (cattle) might not be equally vulnerable to the antibodies that were raised.

Bm86 orthologues

Homologues are genes related by common descent. Orthologues are homologues derived from a single ancestral gene, and typically perform equivalent functions (Koonin, 2005).

Two Bm86 homologues in [*B.*] *R. decoloratus* were found to have 86% and 85% amino acid sequence identity with Bm86 and were designated Bd86-1 and −2, respectively. Native Bd86 protein in *R. decoloratus* midgut was shown by indirect immune-peroxidase staining to react strongly with sera from TickGARD-vaccinated cattle. When challenged with *R. decoloratus* larvae, the weight of engorged female ticks collected from these cattle was reduced by 55.6% and tick egg production by 61%. The vaccination had no effect on challenge infestation with adult female *R. appendiculatus* (Odongo *et al.*, 2007).

Variations in the efficacy of Bm86 vaccination against different isolates of *R. microplus* led to the notion of cloning and expression of Bm86 from local tick strains to eliminate geographic regional differences. Standardizing the expression system from *E. coli*, *Aspergillus nidulans* or *A. niger* to *P. pastoris* was also expected to improve the antigenicity and immunogenicity of the recombinant antigen. The genes encoding Bm86 (*R. microplus*), Ba86 (*R. annulatus*) and Bd86 (*R. decoloratus*) were cloned and expressed in *P. pastoris*. Rabbits were immunized with the recombinant proteins, using Montanide ISA 50 V as the adjuvant, and their sera evaluated by Western blot to demonstrate cross-reactivity between the three orthologues (Canales *et al.*, 2008).

In order to test the cross-reactivity between Bm86 and Ba86 previously demonstrated serologically, cattle were vaccinated with recombinant Ba86 or Bm86 from two different *R. microplus* strains. Ba86 vaccination reduced infestations of *R. annulatus* and *R. microplus* by 71% and 40%, respectively. The two Bm86 proteins were more effective than Ba86 against *R. annulatus* but varied in their efficacy against *R. microplus* (Canales *et al.*, 2009a).

A Bm86 orthologue was cloned from the eggs of laboratory-reared *H. a. anatolicum*, expressed as a fusion protein in *E. coli* and designated rHaa86. The recombinant protein was formulated with Montanide 888 in mineral oil and used to immunize tick-naïve calves three times, 30 days apart. The calves were challenged after another 37 days with unfed adult *H. a. anatolicum*. The calves' antibody titres were confirmed by ELISA and found to peak 124 days after the first vaccination. Vaccinated calves yielded 73.8% fewer engorged female ticks than controls (Azhahianambi *et al.*, 2009). Subsequent work demonstrated that vaccination with rHaa86 could serve as a component in integrated control of *H. a. anatolicum* and the *Theileria annulata* it transmits (Jeyabal *et al.*, 2010).

In the belief that the homologous form of Bm86 in each tick species will be better than heterologous cross-protection, homologues of Bm86 were isolated from *O. savignyi*, *A. variegatum*, *D. reticulatus*, *D. variabilis*, *Haemaphysalis elliptica*, *H. marginatum*, *I. ricinus* and *R. e. evertsi*. These were amplified, which led to the identification of a structurally related protein (see *ATAQ proteins* below) (Nijhof *et al.*, 2010).

Orthologues of the Bm86 gene were isolated from strains of *Hyalomma scupense* (syn. *H detritum*) isolated in Tunisia. The recombinant protein rHd86 from one strain was expressed in *P pastoris* and found to display 35 to 40% nucleotide sequence diversity from Bm86 and

Bm95 proteins. Homologue Hd86 proteins from different *H scupense* strains showed limited intra-specific diversity of 1.7%, indicating its suitability as a vaccine candidate against this tick species (Ben Said *et al.*, 2012a). Further investigation of Bm86 orthologues in *Hyalomma* spp. in Tunisia revealed 60–66% amino acid sequence agreement between Bm86 and Hm86, He86 and Hdr86 proteins from *H. m. marginatum*, *H. excavatum* and *H. dromedarii*, respectively. There was closer agreement with the sequence in the previously expressed Hd86 protein of 91%, 88% and 87%, respectively. This reaffirmed the indication that rHd86 will be a better vaccine candidate against *Hyalomma* spp. than Bm86 (Ben Said *et al.*, 2012b). Phylogenetically, the amino acid sequence variations in Bm86 orthologues from different *Hyalomma* spp. were seen as a tool to augment morphological species identification (Ben Said *et al.*, 2015).

Homologues of the Bm86 gene were found in *R. appendiculatus* and designated Ra86. Analysis of the sequences of different field populations and a laboratory strain indicated that they clustered into four major phylogenetic clades (Kamau *et al.*, 2016). This work did not investigate immunogenetic differences possibly attributable to the genetic variations.

Multiple orthologues of Bm86 with at least three identifiable epidermal growth factor (EGF)-like domains have been discovered in *Ixodes scapularis*. Although upregulated during *Borrelia burgdorferi* infection, RNAi knockdown of the Is86 genes did not seem to affect tick engorgement or *B. burgdorferi* persistence in mice. Immunization of mice with recombinant EGF antigens marginally reduced tick engorgement and skin spirochaete loads, but insufficiently for them to be considered as likely vaccine candidates (Koči *et al.*, 2021).

Bm95

The discovery of sequence variations in the Bm86 locus in *R. microplus* strains from Mexico, Argentina, Venezuela and Cuba and *R. australis* from Australia (García-García *et al.*, 1999) and the appearance of isolates of [*B.*] *R. microplus* that were less susceptible to Bm86 vaccination led to the isolation and cloning from an Argentinean strain of the tick a gene encoding an antigen designated Bm95 and expressing it in *P. pastoris* (García-García *et al.*, 2000). There was an inverse relationship between the efficacy of vaccination with Bm86 and sequence heterogeneity in the Bm86 locus. Diversity in the Bm86 amino acid sequence greater than 2.8% was calculated to confer resistance to vaccination (García-García *et al.*, 1999). Vaccination with Bm95 in Montanide 888 adjuvant protected cattle from infestation with *R. microplus* larvae of the Cuban Bm86-sensitive Camcord, and of the Argentinean Bm86-refractory isolate (García-García *et al.*, 2000).

Bm91

A glycosylated membrane protein was discovered in the salivary gland and gut of adult female [*B. microplus*] *R. australis* and designated Bm91. Partial amino acid sequence data for the protein show striking similarities to that of mammalian carboxydipeptidases or angiotensin-converting enzymes, suggesting that it may have an enzymatic function (Jarmey *et al.*, 1995). It was of relatively low abundance, with approximately 300–400 μg being recovered from 1 kg of semi-engorged adult female ticks. Absence of recognition by sera from cattle exposed to natural tick infestation indicated that this was another example of a concealed antigen (Riding *et al.*, 1994). Cattle were vaccinated either with Bm86 alone or in combination with Bm91 and challenged with [*B. microplus*] *R. australis*. The addition of the Bm91 antigen led to statistically significantly enhanced efficacy over that with Bm86 alone (Willadsen *et al.*, 1996). Knocking out the Bm91 gene by RNAi through injection of dsRNA into freshly moulted and engorged female *R. microplus* reduced gene transcription by 90% in both the unfed and replete female ticks, but had no effect on engorged tick weight, mortality, ovipositioning or egg hatchability (Nijhof *et al.*, 2007).

Ubiquitin

Ubiquitin contributes to several intracellular processes in addition to protein turnover, such as endocytosis, DNA repair, transcription and immunity. It is known to occur in arthropod disease vectors such as mosquitoes, lice and ticks. Among others, ubiquitination regulates the IMD pathway (see section 3.1.4, this volume) in *I. scapularis* (Choy *et al.*, 2013). Another function of ubiquitin is to be attached as a label to a protein destined for destruction in a proteasome, a discovery for which the Nobel Prize in Chemistry was awarded in 2004 (Anon., 2004). The 'ubiquitin machinery' is under the control of a collection of activating, conjugating and ligase enzymes. Ubiquitination involves ubiquitin-activating and -conjugating enzymes and a ubiquitin-protein ligase, and is countered by de-ubiquitinases removing ubiquitin from molecules (Choy *et al.*, 2013). Ubiquitin was identified as the most consistently expressed household gene in *A. americanum* salivary glands and hence the most suitable reference gene (Bullard *et al.*, 2016b).

The p47 enzymatic substrate of the E3 ubiquitin ligase X-linked inhibitor of apoptosis (XIAP) is a positive regulator of the *I. scapularis* IMD network, acting as a molecular rheostat (McClure Carroll *et al.*, 2019). It restricts bacterial colonization: disruption of p47 expression through RNAi increased colonization of *I. scapularis* by *B. burgdorferi* and *A. phagocytophilum* (Severo *et al.*, 2013; McClure Carroll *et al.*, 2019). Silencing the genes encoding, for example, ferritin, subolesin and ubiquitin in *D. variabilis* inhibited infection by *A. marginale*, while injection of ubiquitin dsRNA increased tick mortality (de la Fuente *et al.*, 2007b).

Knocking down the tick homologue of the *D. melanogaster* ubiquitin-63E gene in [*R. microplus*] *R. australis* with 594 bp dsRNA caused differential expression (down-/upregulation) of 280 ESTs, the functions of more than half of which were unknown or hypothetical. Ubiquitin knockdown was associated with changes in proteolytic pathways, as evidenced by the downregulation of several proteases. Gene-silenced ticks did not lay eggs. Refining the gene silencing and limiting the off-target effects with shorter (~100–200 bp) dsRNA meant that the ESTs could be selected more predictably (Lew-Tabor *et al.*, 2011).

Bites by *H. longicornis* were shown by quantitative proteomics to give rise to differentially ubiquinated proteins (DUPs) in rabbit skin. These DUPs were concluded to be involved in protein degradation, metabolic processes and immune responses. Differential ubiquitination of, for example, MHC-II can have a regulating effect on the ubiquitin–proteasome system and the MHC-I and MHC-II antigen-presenting pathways (Wang *et al.*, 2020).

G protein-coupled receptors (GPCRs)

G proteins are a family of guanine nucleotide-binding regulatory proteins that serve an essential role in transducing receptor-generated signals (e.g. olfactory and light sensory signals) across the plasma membrane (Hepler and Gilman, 1992). The GPCRs are cell surface membrane receptors considered as poor antigens for anti-tick vaccines, but little is known about their physiological role in ticks (Brock *et al.*, 2019). Neuropeptides, produced in the arthropod synganglion, are the main ligands of GPCRs, making them candidate targets. The *R. microplus* synganglion transcriptome was analysed to gain information on their encoding gene sequences, in support of research into novel tick control technologies (Guerrero *et al.*, 2016; Waldman *et al.*, 2022).

Kinins are multifunctional neuropeptides that regulate diuresis, feeding and ecdysis in insects but their physiological roles in ticks are unclear. The kinin receptor in *R. microplus* is a GPCR and silencing it reduces the tick's reproductive fitness (Xiong *et al.*, 2019).

RNAi in two strains of unfed female *R. microplus* was used to investigate the function of the leucokinin receptor (LKR), one of the GPCRs. Immunohistochemistry was used on fed female ticks to localize expression of the LKR to the midgut. There were strain differences but gene-silenced ticks were found to spend less time taking a bloodmeal and weighed 30% less, their egg production was 28.3% less, and their egg hatchability was 36.7% compared to 56.9% in unsilenced ticks (Brock *et al.*, 2019).

Bioinformatic analysis of the sequenced genome of *I. scapularis* led to the annotation of a number of neuropeptide GPCR genes. One of these encodes for corazonin, which plays a central role in the tick's physiology and behaviour. The genomic organization is similar to that of the human gonadotropin-releasing hormone (GnRH) receptor gene. An unexpected discovery was that the corazonin receptor gene encodes for two splice variants of the receptor that vary in their amino acid sequences and could have different roles (Hauser *et al.*, 2023).

Octopamine is a neurotransmitter that binds to GPCRs and is found in insects. An amino acid sequence similar to that of the octopamine receptor in insects was found in [*B. microplus*] *R. australis*. Amitraz is a formamidine acaricide and a specific agonist of the octopamine receptor. Emerging resistance to amitraz was suspected of being the result of a mutation in the nucleotide sequence of the octopamine receptor, but this was shown not to be the case (Baxter and Barker, 1999). Subsequent investigations have revealed consistent and strong associations between GPCR mutations and resistance to amitraz in the USA, Latin America and South Africa (Robbertse *et al.*, 2016; Jonsson *et al.*, 2018).

Cystatins

Cystatins are a group of cysteine peptidase inhibitors present in lysosomes and extracellular fluids. In ticks, they modulate blood acquisition and digestion, host immune responses and tick immunity (see sections 3.4, 4.1.1, 4.6.3, 4.6.5, 4.6.8, this volume), all functions that would prevent ticks from feeding if they were to be disabled.

Three novel cystatins were described from *I. persulcatus*. Their transcripts were detected in different tissues and instars, indicating their widespread expression during tick development. Hamsters immunized with a recombinant cystatin from *R. microplus* developed a serologically detectable humoral immune response but were not protected against challenge with adult *I. persulcatus* (Rangel *et al.*, 2017).

Antibodies raised against recombinant *R. microplus* cystatin cross-reacted with *R. appendiculatus* cystatin, and vaccine trials with recombinant cystatins impaired engorgement of *O. moubata* and *I. scapularis* nymphs (Parizi *et al.*, 2020). A novel *R. microplus* cystatin, Rmcystatin-1b, was found to be highly expressed in the midgut of partially and fully engorged female ticks. RNAi-mediated knockdown resulted in increased midgut proteolytic activity. Recombinant Rmcystatin-1b was expressed in *E. coli* and inhibited cysteine peptidases, which included a cathepsin L-like protease. A possible role in interaction with the apicomplexan parasite *Babesia bovis* during its proliferation, preventing deleterious effects to the tick, was suggested for this peptidase (Lu *et al.*, 2020).

Cathepsins

Cathepsins are a group of proteases involved in many cellular processes (see section 4.1.1, this volume). *R. microplus* egg yolk contains an aspartic protease designated *Boophilus* yolk procathepsin (BYC). It contributes to tick embryogenesis by its involvement in the degradation of vitellin. Cattle immunized with either native or recombinant (expressed in *E. coli*) BYC mounted a humoral immune response that offered modest protection against subsequent challenge with [*B.*] *R. microplus* larvae. The authors suggested that BYC be considered as a candidate antigen in a multicomponent vaccine (Leal *et al.*, 2006a, b).

Akirin, subolesin and chimeras

A gene called akirin (from the Japanese 'akiraka ni suru' – 'making things clear') was discovered in *Drosophila melanogaster* by RNAi, shown to act in parallel with the NF-κB transcription factor downstream of the IMD pathway, and to help defend against Gram-negative bacteria. Akirin (AKR) is localized in the nucleus and highly conserved, with two homologues in the human genome. Knockout of both homologues in mice revealed the essential downstream function in TLR, TNF and IL-1β signalling pathways towards production of IL-6 (Goto *et al.*, 2008a, b).

Subolesin (SUB) was discovered in *I. scapularis* larvae by ELI of mice, identified as an endopeptidase and designated 4D8 (Almazán *et al.*, 2003). It is the orthologue (non-identical sequence but similar function) of akirin in insects. The evolutionary history reveals that not only sequence and structure but also function in relation to biological processes and pathogen infection were conserved in AKR and SUB (Artigas-Jerónimo *et al.*, 2018). SUB has since been cloned from 10 tick species representing six genera and was shown by RNAi to play a role in multiple cellular processes. Gene knockdown ticks showed tissue degeneration in guts, salivary glands and reproductive organs. It was given the generic name 'subolesin' from the Latin *suboles*: offspring, progeny (de la Fuente *et al.*, 2006a, 2008) and shown to be involved in tick innate immunity to pathogen infection (Zivkovic *et al.*, 2010b; Moreno-Cid *et al.*, 2013; Naranjo *et al.*, 2013).

The description of a SUB orthologue with conserved epitopes in *A. albopictus* (Canales *et al.*, 2009b) leads one to surmise that SUB/AKR may in future be referred to by a collective name that acknowledges their conserved status in insects and ticks.

Silencing the SUB gene in engorged female *R. microplus* led to the production of abnormal eggs, suggesting a possible role of this protein in embryonic development (Nijhof *et al.*, 2007). RNAi in replete females of three three-host tick species (*A. americanum*, *D. variabilis* and *I. ricinus*) also affected subolesin expression in eggs and larvae (Kocan *et al.*, 2007).

When used as an antigen, SUB induced an immunity which decreased tick survival and reproduction rates, and caused degeneration of gut, salivary gland and reproductive tissues. Conserved protective antigens such as SUB/AKR were considered to show promise for inclusion in a universal vaccine to control arthropod vectors and reduce pathogen transmission, but further research was needed (de la Fuente *et al.*, 2011, 2013; Naranjo *et al.*, 2013).

Silencing the SUB gene impaired the tick's vector capacity for *Anaplasma marginale* and *A. phagocytophilum* (de la Fuente *et al.*, 2006b, 2010). The SUB-induced immune reduction of tick burdens was shown to decrease *Babesia bigemina* infection in vaccinated cattle (Merino *et al.*, 2011). *Hyalomma lusitanicum* infected with *B. bigemina* in Sicily had upregulated levels of SUB. Vaccines using tick proteins involved in vector–pathogen interactions could achieve reductions in both tick burdens and pathogen infection (Zivkovic *et al.*, 2010b; Merino *et al.*, 2013b) but SUB/AKR vaccines had no effect on TBEV infection and transmission (Merino *et al.*, 2013a).

Recombinant SUB expressed by *E. coli* was used to vaccinate rabbits before challenge with *H. longicornis*. Using the usual parameters of replete weight and egg production, the calculated efficacy was 37.4% (Lee *et al.*, 2020). Whereas SUB on its own might lack a convincing protective immune response, its use in combination with other antigen(s) holds promise. A synergistic effect was shown when larvae of *R. microplus* were fed *in vitro* on serum from cattle vaccinated with both Bm86 and SUB, and SUB is a routine inclusion in many experimental tick vaccines (Trentelman *et al.*, 2019; Estrada-Garcia, personal communication, Matanzas, Cuba, 28 March 2022), with the possibility of broadening the efficacy spectrum. There is clearly still some controversy, in that SUB alone was more effective than either Bm86 alone or a SUB/Bm86 combination against natural *R. microplus* infestation (Mendoza-Martinez *et al.*, 2021).

Three separate experiments investigated the immune responses of red deer (*Cervus elaphus*) and white-tailed deer (*Odocoileus virginianus*) to vaccination with either Bm86, SUB and/or mosquito AKR. The assessments were based on antibody responses, control of induced *R. microplus* infestation and antibody response and tick counts after natural tick exposure. Bm86 and SUB were similarly effective (76–83%) against induced *R. microplus* infestations on white-tailed deer. AKR reduced counts of natural infestations of *Hyalomma* spp. and *Rhipicephalus* spp. on red deer by 25–33% 14–20 weeks after immunization (Carreón *et al.*, 2012).

Biosynthetic antibody-binding sites can be connected by amino acid linkers to form a single chain (Huston *et al.*, 1988; Aguilar-Gurrieri *et al.*, 2023). The SUB/AKR chimeras Q38 and Q41 were designed by combining recombinant protective epitopes identified with sera from sheep and rabbits immunized with *I. scapularis* SUB and *Aedes albopictus* AKR. Q38 was the result of combining selected SUB and AKR epitopes with GGGS (glycine, serine) amino acid linkers. In Q41 SUB and AKR were linked by cysteins, forming disulfide bridges. SUB and AKR expressed in *P. pastoris* and the chimeras expressed in *E. coli* were used to vaccinate mice infested with *I. ricinus*, *A. albopictus* and *Phlebotomus perniciosus* in an attempt to control multiple vector species. SUB vaccination had the highest efficacy across all vector species, Q41 the highest efficacy in mosquitoes and Q38 the highest effect on reducing mosquito and sand fly egg production (Moreno-Cid *et al.*, 2013). A Q38 vaccine was 99.9% and 46.4% effective against *I. ricinus* and *D. reticulatus* larvae respectively fed on rabbits (Contreras and de la Fuente, 2016). A wild population of roe deer (*Capreolus capreolus*) in Andalucía was vaccinated once a year with Q38 over a 3 year period, demonstrating an antibody response and a reduction in natural infestation with *H. marginatum*, *H. lusitanicum*, *R. bursa* and *I. ricinus* (Contreras *et al.*, 2020).

BmVDAC

An investigation of the molecular interactions between *R. microplus* midgut cells and *Babesia bigemina* led to the discovery of a mitochondrial voltage-dependent anion-selective channel (VDAC), also known as a mitochondrial porin, and a central component of the apoptosis process. Porins interact with intracellular parasites, regulating the permeability of the outer mitochondrial membrane. The VDAC-encoding gene was identified and sequenced (Rodríguez-Hernández *et al.*, 2012). BmVDAC was shown by RT-PCR to be expressed at higher levels in *R. microplus* when infected with *B. bigemina* and considered to be a potential anti-tick vaccine antigen candidate (Rodríguez-Hernández *et al.*, 2015). The protective effect of recombinant BmVDAC was demonstrated by an 82% efficacy against *R. microplus* infestation on immunized cattle. This effect was moderated, with efficacy of only 34% against ticks on cattle infected with *B. bigemina* (Ortega-Sánchez *et al.*, 2020).

Ferritin-2

Blood-feeding ticks have a copious amount of free (non-haem) iron in their bloodmeals to utilize, detoxify, store and transport. Ferritins are involved in iron metabolism and the intracellular ferritin-1 was first described in *I. ricinus* and *O. moubata*. Secreted ferritin-2 (Fer2) is required for iron transport from the tick gut to ovaries and salivary glands. Silencing of the Fer2 gene impairs the ability of ticks to feed, making it a promising candidate for a tick vaccine (Hajdusek *et al.*, 2009). Fer2 sequences were amplified from *I. ricinus* and *R. microplus*, cloned into the expression vector pET100, expressed in *E. coli* and formulated with Montanide ISA 50 V. Vaccinated rabbits infested with unfed adult *I. ricinus* yielded fewer, lighter and less fertile engorged adult female ticks. Vaccinated cattle were infested with *R. microplus* and *R. annulatus* larvae and protected to a similar level as with Bm86 vaccination (Hajdusek *et al.*, 2010).

Fer2 is also secreted by *H. longicornis* where it was shown to be present in ovaries and eggs. Silencing the Fer2 gene induced a reduction in engorged tick weight, increased mortality and decreased fecundity, demonstrating the crucial role of this protein in blood feeding and reproduction (Galay *et al.*, 2013). Fer2 was extracted from eggs of *H. longicornis* at various stages of embryogenesis and assumed to act as an iron transporter and conserver (Hernandez *et al.*, 2023).

Analysing the Fer2 sequence revealed conserved antigenic regions among various tick species. Fer2 was derived from *I. persulcatus* and shown to have a high iron-binding capacity, lending further support to its possible utility in a vaccine (Githaka *et al.*, 2020).

TROSPA

A midgut receptor for outer surface protein A (TROSPA) has been found in *I. scapularis*, (Pal *et al.*, 2004), *R. annulatus* (Antunes *et al.*, 2012), *I. ricinus* (Figlerowicz *et al.*, 2013) and *R. microplus* (Merino *et al.*, 2013b). TROSPA binds and facilitates midgut colonization and subsequent pathogen transmission to the host (Chmelař *et al.*, 2016). RNA interference with this gene impairs infection of the tick by *B. burgdorferi* (Pal *et al.*, 2004; Figlerowicz *et al.*, 2013) and *B. bigemina* (Antunes *et al.*, 2012; Hajdušek *et al.*, 2013; Merino *et al.*, 2013b), but not *A. marginale* (Merino *et al.*, 2013b). Cattle were vaccinated with recombinant TROSPA, expressed in *E. coli* and formulated with Montanide ISA 50 V, infested with *R. microplus* larvae and coinfected with *A. marginale* and *B. bigemina*. Vaccination did not interfere with tick infestation or egg laying but reduced the amount of *B. bigemina* DNA recovered from collected replete ticks (Merino *et al.*, 2013b).

Paramyosin

Paramyosin is a muscle protein found in a large number of invertebrates and, beyond its structural function, has been implicated in modulation of the host's immune system by inhibiting the classical complement pathway (see section 3.1.3, this volume) and binding of IgG. Recombinant [*B.*] *R. microplus* paramyosin (rBmPRM) was expressed in *E. coli*. Expression analysis indicated the presence of BmPRM in all tested tissues (e.g. fat body and salivary glands) and developmental stages, but not in saliva. It was not yet known if BmPRM binds IgG because it acts as an Fc receptor (see section 3.1.3, this volume; Ferreira *et al.*, 2002).

The IgG response of cattle exposed to natural infestation with *R. microplus* was determined by ELISA, using both recombinant paramyosin (BmPRM) expressed in *E. coli* and salivary gland protein extract used as the antigen. The comparative reactions were more highly correlated in Nelore (Zebu) than in Hereford (European) cattle. The expression of paramyosin was determined by qRT-PCR in various tick stages and tissues and found to be highest in the adult female fat body and the gut in partially engorged adult female ticks. The fact that tick-infested cattle displayed a serological response to what is considered to be a concealed antigen presented an enigma. The authors concluded that BmPRM is an antigen to consider for inclusion in a 'cocktail' vaccine against *R. microplus* (Leal *et al.*, 2013).

After cloning the cDNA encoding paramyosin in *H. longicornis*, the recombinant protein was expressed in *E. coli* and vaccinated into rabbits, providing them with 50% immune protection against tick infestation. The protective epitope was analysed and identified as a peptide and conjugated with keyhole limpet hemocyanin (KLH). The cumulative (engorgement, fertility and fecundity) immunoprotective efficacy of the two vaccines in rabbits challenged with infestation by adult *H. longicornis* was 60.4% and 70.9%, respectively (Wu *et al.*, 2021).

Serpins

Serpins in tick saliva modulate the host's innate immune response by interfering with blood coagulation (see section 3.4.1, this volume) and inflammation (see section 3.4.3, this volume), and the adaptive response by inhibiting T-cell activation and cytokine secretion (see section 4.6.5, this volume). They seem to bridge the gap between secreted and concealed antigens, depending on where the immune confrontation occurs. Clearly, antibodies acting in the host against tick salivary protein at the bite wound are addressing a secreted antigen. But if the effect of the immune response occurs in the tick at the site of the serpin expression before it is secreted, the antigen would be regarded as concealed.

Rapid amplification of cDNA ends (RACE) was used to isolate and clone the cDNA coding for a [*R. microplus*] *R. australis* serpin. The recombinant serpin (rRMS-3) was secreted by *P. pastoris* and demonstrated by qRT-PCR expression analysis to be mainly expressed in the salivary glands of female adult ticks. Only sera from tick-resistant bovines recognized the serpin's B-cell epitope, and semi-engorged ticks fed sheep sera with antibodies to the epitope by capillary tube showed an 81.16% reduction in reproduction capacity (Rodriguez-Valle *et al.*, 2012b).

Serpin 19 is characterized by a reactive centre loop that is 100% conserved in ixodid ticks. The specific reactivity of recombinant *A. americanum* serpin 19 makes it a potential candidate antigen for a universal tick vaccine (Kim *et al.*, 2015b). Serpin 19 was confirmed to be important to *A. americanum* fitness and feeding by mRNA disruption with RNAi. Treated ticks took smaller bloodmeals, were deformed and died during subsequent incubation, bolstering the opinion that it was a potential component of a 'cocktail' tick vaccine (Kim *et al.*, 2016a).

A serpin involved in vitellogenesis (egg yolk formation) was found in *R. haemaphysaloides*, labelled RHS8, and its gene cloned into a pET-30a vector and expressed in *E. coli*. Antiserum against the recombinant rRHS8 was produced in vaccinated mice. Knockdown of the RHS8 gene by RNAi in unfed adult female ticks resulted in reduced engorged weight and egg production and hatchability. RHS8 is worth considering in the development of a control strategy (Xu *et al.*, 2020).

Ribosomal phosphoproteins

Ribosomal phosphoproteins P0, P1 and P2 are located within the 60S ribosomal subunit, are highly conserved between species and considered to play an essential role in protein synthesis. Their phosphorylation could potentially influence their antigenicity. Approximately 15% of patients with systemic lupus erythematosus develop autoantibodies against these ribosomal proteins (Hasler *et al.*, 1991), with ribosomal protein P0 considered the classic lupus antigen (Frampton *et al.*, 2000). Their conserved nature mitigates against their suitability as a vaccine candidate (Hassan *et al.*, 2020), but a relatively poorly conserved 20 amino acid synthetic peptide used as a vaccine in rabbits protects against infestation by *R. sanguineus*, a three-host tick. The calculated efficacy was 90%, based on a reduction in the viability of moulted nymphs and numbers of engorged adults and their egg production (Rodríguez-Mallon *et al.*, 2012).

The vaccine displayed an efficacy of 96%, based on the same criteria, against *R. microplus* (Rodríguez-Mallon *et al.*, 2015), and *Amblyomma mixtum* on rabbits and *I. ricinus* on cattle. The P0 peptide was conjugated with Bm86 and KLH to enhance the spectrum and level of efficacy prior to vaccinating cattle against *R. microplus* (Rodríguez-Mallón *et al.*, 2020a, b). Another combination of P0 was with recombinant *Rhipicephalus haemaphysaloides* subolesin. In vaccinated rabbits challenged with adult *H. longicornis*, the efficacy was 86.5% (Hassan *et al.*, 2020).

For unknown reasons, the P0 conjugated with KLH or Bm86 (with Montanide ISA50 as adjuvant in the latter case) was disappointing when tested against *R. australis* (Mahony, 2021).

ATAQ proteins

Analysis of Bm86 homologues from argasid and ixodid ticks led to the discovery of a novel protein in metastriate ticks, named ATAQ after a part of its signature peptide. ATAQ proteins are structurally related to Bm86, contain multiple EGF-like domains and were shown by qRT-PCR to be expressed both in midguts and Malpighian tubules (Bm86 orthologues are only expressed in tick midguts) and more continuously over the life stages of *R. microplus* and *R. appendiculatus*. The vaccine potential of ATAQ proteins against tick infestations was yet to be evaluated but because they are more conserved than Bm86 orthologues, were thought to possibly confer protection against heterologous tick infestations (Nijhof *et al.*, 2010).

A yeast two-hybrid screening system was used to analyse the protein–protein interactions of Bm86 and ATAQ from *R. microplus*. They were shown to share two (aldehyde and retinol dehydrogenase) interacting partners, but Bm86 was shown to also have a Kunitz-like protein component. The three moieties are all involved in retinol (the alcohol form of vitamin A) metabolism that helps regulate the immune responses (Kiper, 2013). The ATAQ genes of seven Mexican isolates of *R. microplus* were sequenced and found to have a high degree of conservation (98–100% for nucleotides and 97.8–100% for the encoded proteins), but to differ for 20 amino acid sequences from a *R. microplus* isolate from Mozambique. It would be necessary to gather more information on diversity in the ATAQ gene in order to form an opinion on its suitability as a vaccine candidate (del Castillo *et al.*, 2020).

A homologue of *R. microplus* ATAQ was found in *H. longicornis* (rHlATAQ), expressed throughout the midgut and in Malpighian tubule cells and containing multiple EGF-like domains. It was genetically distant from previously reported ATAQ proteins and expressed throughout all life cycle stages, increasing steadily during feeding. *H. longicornis* females fed on rabbits immunized with rHlATAQ took longer to complete their engorgement, weighed more, produced more eggs over a longer period and their eggs took longer to hatch. It was concluded that antibodies against ATAQ might disrupt tick engorgement and ovipositioning (Adjou Moumouni *et al.*, 2023).

Aquaporins

Aquaporins are water channels enabling ticks to deal with a bloodmeal 100 times their body weight, while returning 75% of the ingested water and electrolytes to the host via their saliva. An aquaporin in the gut, rectal sac and salivary glands of *I. ricinus* was identified from a cDNA library and cloned (*Ir*AQP1) for production of dsRNA and subsequent RNAi in unfed adult female ticks. Their feeding was assessed *in vitro*, using a membrane feeding technique (Kröber and Guerin, 2007) and *in vivo* on guinea pigs. Silencing the *Ir*AQP1 gene dramatically affected the volume of blood ingested. It was not lethal, thus ruling out this protein as a potential target (Campbell *et al.*, 2010).

Triosephosphate isomerase (TIM)

Triosephosphate isomerase is a key enzyme in glycolysis and a potential candidate antigen for a vaccine. The TIM homologue gene of *H. longicornis* was found to be expressed in all developmental stages and in all tissues of the unfed adult female. The gene was cloned and inserted into a vector to obtain the recombinant protein. Vaccinated rabbits displayed a humoral immune response confirmed by Western blot, demonstrated by ELISA, and 50.9% efficacy against unfed adult *H. longicornis*, as evidenced by their reduced replete weights, egg production and egg hatchability (Liang *et al.*, 2022).

5.2.6 Epitope diversity

Variable efficacy of various versions of Bm86 as a vaccine against *R. decoloratus*, *R. microplus*, *R. australis* and *R. annulatus* has been one of the stumbling blocks to greater commercial success. The system used for expressing the antigen (*E. coli*, Baculovirus, *Pichia pastoris* or pKLAC2-*Kluyveromyces lactis*) (Tabor, 2021) is no doubt partly to blame. But another problem bedevilling the search for recombinant subunit tick antigens that will offer a wide spectrum of protection is sequence polymorphism in the genes that encode the proteins, and in their amino acids, leading to variable and unsatisfactory vaccine efficacy (García-García *et al.*, 1999, 2000; Cunha *et al.*, 2011).

The midgut Bm86 and Bm85 genes of 30 [*B.*] *R. microplus* strains from Brazil, Argentina, Uruguay, Venezuela and Colombia were sequenced. Variations of up to 3.65% were seen in the nucleotide sequences of the Bm86 gene, and 6.08% in the amino acid sequences of the Bm86 protein. Amino acid sequence variations greater than 2.8% are deemed sufficient to confer vaccine inefficiencies (Sossai *et al.*, 2005). Sequencing the Bm86 cDNA gene from 125 field isolates revealed 3.1–7.4% divergence from the Yeerongpilly reference vaccine antigen, which was thought to account for the poor efficacy of the vaccine in many parts of Mexico (Martínez-Arzate *et al.*, 2019). Bm86 homologues cloned from [*B.*] *R. decoloratus*, sequenced and expressed by *E. coli*, contained two conserved linear peptides that helped to explain the significant reduction in engorged female weight and egg production in *R. decoloratus* ticks fed on Bm86-vaccinated cattle .

Rhipicephalus microplus and *R. annulatus*, both vectors of bovine and equine babesiosis, share midgut Bm86 antigen sequences but with enough amino acid divergence to render vaccine protection ineffective. Bm86 antigens from vaccine strains of *R. australis* and *R. microplus*, Australian Yeerongpilly and Cuban Camcord, compared with Bm86 from South Texas isolates of *R. annulatus* and *R. microplus* ('cattle fever ticks'), displayed 10–10.2% divergence in the amino acid sequences (Freeman *et al.*, 2010).

Ra86 homologues of Bm86 from a laboratory strain and four field isolates of *R. appendiculatus* were sequenced. The laboratory strain contained two alleles, based on amino acid insertions and deletions (indels), and the field isolates three more. The amino acid sequence identity between the sequence types varied from 74 to 97% (Kamau *et al.*, 2016), which is bound to adversely affect the consistency of effect of a putative vaccine in the field.

Considering the multitude of tick species and the plethora of potentially immunogenic structural and secreted epitopes and their different functions, the prospect of a single vaccine that can offer protection on this wide front is daunting (Hassan *et al.*, 2020). It seems inevitable that the successful vaccine will contain several antigens (Parthasarathi *et al.*, 2021). A vaccine composed of three recombinant antigens (*R. microplus* Bm86 and *H. anatolicum* subolesin and tropomyosin), injected into cattle three times over 60 days gave 86.7% protection against challenge with *R. microplus* and 87.2 and 86.2% efficacy against *H. anatolicum* larvae and adults. A significant antibody response against all three antigens was recorded for up to 140 days (Parthasarathi *et al.*, 2023).

Another combination of relatively well-conserved antigens was used to overcome the vulnerability of a single antigen to genomic variability. SUB, calreticulin and cathepsin-L genes of *H. anatolicum* and *R. microplus* were sequenced and analysed for intra- and inter-species homogeneity. Intraspecies sequence homology was >97%, while between species it was >77% and >85% for SUB and calreticulin respectively, and >57% for cathepsin-L. Cattle were vaccinated with the individual recombinant antigens and challenged with newly hatched larvae of the two tick species. The efficacy percentages are summarized in Table 5.2 (Kumar *et al.*, 2017). Although the individual percentages, by antigen or tick species, are disappointing at first glance, it is intriguing to consider what the cumulative (or possibly synergistic) effect of an antigen combination against a multispecies infestation challenge might be in a field situation.

Table 5.2. Summarized efficacy of three recombinant antigens against *H. anatolicum* and *R. microplus* on cattle. Adapted from Kumar *et al.* (2017).

Antigen	% Efficacy	
	H. anatolicum	R. microplus
Subolesin	65.4	54.00
Calreticulin	41.3	37.56
Cathepsin-L	30.2	22.21

5.2.7 A double-barrel approach

Immunity to the vector might imply protection against the pathogens it transmits, but a vaccine that offers protection against both the vector and its transmitted pathogen may be worth considering. A multiantigen vaccine offering broad-spectrum immunity against multiple tick genera seems entirely feasible, but a practical difficulty might be the selection of the pathogen whose antigen(s) should be combined with those of the tick. New technology might allow the nimble approach of ordering small quantities of a bespoke vaccine for a specific geographic region based on the tick(s) and tick-borne disease(s) that prevail there.

Immunoinformatic approaches were taken for the *in silico* design of a multivalent vaccine that would target more than one immunodominant epitope of structural proteins of CCHFV. This would be combined with tick salivary gland subolesin to impart dual activity. Linear and conformational B-cell, helper and cytotoxic T-cell epitopes from the viral proteins were incorporated, with appropriate linkers and adjuvant. The proposed vaccine construct was expected to induce immune protection against both the CCHFV pathogen and its tick vector (Shrivastava *et al.*, 2020).

Alternatively, a vaccine targeting and neutralizing the tick molecules essential for transmission of tick-borne infections will protect against infection and avoid the need for vaccination against every tick-borne pathogen (Brossard and Wikel, 2004). An example of this was the vaccination of cattle with tick proteins involved in vector–pathogen interactions, such as SUB, TROSPA, silk and the Q38 chimera. They were subsequently infected with *Anaplasma marginale* and *Babesia bigemina*, before being infested with *R. microplus* larvae. Vaccination with TROSPA did not affect the tick parameters, whereas Q38, silk and SUB were 75%, 62 and 60% effective. *B. bigemina* transmission was reduced by Q38, TROSPA and SUB and that of *A. marginale* by silk and SUB vaccination (Merino *et al.*, 2013b).

5.3 The Vector Microbiome

Disturbance of the microbiome equilibrium (dysbiosis; see section 2.1.7, this volume) not only causes anomalies in tick development but also impairs the tick's chances of survival and its vector competence (Estrada-Peña and Cabezas-Cruz, 2019; Wu-Chuang *et al.*, 2022). *I. scapularis* larvae infected with *B. burgdorferi* had a smaller microbiome redundancy, with 15.4% fewer functional pathways than uninfected nymphs (Estrada-Peña *et al.*, 2020).

The realization that the tick's gut microbiome might present a hitherto neglected source of hidden antigen was an exciting discovery (Narasimhan and Fikrig, 2015; Wu-Chuang *et al.*, 2022). Vaccines against tick microbiota alter the structure of the microbial community (Fig. 5.3), vector feeding, the functional profile of their microbiome and the development of pathogens in their vectors (Mateos-Hernández *et al.*, 2020, 2021; Maitre *et al.*, 2022), as in the case of *B. afzelii* infection in *I. ricinus* (Wu-Chuang *et al.*, 2023). The functional redundancy of the tick microbiome (15.7–19.2% of pathways provided by more than 100 genera in uninfected *I. scapularis*; Estrada-Peña *et al.*, 2020) provides a sobering background to the selection of vaccine antigens from this potential source.

5.4 The Promise of New Technology

5.4.1 Synthetic antigens

The Q38 and Q41 SUB/AKR chimeras (see section 5.2.5) were not the first examples of biosynthetic epitopes.

Taking note of the sequence variation in recombinant Bm86 (see section 5.2.5), synthetic peptides were designed *in silico* with

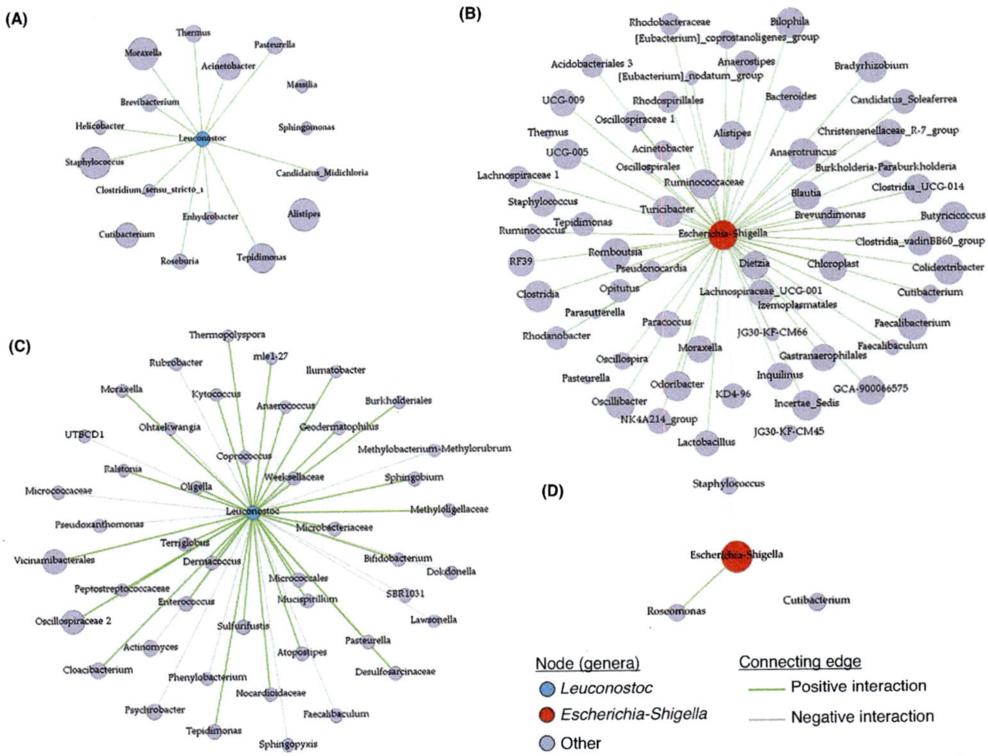

Fig. 5.3. Animals vaccinated against the tick microbiota display an impact on the structure of the tick's microbial community. From Mateos-Hernández *et al.* (2021) under the terms of the Creative Commons Attribution License (CC BY).

selected amino acids, mapping the T and B epitopes of the Bm86 protein, expressed in *Komagataella (Pichia) pastoris* and refined to one candidate. The chosen amino acid sequences of the immunogenic epitopes were found to be conserved in *R. microplus* strains from different parts of the Americas. The synthetic peptide is designated SBm7462® and has been patented in several countries (Patarroyo *et al.*, 2002, 2009, 2020). Tick-naïve calves vaccinated with the recombinant peptide with saponin as adjuvant were challenged with newly hatched *R. microplus* larvae after the vaccination. The efficacy of immunization as assessed by the usually combined parameters of engorged tick numbers, egg production and fertility was 72.5%. The immune response of the vaccinated calves was monitored by ELISA confirmation of IgG production. Peripheral blood mononuclear cells (PBMC) were isolated, cultured and stimulated with concanavalin A for detection of cytokine gene expression. RNA was extracted and cDNA obtained by reverse transcription for quantitative transcription profiling of IL-4, IFN-γ, IL-10, IL-12 and TNF-α expression by qPCR. IL-4 was found to have been upregulated and TNF-α downregulated. The site of action of antibodies to SBm7462 in the tick gut was displayed by immunohistochemistry (Fig. 5.4), and changes in regional lymph node germinal centres were measured by histomorphometry. These results point conclusively to a type two adaptive immune response elicited by SBm7462 (Patarroyo *et al.*, 2020).

Tick subolesin have two different epitope types in addition to the linear B-cell epitope (Prudencio *et al.*, 2010). B-cell-reactive epitopes were identified in the mapped peptide array of SUB from three different tick species. If these epitopes can be related to the protection and efficacy of SUB-based vaccines, it could lead to the design of new chimeras (Contreras *et al.*, 2022).

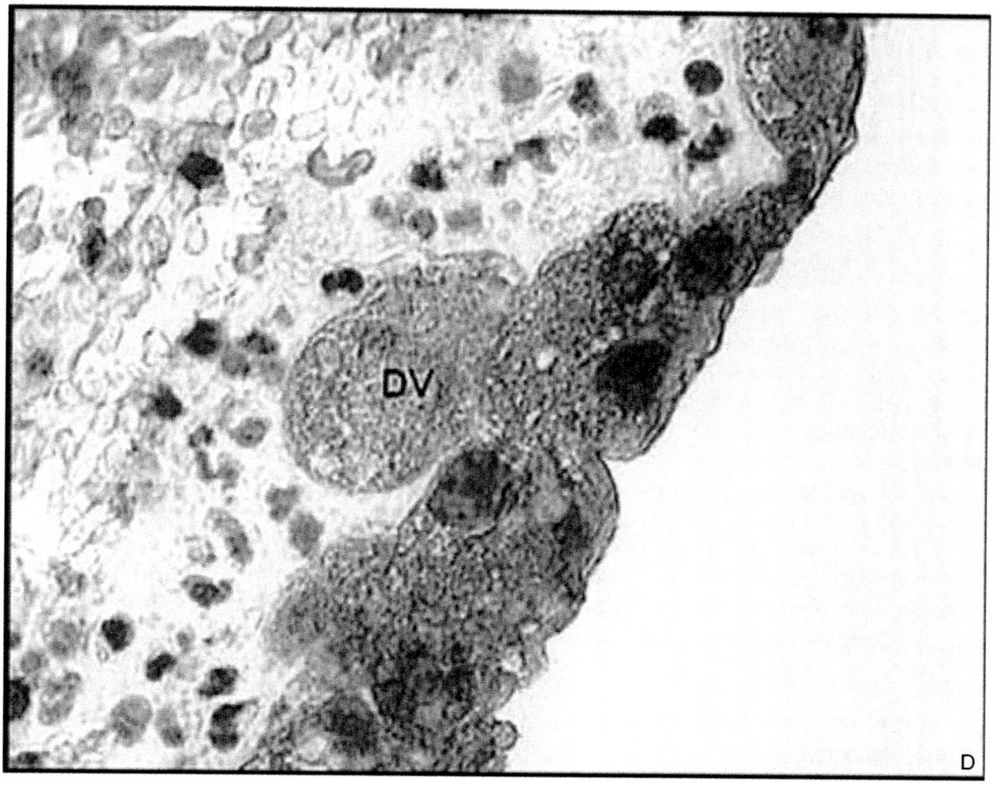

Fig. 5.4. Microphotograph of indirect immunoperoxidase staining of Bm86 protein on gut cells of [*B.*] *R. microplus* feeding on a calf vaccinated with the synthetic peptide SBm7462. From Patarroyo *et al.* (2002) with permission of Elsevier Science B.V.

5.4.2 Antigen delivery and presentation

Exogenous antigens need to be processed and presented to receptors to elicit an immune response. Virus-like particles (VLPs) are structural proteins devoid of native virus genome and are efficiently processed by dendritic cells for presentation by MHC class I molecules to cytotoxic T-lymphocytes, and by MHC class II molecules for activation of T-helper cells. They can also be considered as typical T-cell-independent B-cell antigens. They are thus capable of activation of innate and adaptive immune responses, both humoral and cell mediated. Recombinant VLPs were considered as veterinary immunogens against a variety of pathogens, all of which were viruses at the time (Liu *et al.*, 2012).

DNA tattoo vaccination

The skin is rich in APCs, and dermal delivery of DNA vaccines by tattooing induces higher specific humoral and cellular immune responses than intramuscularly injected DNA. The tattoo procedure causes many minor mechanical injuries followed by haemorrhage, necrosis, inflammation and regeneration, thus stimulating the innate immune system (Pokorna *et al.*, 2008; Quaak *et al.*, 2009). Plasmid DNA vaccines are easier and simpler to produce than recombinant protein and highly flexible with regard to modification of the expression cassette (Van der Berg *et al.*, 2014).

Tattoo vaccination of mice against *B. burgdorferi* induced high IgG titres and provided near total protection against challenge with infected *I. scapularis* nymphs. Tattoo vaccination with four recombinant *I. scapularis* salivary proteins induced low to moderate IgG titres and did not provide protection against infestation (Klouwens *et al.*, 2021). The same antigens will have to be tested by conventional administration before tattoo vaccination against ticks is rejected as a possibility.

Transgenic plants

Plants expressing recombinant immunizing proteins could offer the possibility of delivering the first and booster doses of an oral vaccine with considerable benefits, such as low cost, minimal animal handling and ease of repeated administration.

Three transgenic plant lines expressing the spike protein of transmissible gastroenteritis virus (TGEV) were used to immunize pigs. Expression of the gene products was confirmed by ELISA and Western blotting, while the pigs' TGEV-specific immune responses were determined by ELISA and virus neutralization (Tuboly *et al.*, 2000). Emulating these results against tick infestation in a ruminant might bear investigation.

Oral administration

Recombinant *R. microplus* SUB produced in *E. coli* was mixed with heat-inactivated *Mycobacterium bovis* in phosphate-buffered saline and administered orally to European cross-bred calves. The animals were challenged with an induced infestation of *R. microplus* larvae 3 weeks after the second vaccination. IgG antibody responses were assessed by ELISA and the expression profiles of their genes involved in immunity (complement 3, TNF-α, IL-2, IL-12) were analysed by qRT-PCR. Vaccination reduced the number of engorged female ticks by 51% and the hatchability of the eggs they produced by 30% (Contreras *et al.*, 2019).

The principle of a multivalent (four different epitopes) Semliki Forest virus replicon-based mRNA vaccine (see *Endogenous expression* below) administered orally by way of a *Salmonella typhimurium* mutant was proven in mice and hamsters protected against SARS-CoV-2 infection (Jawalagatti *et al.*, 2022).

Endogenous expression

The concept of transfecting APCs, or muscle or skin cells, with the DNA encoding for an antigen was tested by constructing expression vectors containing the ovalbumin gene alone, or linked to cytokine genes, including granulocyte and macrophage-colony stimulating factor (GM-CSF), IFN-γ, IL-2, IL-4, IL-12 or a sequence encoding nine amino acids of IL-1β, and injecting these into mice. The results indicated that humoral, cytokine and cytotoxic responses to DNA vaccination can be altered by certain cytokine constructs (Maecker *et al.*, 1997).

Prior to this, mouse cells had been successfully transfected *in vitro* with liposome-mediated luciferase messenger RNA (mRNA), resulting in greatly increased luciferase protein expression (Malone *et al.*, 1989). Development and refinement of the technology was well under way, and it had been acknowledged as a promising alternative to conventional vaccines (Scorza and Pardi, 2018), by the time the global human Covid-19 pandemic thrust the concept of endogenously expressed antigens, prompted by mRNA administered by various means, into lay public awareness.

Although the initial use for livestock is likely to be dominated by infectious diseases (Mahony *et al.*, 2024), the relative ease with which virtually any genomic sequence can be designed *in silico*, customized, synthesized and delivered as an mRNA vaccine, for expression of the antigen as an intracellular, secreted, or membrane-bound protein, holds promise for the future immunogenic management of ticks on livestock. Antigen-encoding mRNA vaccines have been shown to elicit antigen-specific humoral and cellular immune responses (Chahal *et al.*, 2016; Maruggi *et al.*, 2019; Abbas *et al.*, 2023).

The risk of antigenic drift or genomic diversity (see section 5.2.5) is justification for using an mRNA that encodes for a well-conserved epitope or multiple epitopes. Covid-19 vaccines have shown efficacy varying from 60% to 95%, attributed to the fact that they encode for epitopes in the virus spike protein which is prone to frequent mutation (Piadel *et al.*, 2022).

Exogenous mRNA is recognized by a variety of innate immune receptors, and cells have a propensity to limit the duration of expression, which limits the stability and activity of conventional mRNA (Chahal *et al.*, 2016; Maruggi *et al.*, 2019). This is potentially advantageous if it provides adjuvant activity, promoting DC maturation and eliciting robust T- and B-cell responses. But this innate immune response might also inhibit antigen expression and negatively affect the immune response (Pardi *et al.*, 2018), as well as possibly inducing toxicity. Ideally, mRNA vaccines need to be delivered intracellularly (Chahal *et al.*, 2016). The mRNA can be encapsulated for protection in a variety of lipid, polymer or dendrimer nanoparticles. The innate immune activation can also be decreased and the protein translation increased by modifying the mRNA nucleosides (Pardi *et al.*, 2018; Scorza and Pardi, 2018). Elimination of exogenous mRNA by the innate immune system can also be circumvented by mRNA replicons (Sethna *et al.*, 1989).

The hypothesis that primary vaccination with the gene for Bm86 with or without the genes for the cytokines GM-CSF and IL-1β would extend the antibody response to a booster vaccination with Bm86 could not be proven in sheep (De Rose *et al.*, 1999). Safety concerns about the possible stable transfection of DNA into somatic or germ cells were allayed by indications that the majority of plasmid DNA injected into skeletal muscle remains at the injection site. Various groups of researchers have attempted to develop a DNA vaccine against tick infestation (Abbas *et al.*, 2023).

Guinea pigs were vaccinated with a 19ISP vaccine and subsequently challenged with *I. scapularis*. Bite wounds displayed early erythema, the ticks' engorgement was curtailed and their transmission of *B. burgdorferi* was impeded. The mRNA in the vaccine encoded 19 *I. scapularis* proteins, known to be expressed in salivary glands, many of them secreted in the bite wound. The nucleoside sequences had been varied and the mRNAs were encapsulated in lipid nanoparticles (Sajid *et al.*, 2021). In a subsequent refinement, the number of mRNAs was reduced to 12, and the 12ISP vaccine shown to provide similar protection. None of the antigens administered individually elicited a protective immunity. Salp14 was the component responsible for the strongest tick bite erythema response. The authors conclude that salivary antigens not included in the 12ISP cocktail might contribute to its efficacy, as may the inclusion of mRNA encoding for hidden gut antigens (Matias *et al.*, 2023). The improved protection elicited by a combination of mRNA-encoded antigens had previously been demonstrated, admittedly for a different pathogen (Freyn *et al.*, 2020).

5.5 Formulating the Vaccine

There appear to be conflicting opinions on the importance of antibody titre level and the extension of titre half-life to enhance vaccine efficacy. In both instances, the simulation models were based on the life history of the single-host tick [*B.*] *R. microplus*. Simulations based on European breed cattle in Australia indicated that control was improved with increases in both antibody titre and titre half-life, but with a flattening off and diminishing returns for antibody titre and linearly increased vaccination efficacy from extended half-life (Floyd *et al.*, 1995). Using vaccination data gathered in Cuba and Brazil, returns from increased titre half-life flattened earlier, and vaccination efficacy improved linearly with increased titre levels (Lodos *et al.*, 2000).

The difference is bound to be one of mathematics, with differences in the models used (TICK2 vs TICKSIM) and the assumptions underpinning these. But it highlights the potential pitfalls in designing a vaccination regime that will be effective against different tick species with single- and multi-host life cycles on the same host, which is the norm rather than the exception.

5.5.1 Enhancing the immune response: the role of adjuvants

The refinement of vaccine antigens, moving from whole organisms to extracts, toxoids, or single proteins or peptides expressed by recombinant technology, has been accompanied by a decline in immunogenicity, which can be remedied by an adjuvant (Brewer, 2006) – an ill-defined substance that non-specifically triggers the innate immune system and accelerates, prolongs and/or enhances the immune response. An adjuvant can cause clustering of antigens, which enhances the activation of B-cells and boosts antibody titres. The migration pattern and cellular uptake of vaccine particles are affected by their size. Large particles remain in tissue at the injection site and have to be transported to the lymph node by monocytes, neutrophils and DC. Smaller particles are taken up more efficiently by DC or can drain directly into lymphatic vessels draining to the lymph nodes (de Veer and Meeusen, 2011).

There are different types of adjuvants, with different modes of action. They can be grouped as aluminium salts, liposomes, emulsions, agonists of the stimulator of interferon genes (STING), TLR ligands, RLR and CLR. Liposomes can encapsulate both the antigen and immunostimulatory molecules, enhancing uptake of antigen and stimulation of immune cells and releasing entrapped antigens slowly over an extended period. Freund's adjuvant is a water-in-oil emulsion either with (complete) or without (incomplete) killed *M. tuberculosis* bacteria. They not only improve antibody titres but also enhance the specific cytotoxic T-lymphocyte response (Wu and Liu, 2021).

Aluminium adjuvants (alum) have been used in human vaccines since the 1920s but until recently, the physicochemical interactions between aluminium compounds and antigens were poorly understood (Brewer, 2006). Dynamic alterations in antigen processing and presentation underlie enhanced DC function induced by alum. *In vitro*, alum induces increased antigen accumulation and presentation and reduces protein degradation by DC (Ghimire *et al.*, 2012). This survey did not find any mention of alum in conjunction with a tick antigen.

Keyhole limpet hemocyanin (KLH) is a copper-containing respiratory protein from the marine gastropod *Megathura crenulata*. Although clinically used for treatment of carcinoma in human medicine, it has also become a generalized vaccine component and carrier of conjugated haptens (Harris and Markl, 1999). KLH was conjugated with the P0 peptide and Bm86 to vaccinate cattle against *R. microplus* (Rodríguez-Mallón *et al.*, 2020a, b; Mahony, 2021).

Heat-inactivated *Mycobacterium bovis* activates the innate immune response through complement three and was used to enhance the protective response to a *R. microplus* SUB vaccine in an oral formulation (Contreras *et al.*, 2019).

The use of nanotechnology offers a new communication medium with the immune system. Nanoparticles mimic the size of microorganisms (bacteria and viruses) and by incorporating key molecules involved in immune processes, nanocarriers can be taken up by the immune cells and modulate their responses (Dacoba *et al.*, 2017). The size, shape and surface properties of mesoporous silica nanoparticles (MSNs) can be manipulated (Frickenstein *et al.*, 2021) and they can be used as self-adjuvanting vaccine carriers with remarkable potential for the delivery of a variety of antigens. The adjuvant effect of nanoparticles results in higher IgG levels than from conventional alum-adsorbed vaccines (Prego *et al.*, 2010). Silica vesicles, one class of MSNs, have been tested as self-adjuvanting vaccine delivery systems targeting infectious and protozoal bovine diseases and [*R. microplus*] *R. australis*. Bm86 expressed by *E. coli* and amplified in recombinant baculovirus was experimentally formulated in silica nanovesicles as carriers, and its distribution pattern in mice demonstrated by fluorescent imaging (Mody *et al.*, 2021).

5.5.2 Duration of effect: the need for a sustained stimulus

In the absence of a boosting effect from natural tick challenge when a concealed tick antigen is used in a vaccine, repeat vaccination is a prerequisite for maintaining a protective immunity. Under extensive production systems, where mustering cattle is a considerable financial impost, a vaccine that will provide prolonged immune cover is needed, reducing the frequency of booster vaccination. There have been several attempts but few have thus far been commercially successful.

Chitosan is a non-toxic linear polysaccharide derived from chitin by deacetylation, found in the exoskeletons of crustaceans and insects, and structurally similar to cellulose. Because of its biocompatibility and biodegradability, chitosan is commonly used for many applications in pharmaceutical and medical fields, such as vaccine delivery systems in both solution and particulate forms (Chua *et al.*, 2012; Duttagupta *et al.*, 2015). A biodegradable vaccine depot with the antigen incorporated into the chitosan component induced antibody titres lasting for up to 55 weeks from a single injection in mice (Chua *et al.*, 2015). An injectable biopolymer providing initial rapid release followed by sustained delivery of a biologically active agent, with chitosan as one of the possible components, was patented in 2017 (Al Kobaisi and Mainwaring, 2017) and tested with Bm86 in cattle against *R. australis*. When challenged with tick larvae 56 days after the vaccination, cattle enjoyed 76.9% protection. Immunoglobulin titres increased dramatically to a booster injection 1 year later, but there was an apparent allergic skin reaction at the booster injection sites (Mahony *et al.*, 2019) which would have a profound negative impact on producer acceptance of this product.

Subcutaneously injected clay nanoparticles formed nodules with loose structures from which conjugated antigen was sustainably released over several weeks. The nanoparticles actively and continuously recruited immune cells and stimulated a stronger immune response than alum or QuilA as alternative adjuvants (Chen *et al.*, 2018).

The synthetic peptide SBm7462 was encapsulated in biodegradable microspheres made from polyesters of lactic and glycolic acids and injected subcutaneously in mice. Although the *in vitro* release profile over 51 days was encouraging, this was not reflected in the immune responses of the mice. IgG titres elicited by the microencapsulated antigen were significantly lower than those resulting from immunization with the antigen emulsified in saponin over a period of 21 weeks (Sales-Junior *et al.*, 2005).

The continued expression of therapeutic proteins for as long as 7 weeks *in vivo* can be advantageous where continuous therapeutic levels of the encoded protein are needed, moderating the need for repeated injections (McCafferty *et al.*, 2021), e.g. therapeutic oncology vaccines (Maine *et al.*, 2021). Messenger RNA replicons function as a mechanism for mRNA self-amplification (Sethna *et al.*, 1989), leading to sustained translation. It has been suggested that an mRNA liquid nanoparticle formulation could enable slow continuous antigen delivery (Abbas *et al.*, 2023). This will clearly be desirable for a concealed-antigen vaccine against tick infestation in cattle. RNA replicons with genetic switches that allow control of timing and magnitude of their translation after *in vivo* delivery would be desirable in the case of vaccines, where a measured dose of antigen is usually preferable. Such a switch was encoded on an RNA replicon derived from Venezuelan equine encephalitis virus, and turned off by the administration of trimethoprim, at a serum level 45-fold below what is used in human therapy (McCafferty *et al.*, 2021).

5.6 Efficacy Testing Methodology

Although a vaccine has to be tested under field conditions to confirm its efficacy, the imperatives of cost, animal ethics and sustainability are strong incentives towards developing and adopting laboratory model and *in vitro* screening and testing methods for the early stages of tick vaccine development. As in the case of chemical acaricides (Holdsworth *et al.*, 2006), the effect of an immune response on parasitic tick survival, feeding, egg production (fecundity) and hatchability (fertility) has to be assessed (Costa *et al.*, 2021) in order to judge a vaccine candidate's suitability. Calculation of the efficacy of a vaccine that incorporates these parameters will need to be standardized in order for thresholds to be set and candidate products compared equitably. The protective antibody titre threshold and the duration of this protective effect also need to be known, as the immune response wanes without stimulation or boosting.

The various methods of evaluation of the effect of chemicals on ticks are well established, but innovation and standardization are required for the variety of ways of exposing the tick to the immune response – *in vitro*, *in vivo*, in the laboratory and in the field, at different life cycle stages.

Agreement on and standardization of test methods will contribute to the ability to collaborate and compare research results on a level playing field. An encouraging attempt towards this goal was a small meeting in Morocco in 2015, giving rise to formation of the cattle tick vaccine consortium (Schetters *et al.*, 2016; Parizi *et al.*, 2023). This was predated by the creation in 1984 of the Ibero-American development programme of science and development (CYTED). Funding of its INCOGARR project (immunogens compatible with integrated management strategies in tick control) commenced in 2017 (Rodríguez-Mallon *et al.*, 2018).

Guinea pigs, rabbits and deer mice were used in early experiments to demonstrate acquired immunity to ticks (Trager, 1939). Rabbits are popular laboratory animals and can yield valuable *in vivo* data in tick vaccine experiments. Vaccination with *A. variegatum* midgut protein fractions was used to demonstrate reduced egg production and hatchability from ticks applied to rabbits' ears and confined with ear bags (Kinyua *et al.*, 2002).

Ornithodoros spp. argasid ticks were fed successfully on the air sac membrane of embryonated chicken eggs to study the transmission of tick-borne pathogens (Burgdorfer and Pickens, 1954; Burgdorfer, 1956). Larvae of [*B. microplus*] *R. australis* were successfully cultivated to the nymphal stage on the air cell membrane of embryonated hens' eggs (Pierce and Pierce, 1956). In one instance, a colony of *O. moubata* was maintained entirely by feeding on the exposed membranes of embryonated hens' eggs (Hood *et al.*, 1976). It remains to be seen if this could be an inexpensive alternative for maintaining laboratory tick colonies and possibly testing the effect of immune products.

Capillary tube artificial feeding of partially engorged *R. microplus* females weighing 25–60 mg has been used to test the effects of immunoglobulins on the tick. The ticks were immobilized with double-sided adhesive tape and microhaematocrit capillary tubes filled with citrated cattle blood placed over their mouthparts. The tubes were replaced every 3 hours and engorgement took ca. 28 hours. The authors suggest that monoclonal antibodies can be used to identify antigens that can be used as vaccine immunogens (Gonsioroski *et al.*, 2012).

In a variation of this method, [*R. microplus*] *R. australis* were exposed either to antibodies or to RNAi achieved by feeding dsRNA. Self-drawn Pasteur pipettes were used instead of capillary tubes. The test ticks were fed blood containing antibodies raised by cattle vaccinated twice 1 month apart with recombinant Bm86. Ticks were fed on 100 μl of this mixture, followed by 100 μl whole blood before incubation for assessment of efficacy, which was calculated at 83%.

A separate experiment of this investigation was the feeding of ubiquitin and Bm86 dsRNA. Knockdown of the two genes was confirmed by qRT-PCR. The ubiquitin dsRNA was highly effective against the ticks,but the effect of the Bm86 dsRNA was minimal (Lew-Tabor *et al.*, 2014). It is difficult to envisage this rather laborious technique being upscaled for screening of large numbers of antigens and their formulations.

Variations in infection levels between ticks make capillary feeding an imperfect method for characterizing the effect of tick–pathogen interventions (Antunes *et al.*, 2014; Bhowmick and Han, 2020).

Amblyomma americanum ticks were successfully fed on defibrinated blood *in vitro* through silicone-coated lens paper membranes in order to collect their cement cones uncontaminated by host skin or hair (Bullard *et al.*, 2016a). This method might lend itself to *in vitro* screening of antigen and vaccine candidates.

5.7 Loss of Vaccine Efficacy

Because immunity to concealed tick antigens is not boosted by natural tick infestation, the induced protective immunity is short-lived (Trimnell *et al.*, 2005). There is also the question of the correlation of antibody titre with resistance to ticks, and the efficacy of anti-tick immunity in the face of varying levels of tick infestation challenge (Leal and Ferreira, 2021). It is easy to envisage the more rapid depletion of protective antibodies by a higher number of blood-sucking ticks in the absence of a boosting stimulus.

Aside from a decline in immunity in the absence of adequate boosting stimuli, possibly hastened by the removal of circulating antibodies by feeding ticks, it seems there are at least two ways in which vaccine efficacy could wane over time, due to repeated use. One is the selection, by vaccination, of tick strains with diverse midgut antigen amino acid sequences, rendering them non-susceptible to host antibodies. The other could be spontaneous antigenic drift due to mutations, the rate of which might be calculated using a mutation fixation index (MFI) for the site where the antigen is expressed. At the turn of the 20th century, the MFI for the Bm86 locus was calculated as between 0.02 and 0.1 amino acids per year. This is higher than the rates of human DNA and RNA mutations.

Because amino acid sequence diversity of up to 2.8% did not result in significant tick strain differences in sensitivity to the Bm86 vaccine, it was surmised that amino acid diversity greater than 2.8% would be needed to affect vaccine efficacy. It was concluded that selection of vaccine-resistant tick strains could take from 200 to 1000 years (García-García *et al.*, 1999). The possibility of repeated exposure to vaccine antibodies accelerating the rate of antigen mutation probably also needs consideration.

References

Abbas, M.N., Jmel, M.A., Mekki, I., Dijkgraaf, I. and Kotsyfakis, M. (2023) Recent advances in tick antigen discovery and anti-tick vaccine development. *International Journal of Molecular Sciences* 24, 4969. DOI: 10.3390/ijms24054969.

Ackerman, S., Floyd, M. and Sonenshine, D.E. (1980) Artificial immunity to *Dermacentor variabilis* (Acari: Ixodidae): Vaccination using tick antigens. *Journal of Medical Entomology* 17/5, 391–397. DOI: 10.1093/jmedent/17.5.391.

Adjou Moumouni, P.F., Naomasa, S., Tuvshintulga, B., Sato, N., Okado, K. *et al.* (2023) Identification and characterization of *Rhipicephalus microplus* ATAQ homolog from *Haemaphysalis longicornis* ticks and its immunogenic potential as an anti-tick vaccine candidate molecule. *Microorganisms* 11, 822. DOI: 10.3390/microorganisms11040822.

Agbede, R.I.S. and Kemp, D.H. (1985) Digestion in the cattle tick *Boophilus microplus*: Light microscope study of the gut cells in nymphs and females. *International Journal for Parasitology* 15/2, 147–157.

Agbede, R.I.S. and Kemp, D.H. (1986) Immunization of cattle against *Boophilus microplus* using extracts derived from adult female ticks: Histopathology of ticks feeding on vaccinated cattle. *International Journal for Parasitology* 16/1, 35–41.

Agbede, R.I.S. and Kemp, D.H. (1987) Ultrastructure of secretory cells in the gut of the cattle-tick *Boophilus microplus*. *International Journal for Parasitology* 17/6, 1089–1098. DOI: 10.1016/0020-7519(87)90161-5.

Aguilar-Gurrieri, C., Barajas, A., Rovirosa, C., Ortiz, R., Urrea, V. *et al.* (2023) Alanine-based spacers promote an efficient antigen processing and presentation in neoantigen polypeptide vaccines. *Cancer Immunology, Immunotherapy* 72/7, 2113–2125. DOI: 10.1007/s00262-023-03409-3.

Ali, A., Parizi, L.F., Guizzo, M.G., Tirloni, L., Seixas, A. *et al.* (2015) Immunoprotective potential of a *Rhipicephalus* (*Boophilus*) *microplus* metalloprotease. *Veterinary Parasitology* 207, 107–114. DOI: 10.1016/j.vetpar.2014.11.007.

Aljamali, M.N., Sauer, J.R. and Essenberg, R.C. (2002) RNA interference: Applicability in tick research. *Experimental and Applied Acarology* 28, 89–96.

Al Kobaisi, M. and Mainwaring, D.E. (2017) Injectable composition for delivery of a biologically active agent. Available at: https://patents.google.com/patent/WO2017177265A1/en (accessed 17 July 2024).

Allen, J.R. and Humphreys, S.J. (1979) Immunisation of guinea pigs and cattle against ticks. *Nature* 280, 491–493.

Almazán, C., Kocan, K.M., Bergman, D.K., Garcia-Garcia, J.C., Blouin, E.F. *et al.* (2003) Identification of protective antigens for the control of *Ixodes scapularis* infestations using cDNA expression library immunization. *Vaccine* 21/13-14, 1492–1501. DOI: 10.1016/s0264-410x(02)00683-7.

Anon. (2004) Nobel prize in chemistry for 2004 for the discovery of ubiquitin-mediated protein degradation. Press release. Royal Swedish Academy of Sciences, Stockholm.

Antunes, S. and Domingos, A. (2023) Tick vaccines and concealed versus exposed antigens. *Pathogens* 12, 374. DOI: 10.3390/pathogens12030374.

Antunes, S., Galindo, R.C., Almazán, C., Rudenko, N., Golovchenko, M. *et al.* (2012) Functional genomics studies of *Rhipicephalus* (*Boophilus*) *annulatus* ticks in response to infection with the cattle protozoan parasite, *Babesia bigemina*. *International Journal for Parasitology* 42/2, 187–195. DOI: 10.1016/j.ijpara.2011.12.003.

Antunes, S., Merino, O., Mosqueda, J., Moreno-Cid, J.A., Bell-Sakyi, L. *et al.* (2014) Tick capillary feeding for the study of proteins involved in tick-pathogen interactions as potential antigens for the control of tick infestation and pathogen infection. *Parasites and Vectors* 7, 42. Available at: http://www.parasitesandvectors.com/content/7/1/42 (accessed 4 January 2025).

Artigas-Jerónimo, S., Villar, M., Cabezas-Cruz, A., Valdés, J.J., Estrada-Peña, A. *et al.* (2018) Functional evolution of subolesin/akirin. *Frontiers in Physiology* 9, 1612. DOI: 10.3389/fphys.2018.01612.

Azhahianambi, P., Ray, D.D., Chaudhuri, P., Gupta, R. and Ghosh, S. (2009) Vaccine efficacy of Bm86 ortholog of *H. a. anatolicum*, rHaa86 expressed in prokaryotic expression system. *Journal of Parasitology Research* 165812. DOI: 10.1155/2009/165812.

Banerjee, D.P., Momin, R.R. and Samantaray, S. (1990) Immunization of cattle (*Bos jndicus* x *Bos taurus*) against *Hyalomma anatolicum anatolicum* using antigens derived from tick salivary gland extracts. *International Journal for Parasitology* 20, 969–972. DOI: 10.1016/0020-7519(90)90037-N.

Baxter, G.D. and Barker, S.C. (1999) Isolation of a cDNA for an octopamine-like, G-protein coupled receptor from the cattle tick, *Boophilus microplus*. *Insect Biochemistry and Molecular Biology* 29, 461–467.

Beaufays, J., Adam, B., Decrem, Y., Prévôt, P.P., Santini, S. *et al.* (2008a) *Ixodes ricinus* tick lipocalins: Identification, cloning, phylogenetic analysis and biochemical characterization. *PLoS One* 3/12, e3941. DOI: 10.1371/journal.pone.0003941.

Beaufays, J., Adam, B., Menten-Dedoyart, C., Fievez, L., Grosjean, A. *et al.* (2008b) Ir-LBP, an *Ixodes ricinus* tick salivary LTB4-binding lipocalin, interferes with host neutrophil function. *PLoS One* 3/12, e3987. DOI: 10.1371/journal.pone.0003987.

Bellgard, M.I., Moolhuijzen, P.M., Guerrero, F.D., Schibeci, D., Rodriguez-Valle, M. *et al.* (2012) CattleTickBase: An integrated internet-based bioinformatics resource for *Rhipicephalus* (*Boophilus*) *microplus*. *International Journal for Parasitology* 42/2, 161–169. DOI: 10.1016/j.ijpara.2011.11.006.

Benitez-Usher, C.A. (1975) Some problems associated with the vaccination of ruminants against helminth infections. PhD thesis, University of Glasgow, Glasgow, UK.

Benitez-Usher, C., Armour, J. and Urquhart, G.M. (1976) Studies on immunisation of suckling calves with dictol. *Veterinary Parasitology* 2/2, 209–222. DOI: 10.1016/0304-4017(76)90076-5.

Ben Said, M., Galai, Y., Canales, M., Nijhof, A.M., Mhadhbi, M. *et al.* (2012a) Hd86, the Bm86 tick protein ortholog in *Hyalomma scupense* (syn. *H. detritum*): Expression in *Pichia pastoris* and analysis of nucleotides and amino acids sequences variations prior to vaccination trials. *Veterinary Parasitology* 183/3-4, 215–223. DOI: 10.1016/j.vetpar.2011.07.049.

Ben Said, M., Galai, Y., Mhadhbi, M., Jedidi, M., de la Fuente, J. *et al.* (2012b) Molecular characterization of Bm86 gene orthologs from *Hyalomma excavatum*, *Hyalomma dromedarii* and *Hyalomma marginatum marginatum* and comparison with a vaccine candidate from *Hyalomma scupense*. *Veterinary Parasitology* 190/1-2, 230–240. DOI: 10.1016/j.vetpar.2012.05.017.

Ben Said, M., Mhadhbi, M., Gharbi, M., Galaï, Y. and Sassi, L. (2015) Molecular and phylogenetic study of Bm86 gene ortholog from *Hyalomma excavatum* tick from Tunisia: Taxonomic and immunologic interest. *Hereditary Genetics* 4/3, 154. DOI: 10.4172/2161-1041.1000154.

Bhakta, S., Choudhury, S., Paul, J. and Bhattacharya, A. (2022) Vaccine development through reverse vaccinology using artificial intelligence and machine learning approach. In: Chatterjee, S. (ed.) *COVID-19: Tackling Global Pandemics through Scientific and Social Tools*. Academic Press, London, pp. 33–49.

Bhowmick, B. and Han, Q. (2020) Understanding tick biology and its implications in anti-tick and transmission blocking vaccines against tick-borne pathogens. *Frontiers in Veterinary Science* 7, 319. DOI: 10.3389/fvets.2020.00319.

Bishop, R., Lambson, B., Wells, C., Pandit, P., Osaso, J. *et al.* (2002) A cement protein of the tick *Rhipicephalus appendiculatus*, located in the secretory *e* cell granules of the type III salivary gland acini, induces strong antibody responses in cattle. *International Journal for Parasitology* 32, 833–842.

Brewer, J.M. (2006) (How) do aluminium adjuvants work? *Immunology Letters* 102/1, 10–15. DOI: 10.1016/j.imlet.2005.08.002.

Brock, C.M., Temeyer, K.B., Tidwell, J., Yang, Y., Blandon, M.A. *et al.* (2019) The leucokinin-like peptide receptor from the cattle fever tick, *Rhipicephalus microplus*, is localized in the midgut periphery and receptor silencing with validated double-stranded RNAs causes a reproductive fitness cost. *International Journal for Parasitology* 49/3-4, 287–299. DOI: 10.1016/j.ijpara.2018.11.006.

Brossard, M.L. and Wikel, S.K. (2004) Tick immunobiology. *Parasitology* 129, S161–S176. DOI: 10.1017/S0031182004004834.

Bullard, R., Allen, P., Chao, C.C., Douglas, J., Das, P. *et al.* (2016a) Structural characterization of tick cement cones collected from *in vivo* and artificial membrane blood-fed lone star ticks (*Amblyomma americanum*). *Ticks & Tick-Borne Diseases* 7/5, 880–892. DOI: 10.1016/j.ttbdis.2016.04.006.

Bullard, R.L., Williams, J. and Karim, S. (2016b) Temporal gene expression analysis and RNA silencing of single and multiple members of gene family in the Lone star tick *Amblyomma americanum*. *PLoS One* 11/2, e0147966. DOI: 10.1371/journal.pone.0147966.

Burgdorfer, W. (1956) The possible role of ticks as vectors of leptospirae. Transmission of *Leptospira pomona* by the argasid tick, *Ornithodoros turicata*, and the persistence of this organism in its tissues. *Experimental Parasitology* 5/6, 571–579.

Burgdorfer, W. and Pickens, E.G. (1954) A technique employing embryonated chicken eggs for the infection of argasid ticks with *Coxiella burnetii*, *Bacterium tularense*, *Leptospira icterohaemorrhagiae*, and western equine encephalitis virus. *Journal of Infectious Diseases* 1, 84–89.

Campbell, E.M., Burdin, M., Hoppler, S. and Bowman, A.S. (2010) Role of an aquaporin in the sheep tick *Ixodes ricinus*: Assessment as a potential control target. *International Journal for Parasitology* 40/1, 15–23. DOI: 10.1016/j.ijpara.2009.06.010.

Canales, M., de la Lastra, J.M.P., Naranjo, V., Nijhof, A.M., Hope, M. *et al.* (2008) Expression of recombinant *Rhipicephalus* (*Boophilus*) *microplus*, *R. annulatus* and *R. decoloratus* Bm86 orthologs as secreted proteins in *Pichia pastoris*. *BMC Biotechnology* 8, 14. DOI: 10.1186/1472-6750-8-14.

Canales, M., Almazán, C., Naranjo, V., Jongejan, F. and Fuente, J. (2009a) Vaccination with recombinant *Boophilus annulatus* Bm86 ortholog protein, Ba86, protects cattle against *B. annulatus* and *B. microplus* infestations. *BMC Biotechnology* 9, 29. DOI: 10.1186/1472-6750-9-29.

Canales, M., Naranjo, V., Almazán, C., Molina, R., Tsuruta, S.A. *et al.* (2009b) Conservation and immunogenicity of the mosquito ortholog of the tick-protective antigen, subolesin. *Parasitology Research* 105/1, 97–111. DOI: 10.1007/s00436-009-1368-2.

Carreón, D., de la Lastra, J.M.P., Almazán, C., Canales, M., Ruiz-Fons, F. *et al.* (2012) Vaccination with BM86, subolesin and akirin protective antigens for the control of tick infestations in white tailed deer and red deer. *Vaccine* 30, 273–279. DOI: 10.1016/j.vaccine.2011.10.099.

Černý, J., Lynn, G., Ponte, K., Ledizet, M., Narasimhan, S. *et al.* (2020) Fractionation of tick saliva reveals proteins associated with the development of acquired resistance to *Ixodes scapularis*. *Vaccine* 38/51, 8121–8129. DOI: 10.1016/j.vaccine.2020.10.087.

Chahal, J.S., Khan, O.F., Cooper, C.L., McPartlan, J.S., Tsosie, J.K. *et al.* (2016) Dendrimer-RNA nanoparticles generate protective immunity against lethal Ebola, H1N1 influenza, and *Toxoplasma gondii* challenges with a single dose. *Proceedings of the National Academy of Sciences of the USA* 113, E4133–E4142. DOI: 10.1073/pnas.1600299113.

Chapman, H.D. (2014) Milestones in avian coccidiosis research: A review. *Poultry Science* 93(3), 501–511. DOI: 10.3382/ps.2013-03634.

Chen, W., Zuo, H., Li, B., Duan, C., Rolfe, B. *et al.* (2018) Clay nanoparticles elicit long-term immune responses by forming biodegradable depots for sustained antigen stimulation. *Small* 14/19, 1704465. DOI: 10.1002/smll.201704465.

Cheng, P.H. (2010) Biochemical and molecular characterization of putative immunoprotective molecules of the soft tick, *Ornithodoros savignyi* Audouin (1827). PhD thesis, University of Pretoria, Pretoria, South Africa.

Cheng, P.H., Mans, B.J., Neitz, A.W. and Gaspar, A.R. (2010) Savicalin, a lipocalin from hemocytes of the soft tick, *Ornithodoros savignyi*. *Experimental & Applied Acarology* 52, 313–326.

Chmelař, J., Kotál, J., Karim, S., Kopacek, P., Francischetti, I.M. *et al.* (2016) Sialomes and mialomes: A systems-biology view of tick tissues and tick–host interactions. *Trends in Parasitology* 32/3, 242–254. DOI: 10.1016/j.pt.2015.10.002.

Choy, A., Severo, M.S., Sun, R., Girke, T., Gillespie, J.J. *et al.* (2013) Decoding the ubiquitin-mediated pathway of arthropod disease vectors. *PLoS One* 8/10, e78077. DOI: 10.1371/journal.pone.0078077.

Chua, B.Y., Al Kobaisi, M., Zeng, W., Mainwaring, D. and Jackson, D.C. (2012) Chitosan microparticles and nanoparticles as biocompatible delivery vehicles for peptide and protein-based immunocontraceptive vaccines. *Molecular Pharmaceutics* 9/1, 81–90. DOI: 10.1021/mp200264m.

Chua, B.Y., Sekiya, T., Al Kobaisi, M., Short, K.R., Mainwaring, D. *et al.* (2015) A single dose biodegradable vaccine depot that induces persistently high levels of antibody over a year. *Biomaterials* 53, 50–57. DOI: 10.1016/j.biomaterials.2015.02.066.

Chung, J.M.-W. (2001) Expression of a tick toxin for the development of a canine vaccine. MSc thesis, University of Technology, Sydney, Australia.

Contreras, M. and de la Fuente, J. (2016) Control of *Ixodes ricinus* and *Dermacentor reticulatus* tick infestations in rabbits vaccinated with the Q38 Subolesin/Akirin chimera. *Vaccine* 34/27, 3010–3013. DOI: 10.1016/j.vaccine.2016.04.092.

Contreras, M., Kasaija, P.D., Merino, O., Cruz-Hernandez, N.I., Gortazar, C. *et al.* (2019) Oral vaccination with a formulation combining *Rhipicephalus microplus* subolesin with heat inactivated *Mycobacterium bovis* reduces tick infestations in cattle. *Frontiers in Cellular and Infection Microbiology* 9, 45. DOI: 10.3389/fcimb.2019.00045.

Contreras, M., San José, C., Estrada-Peña, A., Talavera, V., Rayas, E. *et al.* (2020) Control of tick infestations in wild roe deer (*Capreolus capreolus*) vaccinated with the Q38 Subolesin/Akirin chimera. *Vaccine* 38/41, 6450–6454. DOI: 10.1016/j.vaccine.2020.07.062.

Contreras, M., Kasaija, P.D., Kabi, F., Mugerwa, S. and Fuente, J. (2022) The correlation between subolesin-reactive epitopes and vaccine efficacy. *Vaccines* 10, 1327. DOI: 10.3390/vaccines10081327.

Cornwell, R.L. (1961) Observations on calves vaccinated with irradiated larvae of *Dictyocaulus viviparus*. Serum antibody titre, respiratory rate and response to challenge. *Journal of Comparative Pathology and Therapeutics* 71/2, 191–200.

Costa, G.C.A., Ribeiro, I.C.T., Melo-Junior, O., Gontijo, N.F., Sant'Anna, M.R. *et al.* (2021) *Amblyomma sculptum* salivary protease inhibitors as potential anti-tick vaccines. *Frontiers in Immunology* 11, 611104. DOI: 10.3389/fimmu.2020.611104.

Crause, J.C., Wyngaardt, S., Gothe, R. and Neitz, A.W.H. (1994) A shared epitope found in the major paralysis inducing tick species of Africa. *Experimental & Applied Acarology* 18, 51–59.

Cunha, R.C., Andreotti, R. and Leite, F.B.L. (2011) *Rhipicephalus* (*Boophilus*) *microplus*: Expression and characterization of Bm86-GC in *Pichia pastoris*. *Revista Brasileira de Parasitologia Veterinária* 20/2, 103–110.

Dacoba, T.G., Olivera, A., Torres, D., Crecente-Campo, J. and Alonso, M.J. (2017) Modulating the immune system through nanotechnology. *Seminars in Immunology* 34, 78–102. DOI: 10.1016/j.smim.2017.09.007.

De Groot, A.S., Nene, V., Hegde, N.R., Srikumaran, S., Rayner, J. *et al.* (2003) T cell epitope identification for bovine vaccines: An epitope mapping method for BoLA A-11. *International Journal for Parasitology* 33/5-6, 641–653. DOI: 10.1016/s0020-7519(03)00051-1.

de la Fuente, J. (2021) Translational biotechnology for the control of ticks and tick-borne diseases. *Ticks & Tick-Borne Diseases* 12, 101738. DOI: 10.1016/j.ttbdis.2021.101738.

de la Fuente, J. and Kocan, K.M. (2022) The impact of RNA interference in tick research. *Pathogens* 11, 827. DOI: 10.3390/pathogens11080827.

de La Fuente, J., Rodríguez, M., Redondo, M., Montero, C., García-García, J. *et al.* (1998) Field studies and cost-effectiveness analysis of vaccination with Gavac[tm] against the cattle tick *Boophilus microplus*. *Vaccine* 16/4, 366–373.

de La Fuente, J., Rodnguez, M., Montero, C., Redondo, M., Garcıa-Garcıa, J.C. *et al.* (1999) Vaccination against ticks (*Boophilus* spp.): The experience with the bm86-based vaccine gavac. *Genetic Analysis: Biomolecular Engineering* 15, 143–148.

de la Fuente, J., Almazán, C., Blas-Machado, U., Naranjo, V., Mangold, A.J. *et al.* (2006a) The tick protective antigen, 4D8, is a conserved protein involved in modulation of tick blood ingestion and reproduction. *Vaccine* 24/19, 4082–4095. DOI: 10.1016/j.vaccine.2006.02.046.

de la Fuente, J., Almazán, C., Blouin, E.F., Naranjo, V. and Kocan, K.M. (2006b) Reduction of tick infections with *Anaplasma marginale* and *A phagocytophilum* by targeting the tick protective antigen subolesin. *Parasitology Research* 100, 85–91.

de la Fuente, J., Almazán, C., Canales, M., Lastra, J.M.P., Kocan, K.M. *et al.* (2007a) A ten-year review of commercial vaccine performance for control of tick infestations on cattle. *Animal Health Research Reviews* 8/1, 23–28. DOI: 10.1017/S1466252307001193.

de la Fuente, J., Blouin, E.F., Manzano-Roman, R., Naranjo, V., Almazán, C. *et al.* (2007b) Functional genomic studies of tick cells in response to infection with the cattle pathogen, *Anaplasma marginale*. *Genomics* 90/6, 712–722. DOI: 10.1016/j.ygeno.2007.08.009.

de la Fuente, J., Maritz-Olivier, C., Naranjo, V., Ayoubi, P., Nijhof, A.M. *et al.* (2008) Evidence of the role of tick subolesin in gene expression. *BMC Genomics* 9, 372. DOI: 10.1186/1471-2164-9-372.

de la Fuente, J., Kocan, K.M., Blouin, E.F., Zivkovic, Z., Naranjo, V. *et al.* (2010) Functional genomics and evolution of tick–*Anaplasma* interactions and vaccine development. *Veterinary Parasitology* 167, 175–186. DOI: 10.1016/j.vetpar.2009.09.019.

de la Fuente, J., Moreno-Cid, J.A., Canales, M., Villar, M., Lastra, J.M.P. *et al.* (2011) Targeting arthropod subolesin/akirin for the development of a universal vaccine for control of vector infestations and pathogen transmission. *Veterinary Parasitology* 181/1, 17–22. DOI: 10.1016/j.vetpar.2011.04.018.

de la Fuente, J., Moreno-Cid, J.A., Galindo, R.C., Almazan, C., Kocan, K.M. *et al.* (2013) Subolesin/Akirin vaccines for the control of arthropod vectors and vectorborne pathogens. *Transboundary and Emerging Diseases* 60(Suppl 2), 172–178. DOI: 10.1111/tbed.12146.

de la Fuente, J., Contreras, M., Estrada-Peña, A. and Cabezas-Cruz, A. (2017) Targeting a global health problem: Vaccine design and challenges for the control of tick-borne diseases. *Vaccine* 35/38, 5089–5094. DOI: 10.1016/j.vaccine.2017.07.097.

del Castillo, S.M.L.-C., Hernández-Ortiz, R., Gómez-Romero, N., Martínez-Velázquez, M., Castro-Saines, E. *et al.* (2020) Genetic diversity of the ATAQ gene in *Rhipicephalus microplus* collected in Mexico and implications as anti-tick vaccine. *Parasitology Research* 119, 3523–3529. DOI: 10.1007/s00436-020-06773-6.

De Rose, R., McKenna, R.V., Cobon, G., Tennent, J., Zakrzewski, H. *et al.* (1999) Bm86 antigen induces a protective immune response against *Boophilus microplus* following DNA and protein vaccination in sheep. *Veterinary Immunology and Immunopathology* 71, 151–160. DOI: 10.1016/s0165-2427(99)00038-0.

de Veer, M.J. and Meeusen, E. (2011) New developments in vaccine research – unveiling the secret of vaccine adjuvants. *Discovery Medicine* 12/4, 195–204.

de Vos, A.J. and Jorgensen, W.K. (1992) Protection of cattle against babesiosis in tropical and subtropical countries with a live, frozen vaccine. In: Fivaz, B., Petney, T. and Horak, I. (eds) *Tick Vector Biology*. Springer, Berlin, pp. 159–174.

de Vos, S., Zeinstra, L., Taoufik, A., Willadsen, P. and Jongejan, F. (2001) Evidence for the utility of the Bm86 antigen from *Boophilus microplus* in vaccination against other tick species. *Experimental & Applied Acarology* 25/3, 245–261.

Duttagupta, D.S., Jadhav, V.M. and Kadam, V.J. (2015) Chitosan: A propitious biopolymer for drug delivery. *Current Drug Delivery* 12, 369–381.

Estrada-Peña, A. and Cabezas-Cruz, A. (2019) Towards the integrative analysis of tick microbiome. *Ticks & Tick-Borne Diseases* 10/1, 34–35. DOI: 10.1016/j.ttbdis.2018.08.017.

Estrada-Peña, A., Cabezas-Cruz, A. and Obregon, D. (2020) Behind taxonomic variability: The functional redundancy in the tick microbiome. *Microorganisms* 8/11, 1829. DOI: 10.3390/microorganisms8111829.

Ferreira, C.A.S., Barbosa, M.C., Silveira, T.C., Valenzuela, J.G., Da Silva Vaz, I. *et al.* (2002) cDNA cloning, expression and characterization of a *Boophilus microplus* paramyosin. *Parasitology* 125/3, 265–274. DOI: 10.1017/s0031182002002019.

Figlerowicz, M., Urbanowicz, A., Lewandowski, D., Jodynis-Liebert, J. and Sadowski, C. (2013) Functional insights into recombinant TROSPA protein from *Ixodes ricinus*. *PLoS One* 8/10, e76848. DOI: 10.1371/journal.pone.0076848.

Floyd, R.B., Sutherst, R.W. and Hungerford, J. (1995) Modelling the field efficacy of a genetically engineered vaccine against the cattle tick, *Boophilus microplus*. *International Journal for Parasitology* 25/3, 285–291. DOI: 10.1016/0020-7519(94)00084-2.

Fogaça, A.C., Sousa, G., Pavanelo, D.B., Esteves, E., Martins, L.A. *et al.* (2021) Tick immune system: What is known, the interconnections, the gaps, and the challenges. *Frontiers in Immunology* 12, 628054. DOI: 10.3389/fimmu.2021.628054.

Frampton, G., Moriya, S., Pearson, J.D., Isenberg, D.A., Ward, F.J. *et al.* (2000) Identification of candidate endothelial cell autoantigens in systemic lupus erythematosus using a molecular cloning strategy: A role for ribosomal P protein P0 as an endothelial cell autoantigen. *Rheumatology* 39, 1114–1120.

Francischetti, I.M., Sá-Nunes, A., Mans, B.J., Santos, I.M. and Ribeiro, J.M.C. (2009) The role of saliva in tick feeding. *Frontiers in Bioscience* 14, 2051–2088.

Francischetti, I.M.B., Anderson, J.M., Manoukis, N., Pham, V.M. and Ribeiro, J.M.C. (2011) An insight into the sialotranscriptome and proteome of the coarse bontlegged tick, *Hyalomma marginatum rufipes*. *Journal of Proteomics* 74/12, 2892–2908. DOI: 10.1016/j.jprot.2011.07.015.

Freeman, J.M., Davey, R.B., Kappmeyer, L.S., Kammlah, D.M. and Olafson, P.U. (2010) Bm86 midgut protein sequence variation in South Texas cattle fever ticks. *Parasites and Vectors* 3, 101.

Freyn, A.W., da Silva, J.R., Rosado, V.C., Bliss, C.M., Pine, M. *et al.* (2020) A multi-targeting, nucleoside-modified mRNA influenza virus vaccine provides broad protection in mice. *Molecular Therapy* 28/7, 1569–1584. DOI: 10.1016/j.ymthe.2020.04.018.

Frickenstein, A.N., Hagood, J.M., Britten, C.N., Abbott, B.S., McNally, M.W. *et al.* (2021) *Mesoporous silica* nanoparticles: Properties and strategies for enhancing clinical effect. *Pharmaceutics* 13, 570. DOI: 10.3390/pharmaceutics13040570.

Galay, R.L., Aung, K.M., Umemiya-Shirafuji, R., Maeda, H., Matsuo, T. *et al.* (2013) Multiple ferritins are vital to successful blood feeding and reproduction of the hard tick *Haemaphysalis longicornis*. *Journal of Experimental Biology* 216/10, 1905–1915. DOI: 10.1242/jeb.081240.

García-García, J.C., Gonzalez, I.L., González, D.M., Valdés, M., Méndez, L. *et al.* (1999) Sequence variations in the *Boophilus microplus* Bm86 locus and implications for immunoprotection in cattle vaccinated with this antigen. *Experimental & Applied Acarology* 23, 883–895.

García-García, J.C., Montero, C., Redondo, M., Vargas, M., Canales, M. *et al.* (2000) Control of ticks resistant to immunization with Bm86 in cattle vaccinated with the recombinant antigen Bm95 isolated from the cattle tick, *Boophilus microplus*. *Vaccine* 18/21, 2275–2287. DOI: 10.1016/s0264-410x(99)00548-4.

Ghimire, T.R., Benson, R.A., Garside, P. and Brewer, J.M. (2012) Alum increases antigen uptake, reduces antigen degradation and sustains antigen presentation by DCs *in vitro*. *Immunology Letters* 147/1-2, 55–62. DOI: 10.1016/j.imlet.2012.06.002.

Giachetto, P.F., Cunha, R.C., Nhani, A., Garcia, M.V., Ferro, J.A. *et al.* (2020) Gene expression in the salivary gland of *Rhipicephalus* (*Boophilus*) *microplus* fed on tick-susceptible and tick-resistant hosts. *Frontiers in Cellular and Infection Microbiology* 9, 477. DOI: 10.3389/fcimb.2019.00477.

Githaka, N.W.O., Konnai, S., Isezaki, M., Goto, S., Xavier, M.A. *et al.* (2020) Identification and functional analysis of ferritin 2 from the Taiga tick *Ixodes persulcatus* schulze. *Ticks & Tick-Borne Diseases* 11/6, 101547. DOI: 10.1016/j.ttbdis.2020.101547.

Gonsioroski, A.V., Bezerra, I.A., Utiumi, K.U., Driemeier, D., Farias, S.E. *et al.* (2012) Anti-tick monoclonal antibody applied by artificial capillary feeding in *Rhipicephalus* (*Boophilus*) *microplus* females. *Experimental Parasitology* 130/4, 359–363. DOI: 10.1016/j.exppara.2012.02.006.

Goodswen, S.J., Kennedy, P.J. and Ellis, J.T. (2012) A guide to *in silico* vaccine discovery for eukaryotic pathogens. *Briefings in Bioinformatics* 14/6, 753–774. DOI: 10.1093/bib/bbs066.

Goodswen, S.J., Kennedy, P.J. and Ellis, J.T. (2013) A novel strategy for classifying the output from an *in silico* vaccine discovery pipeline for eukaryotic pathogens using machine learning algorithms. *BMC Bioinformatics* 14, 315. DOI: 10.1186/1471-2105-14-315.

Goodswen, S.J., Kennedy, P.J. and Ellis, J.T. (2014a) Enhancing *in silico* protein-based vaccine discovery for eukaryotic pathogens using predicted peptide-MHC binding and peptide conservation scores. *PLoS One* 9/12, e115745. DOI: 10.1371/journal.pone.0115745.

Goodswen, S.J., Kennedy, P.J. and Ellis, J.T. (2014b) Vacceed: A high-throughput *in silico* vaccine candidate discovery pipeline for eukaryotic pathogens based on reverse vaccinology. *Bioinformatics* 30/16, 2381–2383. DOI: 10.1093/bioinformatics/btu300.

Goodswen, S.J., Kennedy, P.J. and Ellis, J.T. (2023) A guide to current methodology and usage of reverse vaccinology towards *in silico* vaccine discovery. *FEMS Microbiology Reviews* 47/2, fuad004.

Goto, A., Matsushita, K., Gesellchen, V., Chamy, L.E., Kuttenkeuler, D. *et al.* (2008a) Akirins are highly conserved nuclear proteins required for NF-κB-dependent gene expression in drosophila and mice. *Nature Immunology* 9, 97–104.

Goto, A., Matsushita, K., Gesellchen, V., Chamy, L.E., Kuttenkeuler, D. *et al.* (2008b) Erratum: Akirins are highly conserved nuclear proteins required for NF-κB-dependent gene expression in drosophila and mice. *Nature Immunology* 9, 216. DOI: 10.1038/ni0208-216.

Guerrero, F.D., Kellogg, A., Ogrey, A.N., Heekin, A.M., Barrero, R. *et al.* (2016) Prediction of G protein-coupled receptor encoding sequences from the synganglion transcriptome of the cattle tick, *Rhipicephalus microplus*. *Ticks & Tick-Borne Diseases* 7/5, 670–677. DOI: 10.1016/j.ttbdis.2016.02.014.

Guizzo, M.G., Mans, B., Pienaar, R. and Ribeiro, J.M.C. (2023) A comparison of illumina and PacBio methods to build tick salivary gland transcriptomes confirms large expression of lipocalins and other salivary protein families that are not represented in available tick genomes. *Ticks & Tick-Borne Diseases* 14/6, 102209. DOI: 10.1016/j.ttbdis.2023.102209.

Hajdusek, O., Sojka, D., Kopacek, P., Buresova, V., Franta, Z. *et al.* (2009) Knockdown of proteins involved in iron metabolism limits tick reproduction and development. *Proceedings of the National Academy of Sciences of the USA* 106/4, 1033–1038. DOI: 10.1073/pnas.0807961106.

Hajdusek, O., Almazán, C., Loosova, G., Villar, M., Canales, M. *et al.* (2010) Characterization of ferritin 2 for the control of tick infestations. *Vaccine* 28, 2993–2998. DOI: 10.1016/j.vaccine.2010.02.008.

Hajdušek, O., Šíma, R., Ayllón, N., Jalovecká, M., Perner, J. *et al.* (2013) Interaction of the tick immune system with transmitted pathogens. *Frontiers in Cellular and Infection Microbiology* 3/26, 1–15. DOI: 10.3389/fcimb.2013.00026.

Hall-Mendelin, S., Craig, S.B., Hall, R.A., O'donoghue, P., Atwell, R.B. *et al.* (2011) Tick paralysis in Australia caused by *Ixodes holocyclus* Neumann. *Annals of Tropical Medicine and Parasitology* 105/2, 95–106. DOI: 10.1179/136485911X12899838413628.

Harris, J.R. and Markl, J. (1999) Keyhole limpet hemocyanin (KLH): A biomedical review. *Micron* 30/6, 597–623. DOI: 10.1016/S0968-4328(99)00036-0.

Hasler, P., Brot, N., Weissbach, H., Parnassa, A.P. and Elkon, K.B. (1991) Ribosomal proteins P0, P1, and P2 are phosphorylated by casein kinase II at their conserved carboxyl termini. *Journal of Biological Chemistry* 266/21, 13815–13820.

Hassan, I.A., Wang, Y., Zhou, Y., Cao, J., Zhang, H. *et al.* (2020) Cross protection induced by combined Subolesin-based DNA and protein immunizations against adult *Haemaphysalis longicornis*. *Vaccine* 38/4, 907–915. DOI: 10.1016/j.vaccine.2019.10.076.

Hauser, F., Pallesen, M., Lehnhof, J., Li, S., Lind, A. *et al.* (2023) A corazonin G protein-coupled receptor gene in the tick *Ixodes scapularis* yields two splice variants, each coding for A specific corazonin receptor. *Biochemical and Biophysical Research Communications* 666, 162–169. DOI: 10.1016/j.bbrc.2023.04.087.

Havlíková, S., Roller, L., Koči, J., Trimnell, A.R., Kazimírová, M. *et al.* (2009) Functional role of 64P, the candidate transmission-blocking vaccine antigen from the tick, *Rhipicephalus appendiculatus*. *International Journal for Parasitology* 39/13, 1485–1494. DOI: 10.1016/j.ijpara.2009.05.005.

Hepler, J.R. and Gilman, A.G. (1992) G proteins. *Trends in Biochemical Sciences* 17, 383–387.

Hernandez, E.P., Shimazaki, K., Niihara, H., Umemiya-Shirafuji, R., Fujisaki, K. *et al.* (2023) Localization of secreted ferritin (FER2) in the embryos of the tick *Haemaphysalis longicornis*. *Parasites and Vectors* 16/1, 42. DOI: 10.1186/s13071-023-05669-5.

Holdsworth, P.A., Kemp, D., Green, P., Peter, R.J., Bruin, C. *et al.* (2006) World Association for the Advancement of Veterinary Parasitology (W.A.A.V.P.) guidelines for evaluating the efficacy of acaricides against ticks (Ixodidae) on ruminants. *Veterinary Parasitology* 136/1, 29–43. DOI: 10.1016/j.vetpar.2005.11.011.

Hollmann, T., Kim, T.K., Tirloni, L., Radulović, Ž.M., Pinto, A.F. *et al.* (2018) Identification and characterization of proteins in the *Amblyomma americanum* tick cement cone. *International Journal for Parasitology* 48/3–4, 211–224. DOI: 10.1016/j.ijpara.2017.08.018.

Hood, S., Edelsten, R.M. and Branagan, D. (1976) The maintenance of the argasid tick *Ornithodoros moubata* (Murray) on embryonated hen eggs. *Tropical Animal Health and Production* 8/3, 163–167.

Hope, M., Jiang, X., Gough, J., Cadogan, L., Josh, P. *et al.* (2010) Experimental vaccination of sheep and cattle against tick infestation using recombinant 5'-nucleotidase. *Parasite Immunology* 32, 135–142. DOI: 10.1111/j.1365-3024.2009.01168.x.

Huston, J.S., Levinson, D., Mudgett-Hunter, M., Tai, M.S., Novotný, J. *et al.* (1988) Protein engineering of antibody binding sites: recovery of specific activity in an anti-digoxin single-chain Fv analogue produced in *Escherichia coli*. *Proceedings of the National Academy of Sciences USA* 85/16, 5879–5883. DOI: 10.1073/pnas.85.16.5879.

Hynes, A.P., Villion, M. and Moineau, S. (2014) Adaptation in bacterial CRISPR-Cas immunity can be driven by defective phages. *Nature Communications* 5, 4399. DOI: 10.1038/ncomms5399.

Irvin, A.D. (ed.) (1985) Immunization against theileriosis in Africa. In: *Proceedings of a Joint Workshop, International Laboratory for Research on Animal Diseases and Food and Agriculture Organization of the United Nations,* Nairobi, October 1-5, 1984.

Jarmey, J.M., Riding, G.A., Pearson, R.D., McKenna, R.V. and Willadsen, P. (1995) Carboxydipeptidase from *Boophilus microplus*: A 'concealed' antigen with similarity to angiotensin-converting enzyme. *Insect Biochemistry and Molecular Biology* 25/9, 969–974.

Jasinskas, A., Jaworski, D.C. and Barbour, A.G. (2000) *Amblyomma americanum*: Specific uptake of immunoglobulins into tick hemolymph during feeding. *Experimental Parasitology* 96, 213–221. DOI: 10.1006/expr.2000.4567.

Jawalagatti, V., Kirthika, P., Hewawaduge, C., Yang, M.S., Park, J.Y. *et al.* (2022) Bacteria-enabled oral delivery of a replicon-based mRNA vaccine candidate protects against ancestral and delta variant SARS-coV-2. *Molecular Therapy* 30/5, 1926–1940. DOI: 10.1016/j.ymthe.2022.01.042.

Jeyabal, L., Azhahianambi, P., Susitha, K., Ray, D.D., Chaudhuri, P. *et al.* (2010) Efficacy of rHaa86, an orthologue of Bm86, against challenge infestations of *Hyalomma anatolicum anatolicum*. *Transboundary and Emerging Diseases* 57/1-2, 96–102. DOI: 10.1111/j.1865-1682.2010.01107.x.

Johnston, L.A.Y., Kemp, D.H. and Pearson, R.D. (1986) Immunization of cattle against *Boophilus microplus* using extracts derived from adult female ticks: Effects of induced immunity on tick populations. *International Journal for Parasitology* 16/1, 27–34.

Jongejan, F., Nene, V., Fuente, J., Pain, A. and Willadsen, P. (2007) Advances in the genomics of ticks and tick-borne pathogens. *Trends in Parasitology* 23/9, 391–396. DOI: 10.1016/j.pt.2007.07.004.

Jonsson, N.N., Matschoss, A.L., Pepper, P., Green, P.E., Albrecht, M.S. *et al.* (2000) Evaluation of tickGARD^{PLUS}, a novel vaccine against *Boophilus microplus*, in lactating Holstein-Friesian cows. *Veterinary Parasitology* 88, 275–285.

Jonsson, N.N., Piper, E.K. and Constantinoiu, C.C. (2014) Host resistance in cattle to infestation with the cattle tick *Rhipicephalus microplus*. *Parasite Immunology* 36/11, 553–559. DOI: 10.1111/pim.12140.

Jonsson, N.N., Klafke, G.M., Corley, S.W., Tidwell, J., Berry, C.M. *et al.* (2018) Molecular biology of amitraz resistance in cattle ticks of the genus *Rhipicephalus*. *Frontiers in Bioscience* 23/2, 796–810. DOI: 10.2741/4617.

Kamau, L.M., Skilton, R.A., Githaka, N., Kiara, H., Kabiru, E. *et al.* (2016) Extensive polymorphism of Ra86 genes in field populations of *Rhipicephalus appendiculatus* from Kenya. *Ticks & Tick-Borne Diseases* 7/5, 772–781. DOI: 10.1016/j.ttbdis.2016.03.011.

Kelly, K. (2018) What are reasonable expectations of ovine toxoplasmosis vaccine? In: *Proceedings of Australian Small Animal Veterinarians, Sheep Camelid and Goat Veterinarians, and Australian Veterinary Behaviour Interest Group Conference*, Melbourne, pp. 242–247.

Kemp, D.H., Agbede, R.I.S., Johnston, L.A.Y. and Gough, J.M. (1986) Immunization of cattle against *Boophilus microplus* using extracts derived from adult female ticks: Feeding and survival of the parasite on vaccinated cattle. *International Journal for Parasitology* 16/2, 115–120.

Kim, T.K., Ibelli, A.M.G. and Mulenga, A. (2015a) *Amblyomma americanum* tick calreticulin binds C1q but does not inhibit activation of the classical complement cascade. *Ticks & Tick-Borne Diseases* 6/1, 91–101. DOI: 10.1016/j.ttbdis.2014.10.002.

Kim, T.K., Tirloni, L., Radulovic, Z., Lewis, L., Bakshi, M. *et al.* (2015b) Conserved *Amblyomma americanum* tick Serpin19, an inhibitor of blood clotting factors Xa and XIa, trypsin and plasmin, has anti-haemostatic functions. *International Journal for Parasitology* 45/9-12, 613–627. DOI: 10.1016/j.ijpara.2015.03.009.

Kim, T.K., Radulovic, Z. and Mulenga, A. (2016a) Target validation of highly conserved *Amblyomma americanum* tick saliva serine protease inhibitor 19. *Ticks & Tick-Borne Diseases* 7/3, 405–414. DOI: 10.1016/j.ttbdis.2015.12.017.

Kim, T.K., Tirloni, L., Pinto, A.F., Moresco, J., Yates III, J.R. *et al.* (2016b) *Ixodes scapularis* tick saliva proteins sequentially secreted every 24 h during blood feeding. *PLoS Neglected Tropical Diseases* 10/1, e0004323. DOI: 10.1371/journal.pntd.0004323.

Kinyua, J.K., Osir, E.O., Ogoyi, D.O. and Nguu, E.K. (2002) Characterization of protective antigens from the midgut of *Amblyomma variegatum* ticks. *Experimental & Applied Acarology* 26, 101–113.

Kiper, I. (2013) Two-hybrid analysis and functional annotation of Bm86 and ATAQ from *Rhipicephalus microplus*. MSc thesis, University of Pretoria, Pretoria, South Africa.

Klouwens, M.J., Trentelman, J.J.A., Wagemakers, A., Ersoz, J.I., Bins, A.D. *et al.* (2021) Tick-tattoo: DNA vaccination against *B. burgdorferi* or *Ixodes scapularis* tick proteins. *Frontiers in Immunology* 12, 615011. DOI: 10.3389/fimmu.2021.615011.

Kocan, K.M., Manzano-Roman, R. and Fuente, J. (2007) Transovarial silencing of the subolesin gene in three-host ixodid tick species after injection of replete females with subolesin dsRNA. *Parasitology Research* 100, 1411–1415. DOI: 10.1007/s00436-007-0483-1.

Koči, J., Bista, S., Chirania, P., Yang, X., Kitsou, C. *et al.* (2021) Antibodies against EGF-like domains in *Ixodes scapularis* BM86 orthologs impact tick feeding and survival of *Borrelia burgdorferi*. *Scientific Reports* 11/1, 6095. DOI: 10.1038/s41598-021-85624-5.

Konnai, S., Nishikado, H., Yamada, S., Imamura, S., Ito, T. *et al.* (2011) Molecular identification and expression analysis of lipocalins from blood feeding taiga tick, *Ixodes persulcatus* Schulze. *Experimental Parasitology* 127/2, 467–474. DOI: 10.1016/j.exppara.2010.10.002.

Koonin, E.V. (2005) Orthologs, paralogs, and evolutionary genomics. *Annual Review of Genetics* 39, 309–338. DOI: 10.1146/annurev.genet.39.073003.114725.
Kröber, T. and Guerin, P.M. (2007) *In vitro* feeding assays for hard ticks. *Trends in Parasitology* 23/9, 445–449. DOI: 10.1016/j.pt.2007.07.010.
Kumar, B., Manjunathachar, H.V., Nagar, G., Ravikumar, G., Fuente, J. *et al.* (2017) Functional characterization of candidate antigens of *Hyalomma anatolicum* and evaluation of its cross-protective efficacy against *Rhipicephalus microplus*. *Vaccine* 35/42, 5682–5692. DOI: 10.1016/j.vaccine.2017.08.049.
Labuda, M., Trimnell, A.R., Ličková, M., Kazimírová, M., Davies, G.M. *et al.* (2006) An antivector vaccine protects against a lethal vector-borne pathogen. *PLoS Pathogens* 2/4, e27. DOI: 10.1371/journal.ppat.0020027.
Leal, A.T., Pohl, P.C., Ferreira, C.A., Nascimento-Silva, M.C., Sorgine, M.H. *et al.* (2006a) Purification and antigenicity of two recombinant forms of *Boophilus microplus* yolk pro-cathepsin expressed in inclusion bodies. *Protein Expression and Purification* 45/1, 107–114. DOI: 10.1016/j.pep.2005.07.009.
Leal, A.T., Seixas, A., Pohl, P.C., Ferreira, C.A., Logullo, C. *et al.* (2006b) Vaccination of bovines with recombinant *Boophilus* yolk pro-cathepsin. *Veterinary Immunology and Immunopathology* 114/3-4, 341–345. DOI: 10.1016/j.vetimm.2006.08.011.
Leal, B.F. and Ferreira, C.A.S. (2021) Ticks and antibodies: May parasite density and tick evasion influence the outcomes following immunization protocols?. *Veterinary Parasitology* 300, 109610. DOI: 10.1016/j.vetpar.2021.109610.
Leal, B.F., Seixas, A., Mattos, R.T., Coutinho, M.L., Masuda, A. *et al.* (2013) Tissue expression and the host's immunological recognition of a *Rhipicephalus microplus* paramyosin. *Veterinary Parasitology* 197/1-2, 304–311. DOI: 10.1016/j.vetpar.2013.06.020.
Lee, S.H., Li, J., Moumouni, P.F.A., Okado, K., Zheng, W. *et al.* (2020) Subolesin vaccination inhibits blood feeding and reproduction of *Haemaphysalis longicornis* in rabbits. *Parasites and Vectors* 13, 478. DOI: 10.1186/s13071-020-04359-w.
Lew-Tabor, A.E. and Rodriguez-Valle, M. (2016) A review of reverse vaccinology approaches for the development of vaccines against ticks and tick-borne diseases. *Ticks & Tick-Borne Diseases* 7, 573–585. DOI: 10.1016/j.ttbdis.2015.12.012.
Lew-Tabor, A.E., Kurscheid, S., Barrero, R., Gondro, C., Moolhuijzen, P.M. *et al.* (2011) Gene expression evidence for off-target effects caused by RNA interference-mediated gene silencing of ubiquitin-63E in the cattle tick *Rhipicephalus microplus*. *International Journal for Parasitology* 41/9, 1001–1014. DOI: 10.1016/j.ijpara.2011.05.003.
Lew-Tabor, A.E., Bruyeres, A.G., Zhang, B. and Rodriguez-Valle, M. (2014) *Rhipicephalus* (*Boophilus*) *microplus* tick in vitro feeding methods for functional (dsRNA) and vaccine candidate (antibody) screening. *Ticks & Tick-Borne Diseases* 5/5, 500–510. DOI: 10.1016/j.ttbdis.2014.03.005.
Liang, N., Dong, H.M., Fan, X.Y., Wu, Y.X., Yang, F. *et al.* (2022) Characterization and evaluation of a new triosephosphate isomerase homologue from *Haemaphysalis longicornis* as a candidate vaccine against tick infection. *Ticks & Tick-Borne Diseases* 13/4, 101968. DOI: 10.1016/j.ttbdis.2022.101968.
Liu, F., Ge, S., Li, L., Wu, X., Liu, Z. *et al.* (2012) Virus-like particles: Potential veterinary vaccine immunogens. *Research in Veterinary Science* 93/2, 553–559. DOI: 10.1016/j.rvsc.2011.10.018.
Lodos, J., Boue, O. and Fuente, J. (2000) A model to simulate the effect of vaccination against *Boophilus* ticks on cattle. *Veterinary Parasitology* 87, 315–326. DOI: 10.1016/S0304-4017(99)00187-9.
Lu, S., Rocha, L.A., Torquato, R.J., Junior, I.D.S.V., Florin-Christensen, M. *et al.* (2020) A novel type 1 cystatin involved in the regulation of *Rhipicephalus microplus* midgut cysteine proteases. *Ticks & Tick-Borne Diseases* 11/3, 101374. DOI: 10.1016/j.ttbdis.2020.101374.
Lynn, G.E., Černý, J., Kurokawa, C., Diktaş, H., Matias, J. *et al.* (2022) Immunization of guinea pigs with cement extract induces resistance against *Ixodes scapularis* ticks. *Ticks & Tick-Borne Diseases* 13/6, 102017. DOI: 10.1016/j.ttbdis.2022.102017.
Maecker, H.T., Umetsu, D.T., DeKruyff, R.H. and Levy, S. (1997) DNA vaccination with cytokine fusion constructs biases the immune response to ovalbumin. *Vaccine* 15/15, 1687–1696. DOI: 10.1016/S0264-410X(97)00088-1.
Mahony, T.J. (2021) Evaluation of anti-tick vaccines for tick immunological control in cattle. MLA final report B.AHE.2026. Available at: https://www.mla.com.au/research-and-development/search-rd-reports/?q=%22b.ahe.2026%22&sort=1 (accessed 17 July 2024).
Mahony, T.J., Al Kobaisi, M. and Mainwaring, D. (2019) Testing and verification of a single-dose cattle tick vaccine. MLA final report B.AHE.0316. Available at: https://www.mla.com.au/research-and-development/search-rd-reports/?q=%22b.ahe.0316%22&sort=1 (accessed 17 July 2024).

Mahony, T.J., Briody, T.E. and Ommeh, S.C. (2024) Can the revolution in mRNA-based vaccine technologies solve the intractable health issues of current ruminant production systems? *Vaccines* 12, 152. DOI: 10.3390/vaccines12020152.

Maine, C.J., Richard, G., Spasova, D.S., Miyake-Stoner, S.J., Sparks, J. *et al.* (2021) Self-replicating RNAs drive protective anti-tumor T cell responses to neoantigen vaccine targets in a combinatorial approach. *Molecular Therapy* 29/3, 1187–1198. DOI: 10.1016/j.ymthe.2020.11.027.

Maitre, A., Wu-Chuang, A., Aželytė, J., Palinauskas, V., Mateos-Hernández, L. *et al.* (2022) Vector microbiota manipulation by host antibodies: The forgotten strategy to develop transmission-blocking vaccines. *Parasites and Vectors* 15, 4. DOI: 10.1186/s13071-021-05122-5.

Malone, R.W., Felgner, P.L. and Verma, I.M. (1989) Cationic liposome-mediated RNA transfection. *Proceedings of the National Academy of Sciences USA* 86, 6077–6081.

Mans, B.J., Louw, A.I. and Neitz, A.W.H. (2003) The major tick salivary gland proteins and toxins from the soft tick, *Ornithodoros savignyi*, are part of the tick lipocalin family: Implications for the origins of tick toxicoses. *Molecular Biology and Evolution* 20/7, 1158–1167. DOI: 10.1093/molbev/msg126.

Martínez-Arzate, S.G., Sánchez-Bermúdez, J.C., Sotelo-Gómez, S., Diaz-Albiter, H.M., Hegazy-Hassan, W. *et al.* (2019) Genetic diversity of Bm86 sequences in *Rhipicephalus* (*Boophilus*) *microplus* ticks from Mexico: Analysis of haplotype distribution patterns. *BMC Genetics* 20, 56. DOI: 10.1186/s12863-019-0754-8.

Maruggi, G., Zhang, C., Li, J., Ulmer, J.B. and Yu, D. (2019) mRNA as a transformative technology for vaccine development to control infectious diseases. *Molecular Therapy* 27/4, 757–772.

Maruyama, S.R., Anatriello, E., Anderson, J.M., Ribeiro, J.M., Brandão, L.G. *et al.* (2010) The expression of genes coding for distinct types of glycine-rich proteins varies according to the biology of three metastriate ticks, *Rhipicephalus* (*Boophilus*) *microplus*, *Rhipicephalus sanguineus* and *Amblyomma cajennense*. *BMC Genomics* 11, 363. Available at: http://www.biomedcentral.com/1471-2164/11/363 (accessed 4 January 2025).

Masina, S. (1999) The sequence, expression and immunological characterisation of the HT-1 neurotoxin from the Australian paralysis tick *Ixodes holocyclus*. PhD thesis, University of Technology, Sydney, Australia.

Masina, S. and Broady, K.W. (1999) Tick paralysis: Development of a vaccine. *International Journal for Parasitology* 29, 535–541.

Mateos-Hernández, L., Obregón, D., Maye, J., Borneres, J., Versille, N. *et al.* (2020) Anti-tick microbiota vaccine impacts *Ixodes ricinus* performance during feeding. *Vaccines* 8/4, 702. DOI: 10.3390/vaccines8040702.

Mateos-Hernández, L., Obregón, D., Wu-Chuang, A., Maye, J., Bornères, J. *et al.* (2021) Anti-microbiota vaccines modulate the tick microbiome in a taxon-specific manner. *Frontiers in Immunology* 12, 704621. DOI: 10.3389/fimmu.2021.704621.

Matias, J., Cui, Y., Tang, X., Sajid, A., Arora, G. *et al.* (2023) Specific mRNA lipid nanoparticles and acquired resistance to ticks. *Vaccine* 41, 4996–5002. DOI: 10.1016/j.vaccine.2023.06.081.

McCafferty, S., De Temmerman, J., Kitada, T., Becraft, J.R., Weiss, R. *et al.* (2021) *In vivo* validation of a reversible small molecule-based switch for synthetic self-amplifying mRNA regulation. *Molecular Therapy* 29/3, 1164–1173. DOI: 10.1016/j.ymthe.2020.11.010.

McClure Carroll, E.E., Wang, X., Shaw, D.K., O'Neal, A.J., Oliva Chávez, A.S. *et al.* (2019) p47 licenses activation of the immune deficiency pathway in the tick *Ixodes scapularis*. *Proceedings of the National Academy of Sciences USA* 116/1, 205–210.

Meeusen, E.N., Walker, J., Peters, A., Pastoret, P.P. and Jungersen, G. (2007) Current status of veterinary vaccines. *Clinical Microbiology Reviews* 2013, 489–510. DOI: 10.1128/CMR.00005-07.

Meeusen, E.N., de Veer, M., Hertzog, P.J., Stear, M.J., Mallard, B.A. *et al.* (2013) New approaches to innate immunity in livestock and the potential for manipulation - review. MLA final report B.BSC.0321. Available at: https://www.mla.com.au/research-and-development/search-rd-reports/?q=b.bsc.0321&sort=1 (accessed 15 October 2023).

Mendoza-Martinez, N., Alonso-Diaz, M.A., Merino, O., Fernandez-Salas, A. and Lagunes-Quintanilla, R. (2021) Protective efficacy of the peptide subolesin antigen against the cattle tick *Rhipicephalus microplus* under natural infestation. *Veterinary Parasitology* 299, 109577. DOI: 10.1016/j.vetpar.2021.109577.

Merino, O., Almazán, C., Canales, M., Villar, M., Moreno-Cid, J.A. *et al.* (2011) Targeting the tick protective antigen subolesin reduces vector infestations and pathogen infection by *Anaplasma marginale* and *Babesia bigemina*. *Vaccine* 29, 8575–8579. DOI: 10.1016/j.vaccine.2011.09.023.

Merino, O., Alberdi, P., Perez de la Lastra, J.M. and de la Fuente, J. (2013a) Tick vaccines and the control of tick-borne pathogens. *Frontiers in Cellular and Infection Microbiology* 3, 30. DOI: 10.3389/fcimb.2013.00030.

Merino, O., Antunes, S., Mosqueda, J., Moreno-Cid, J.A., Lastra, J.M.P. *et al.* (2013b) Vaccination with proteins involved in tick-pathogen interactions reduces vector infestations and pathogen infection. *Vaccine* 31/49, 5889–5896. DOI: 10.1016/j.vaccine.2013.09.037.

Mody, K.T., Zhang, B., Li, X., Fletcher, N.L., Akhter, D.T. *et al.* (2021) Characterization of the biodistribution of a silica vesicle nanovaccine carrying a *Rhipicephalus* (*Boophilus*) *microplus* protective antigen with *in vivo* live animal imaging. *Frontiers in Bioengineering and Biotechnology* 8, 606652. DOI: 10.3389/fbioe.2020.606652.

Moreno-Cid, J.A., de la Lastra, J.M.P., Villar, M., Jiménez, M., Pinal, R. *et al.* (2013) Control of multiple arthropod vector infestations with subolesin/akirin vaccines. *Vaccine* 31/8, 1187–1196. DOI: 10.1016/j.vaccine.2012.12.073.

Naranjo, V., Ayllon, N., Perez de la Lastra, J.M., Galindo, R.C., Kocan, K.M. *et al.* (2013) Reciprocal regulation of NF-kB (Relish) and subolesin in the tick vector, *Ixodes scapularis*. *PLoS One* 8/6, e65915. DOI: 10.1371/journal.pone.0065915.

Narasimhan, S. and Fikrig, E. (2015) Tick microbiome: The force within. *Trends in Parasitology* 31/7L, 315–323. DOI: 10.1016/j.pt.2015.03.010.

Nene, V., Lee, D., Quackenbush, J., Skilton, R., Mwaura, S. *et al.* (2002) AvGI, an index of genes transcribed in the salivary glands of the ixodid tick *Amblyomma variegatum*. *International Journal for Parasitology* 32, 1447–1456.

Nene, V., Lee, D., Kang'a, S., Skilton, R., Shah, T. *et al.* (2004) Genes transcribed in the salivary glands of female *Rhipicephalus appendiculatus* ticks infected with *Theileria parva*. *Insect Biochemistry and Molecular Biology* 34/10, 1117–1128. DOI: 10.1016/j.ibmb.2004.07.002.

Nijhof, A.M., Taoufik, A., de la Fuente, J., Kocan, K.M., de Vries, E. *et al.* (2007) Gene silencing of the tick protective antigens, Bm86, Bm91 and subolesin, in the one-host tick *Boophilus microplus* by RNA interference. *International Journal for Parasitology* 37/6, 653–662. DOI: 10.1016/j.ijpara.2006.11.005.

Nijhof, A.M., Balk, J.A., Postigo, M., Rhebergen, A.M., Taoufik, A. *et al.* (2010) Bm86 homologues and novel ATAQ proteins with multiple epidermal growth factor (EGF)-like domains from hard and soft ticks. *International Journal for Parasitology* 40, 1587–1597. DOI: 10.1016/j.ijpara.2010.06.003.

Nuttall, P.A., Trimnell, A.R., Kazimirova, M. and Labuda, M. (2006) Exposed and concealed antigens as vaccine targets for controlling ticks and tick-borne diseases. *Parasite Immunology* 28, 155–163. DOI: 10.1111/j.1365-3024.2006.00806.x.

Odongo, D., Kamau, L., Skilton, R., Mwaura, S., Nitsch, C. *et al.* (2007) Vaccination of cattle with TickGARD induces cross-reactive antibodies binding to conserved linear peptides of Bm86 homologues in *Boophilus decoloratus*. *Vaccine* 25/7, 1287–1296. DOI: 10.1016/j.vaccine.2006.09.085.

Olds, C.L., Mwaura, S., Odongo, D.O., Scoles, G.A., Bishop, R. *et al.* (2016) Induction of humoral immune response to multiple recombinant *Rhipicephalus appendiculatus* antigens and their effect on tick feeding success and pathogen transmission. *Parasites and Vectors* 9/1, 484. DOI: 10.1186/s13071-016-1774-0.

Opdebeeck, J.P., Wong, J.Y.M., Jackson, L.A. and Dobson, C. (1988) Vaccines to protect Hereford cattle against the cattle tick, *Boophilus microplus*. *Immunology* 63, 363–367.

Ortega-Sánchez, R., Camacho-Nuez, M., Castañeda-Ortiz, E.J., Martínez-Benítez, M.B., Hernández-Silva, D.J. *et al.* (2020) Vaccine efficacy of recombinant BmVDAC on *Rhipicephalus microplus* fed on *Babesia*-infected and uninfected cattle. *Vaccine* 38/19, 3618–3625. DOI: 10.1016/j.vaccine.2019.12.040.

Paesen, G.C., Adams, P.L., Nuttall, P.A. and Stuart, D.L. (2000) Review. Tick histamine-binding proteins: Lipocalins with a second binding cavity. *Biochimica et Biophysica Acta* 1482, 92–101.

Pal, U., Li, X., Wang, T., Montgomery, R.R., Ramamoorthi, N. *et al.* (2004) TROSPA, an *Ixodes scapularis* receptor for *Borrelia burgdorferi*. *Cell* 119/4, 457–468. DOI: 10.1016/j.cell.2004.10.027.

Pardi, N., Hogan, M.J., Porter, F.W. and Weissman, D. (2018) mRNA vaccines – a new era in vaccinology. *Nature Reviews Drug Discovery* 17/4, 261–279. DOI: 10.1038/nrd.2017.243.

Parizi, L.F., Rangel, C.K., Sabadin, G.A., Saggin, B.F., Kiio, I. *et al.* (2020) *Rhipicephalus microplus* cystatin as a potential cross-protective tick vaccine against *Rhipicephalus appendiculatus*. *Ticks & Tick-Borne Diseases* 11, 101378. DOI: 10.1016/j.ttbdis.2020.101378.

Parizi, L.F., Githaka, N.W.O., Logullo, C., Zhou, J., Onuma, M. *et al.* (2023) Universal tick vaccines: Candidates and remaining challenges. *Animals* 13, 2031. DOI: 10.3390/ani13122031.

Parthasarathi, B.C., Kumar, B. and Ghosh, S. (2021) Current status and future prospects of multi-antigen tick vaccine. *Journal of Vector-Borne Diseases* 58, 183–192.

Parthasarathi, B.C., Kumar, B., Bhure, S.K., Sharma, A.K., Kumar, S. *et al.* (2023) Co-immunization efficacy of recombinant antigens against *Rhipicephalus microplus* and *Hyalomma anatolicum* tick infestations. *Pathogens* 12/3, 43.3. DOI: 10.3390/pathogens12030433.

Patarroyo, J.H., Portela, R.W., de Castro, R.O., Pimentel, J.C., Guzman, F. *et al.* (2002) Immunization of cattle with synthetic peptides derived from the *Boophilus microplus* gut protein (Bm86). *Veterinary Immunology and Immunopathology* 88, 163–172.

Patarroyo, J.H., Vargas, M.I., González, C.Z., Guzmán, F., Martins-Filho, O.A. *et al.* (2009) Immune response of bovines stimulated by synthetic vaccine SBm7462 against *Rhipicephalus* (*Boophilus*) *microplus*. *Veterinary Parasitology* 166/3–4, 333–339. DOI: 10.1016/j.vetpar.2009.09.036.

Patarroyo, J. H., De Sousa Neves, E., Fidelis, C. F., Tafur-Gómez, G.A., Araujo, L. *et al.* (2020) Bovine immunisation with a recombinant peptide derived from synthetic SBm7462(R) (Bm86 epitope construct) immunogen for *Rhipicephalus microplus* control. *Ticks & Tick-Borne Diseases* 11/5: 101461. DOI: 10.1016/j.ttbdis.2020.101461

Pérez-Sánchez, R., Carnero-Morán, A., Luz Valero, M. and Oleaga, A. (2022) A proteomics informed by transcriptomics insight into the proteome of *Ornithodoros erraticus* adult tick saliva. *Parasites and Vectors* 15/1, 1. DOI: 10.1186/s13071-021-05118-1.

Piadel, K., Haybatollahi, A., Dalgleish, A.G. and Smith, P.L. (2022) Selection and T-cell antigenicity of synthetic long peptides derived from SARS-CoV-2. *Journal of General Virology* 103/1, 001698. DOI: 10.1099/jgv.0.001698.

Pierce, A.E. and Pierce, M.H. (1956) A note on the cultivation of *Boophilus microplus* (Canestrini, 1887) (Ixodidae: Acarina) on the embryonated hen egg. *Australian Veterinary Journal* 32/6, 144–146.

Pipano, E., Alekceev, E., Galker, F., Fish, L., Samish, M. *et al.* (2003) Immunity against *Boophilus annulatus* induced by the Bm86 (tick-GARD) vaccine. *Experimental & Applied Acarology* 29/1-2, 141–149.

Pokorna, D., Rubio, I. and Müller, M. (2008) DNA-vaccination via tattooing induces stronger humoral and cellular immune responses than intramuscular delivery supported by molecular adjuvants. *Genetic Vaccines and Therapy* 6, 4. DOI: 10.1186/1479-0556-6-4.

Prego, C., Paolicelli, P., Díaz, B., Vicente, S., Sánchez, A. *et al.* (2010) Chitosan-based nanoparticles for improving immunization against hepatitis B infection. *Vaccine* 28/14, 2607–2614. DOI: 10.1016/j.vaccine.2010.01.011.

Prudencio, C.R., Perez de la Lastra, J.M., Canales, M., Villar, M. and de la Fuente, J. (2010) Mapping protective epitopes in the tick and mosquito subolesin ortholog proteins. *Vaccine* 28/33, 5398–5406. DOI: 10.1016/j.vaccine.2010.06.021.

Quaak, S.G.L., van den Berg, J.H., Oosterhuis, K., Beijnen, J.H., Haanen, J.B. *et al.* (2009) DNA tattoo vaccination: Effect on plasmid purity and transfection efficiency of different topoisoforms. *Journal of Controlled Release* 139/2, 153–159. DOI: 10.1016/j.jconrel.2009.06.033.

Rand, K.N., Moore, T., Sriskantha, A., Spring, K., Tellam, R. *et al.* (1989) Cloning and expression of a protective antigen from the cattle tick *Boophilus microplus*. *Proceedings of the National Academy of Sciences USA* 86, 9657–9661.

Rangel, C.K., Parizi, L.F., Sabadin, G.A., Costa, E.P., Romeiro, N.C. *et al.* (2017) Molecular and structural characterization of novel cystatins from the taiga tick *Ixodes persulcatus*. *Ticks & Tick-Borne Diseases* 8/3, 432–441. DOI: 10.1016/j.ttbdis.2017.01.007.

Riding, G.A., Jarmey, J., McKenna, R.V., Pearson, R., Cobon, G.S. *et al.* (1994) A protective 'concealed' antigen from *Boophilus microplus*. Purification, localization, and possible function. *Journal of Immunology* 153/11, 5158–5166. DOI: 10.4049/jimmunol.153.11.5158.

Robbertse, L., Baron, S., Van der Merwe, N.A., Madder, M., Stoltsz, W.H. *et al.* (2016) Genetic diversity, acaricide resistance status and evolutionary potential of a *Rhipicephalus microplus* population from a disease-controlled cattle farming area in South Africa. *Ticks & Tick-Borne Diseases* 7/4, 595–603. DOI: 10.1016/j.ttbdis.2016.02.018.

Rodríguez, M., Rubiera, R., Penichet, M., Montesinos, R., Cremata, J. *et al.* (1994) High level expression of the *B. microplus* Bm86 antigen in the yeast *Pichia pastoris* forming highly immunogenic particles for cattle. *Journal of Biotechnology* 33, 135–146.

Rodriguez, M., Massard, C.L., da Fonseca, A.H., Ramos, N.F., Machado, H. *et al.* (1995a) Effect of vaccination with a recombinant Bm86 antigen preparation on natural infestations of *Boophilus microplus* in grazing dairy and beef pure and cross-bred cattle in Brazil. *Vaccine* 13/18, 1804–1808. DOI: 10.1016/0264-410X(95)00119-L.

Rodriguez, M., Penichet, M.L., Mouris, A.E., Labarta, V., Luaces, L.L. *et al.* (1995b) Control of *Boophilus microplus* populations in grazing cattle vaccinated with a recombinant Bm86 antigen preparation. *Veterinary Parasitology* 57/4, 339–349. DOI: 10.1016/0304-4017(94)00678-6.

Rodríguez-Hernández, E., Mosqueda, J., Alvarez-Sánchez, M.E., Neri, A.F., Mendoza-Hernández, G. *et al.* (2012) The identification of a VDAC-like protein involved in the interaction of *Babesia bigemina* sexual stages with *Rhipicephalus microplus* midgut cells. *Veterinary Parasitology* 187/3-4, 538–541. DOI: 10.1016/j.vetpar.2012.01.028.

Rodríguez-Hernández, E., Mosqueda, J., León-Ávila, G., Castañeda-Ortiz, E.J., Álvarez-Sánchez, M.E. *et al.* (2015) BmVDAC upregulation in the midgut of *Rhipicephalus microplus*, during infection with *Babesia bigemina*. *Veterinary Parasitology* 212/3-4, 368–374. DOI: 10.1016/j.vetpar.2015.06.016.

Rodríguez-Mallon, A., Fernández, E., Encinosa, P.E., Bello, Y., Méndez-Pérez, L. *et al.* (2012) A novel tick antigen shows high vaccine efficacy against the dog tick, *Rhipicephalus sanguineus*. *Vaccine* 30, 1782–1789. DOI: 10.1016/j.vaccine.2012.01.011.

Rodríguez-Mallon, A., Encinosa, P.E., Méndez-Pérez, L., Bello, Y., Fernández, R.R. *et al.* (2015) High efficacy of a 20 amino acid peptide of the acidic ribosomal protein P0 against the cattle tick, *Rhipicephalus microplus*. *Ticks & Tick-Borne Diseases* 6/4, 530–537. DOI: 10.1016/j.ttbdis.2015.04.007.

Rodríguez-Mallon, A., Anadón, J.L., Pérez, A.A.L., Bechara, G.H., Machado, R.Z. *et al.* (2018) CYTED network to develop an immunogen compatible with integrated management strategies for tick control in cattle. *Vaccine* 36/45, 6581–6586. DOI: 10.1016/j.vaccine.2018.09.064.

Rodríguez-Mallón, A., Encinosa Guzmán, P.E., Bello Soto, Y., Rosales Perdomo, K., Montero Espinosa, C. *et al.* (2020a) A chemical conjugate of the tick P0 peptide is efficacious against *Amblyomma mixtum*. *Transboundary and Emerging Diseases* 67, 175–177. DOI: 10.1111/tbed.13455.

Rodríguez-Mallón, A., Javier González, L., Encinosa Guzmán, P.E., Bechara, G.H., Sanches, G.S. *et al.* (2020b) Functional and mass spectrometric evaluation of an anti-tick antigen based on the p0 peptide conjugated to Bm86 protein. *Pathogens* 9, 513. DOI: 10.3390/pathogens9060513.

Rodriguez-Valle, M.R., Mèndez, L., Valdez, M., Redondo, M., Espinosa, C.M. *et al.* (2004) Integrated control of *Boophilus microplus* ticks in Cuba based on vaccination with the anti-tick vaccine Gavac™. *Experimental & Applied Acarology* 34, 375–382.

Rodríguez-Valle, M., Taoufik, A., Valdés, M., Montero, C., Hassan, I. *et al.* (2012a) Efficacy of *Rhipicephalus* (*Boophilus*) *microplus* Bm86 against *Hyalomma dromedarii* and *Amblyomma cajennense* tick infestations in camels and cattle. *Vaccine* 30, 3453–3458. DOI: 10.1016/j.vaccine.2012.03.020.

Rodriguez-Valle, M., Vance, M., Moolhuijzen, P.M., Tao, X. and Lew-Tabor, A.E. (2012b) Differential recognition by tick-resistant cattle of the recombinantly expressed *Rhipicephalus microplus* serine protease inhibitor-3 (RMS-3). *Ticks & Tick-Borne Diseases* 3/3, 159–169. DOI: 10.1016/j.ttbdis.2012.03.002.

Rodriguez-Valle, M., Moolhuijzen, P., Barrero, R.A., Ong, C.T., Busch, G. *et al.* (2018) Transcriptome and toxin family analysis of the paralysis tick, *Ixodes holocyclus*. *International Journal for Parasitology* 48, 71–82. DOI: 10.1016/j.ijpara.2017.07.007.

Rodriguez-Valle, M., McAlister, S., Moolhuijzen, P.M., Booth, M., Agnew, K. *et al.* (2021) Immunomic investigation of holocyclotoxins to produce the first protective anti-venom vaccine against the Australian paralysis tick, *Ixodes holocyclus*. *Frontiers in Immunology* 12, 744795. DOI: 10.3389/fimmu.2021.744795.

Saimo, M., Odongo, D.O., Mwaura, S., Vlak, J.M., Musoke, A.J. *et al.* (2011) Recombinant *Rhipicephalus appendiculatus* gut (Ra86) and salivary gland cement (Trp64) proteins as candidate antigens for inclusion in tick vaccines: Protective effects of ra86 on infestation with adult *R. appendiculatus*. *Vaccine: Development and Therapy* 1, 15–23. DOI: 10.2147/VDT.S20827.

Sajid, A., Matias, J., Arora, G., Kurokawa, C., DePonte, K. *et al.* (2021) mRNA vaccination induces tick resistance and prevents transmission of the Lyme disease agent. *Science Translational Medicine* 13, eabj9827.

Sales-Junior, P.A., Guzman, F., Vargas, M.I., Sossai, S., González, C.Z.L. *et al.* (2005) Use of biodegradable PLGA microspheres as a slow release delivery system for the *Boophilus microplus* synthetic vaccine SBm7462. *Veterinary Immunology and Immunopathology* 107/3-4, 281–290. DOI: 10.1016/j.vetimm.2005.05.004.

Schetters, T., Bishop, R., Crampton, M., Kopáček, P., Lew-Tabor, A. *et al.* (2016) Cattle tick vaccine researchers join forces in CATVAC. *Parasites and Vectors* 9, 105. DOI: 10.1186/s13071-016-1386-8.

Scorza, F.B. and Pardi, N. (2018) New kids on the block: RNA-based influenza virus vaccines. *Vaccines* 6, 20. DOI: 10.3390/vaccines6020020.

Sethna, P.B., Hung, S.-L. and Brian, D.A. (1989) Coronavirus subgenomic minus-strand RNAs and the potential for mRNA replicons. *Proceedings of the National Academy of Science USA* 86, 5626–5630.

Severo, M.S., Choy, A., Stephens, K.D., Sakhon, O.S., Chen, G. *et al.* (2013) The E3 ubiquitin ligase XIAP restricts *Anaplasma phagocytophilum* colonization of *Ixodes scapularis* ticks. *Journal of Infectious Diseases* 208/11, 1830–1840. DOI: 10.1093/infdis/jit380.

Shrivastava, N., Verma, A. and Dash, P.K. (2020) Identification of functional epitopes of structural proteins and in-silico designing of dual acting multiepitope anti-tick vaccine against emerging Crimean-Congo hemorrhagic fever virus. *European Journal of Pharmaceutical Sciences* 151, 105396. DOI: 10.1016/j.ejps.2020.105396.

Smith, W.D. (1993) Protection in lambs immunised with *Haemonchus contortus* gut membrane proteins. *Research in Veterinary Science* 54/1, 94–101.

Smith, W.D. and Smith, S.K. (1993) Evaluation of aspects of the protection afforded to sheep immunised with a gut membrane protein of *Haemonchus contortus*. *Research in Veterinary Science* 55/1, 1–9.

Smith, W.D., Smith, S.K. and Murray, J.M. (1994) Protection studies with integral membrane fractions of *Haemonchus contortus*. *Parasite Immunology* 16/5, 231–241.

Smith, W.D., Van Wyk, J.A. and Van Strijp, M.F. (2001) Preliminary observations on the potential of gut membrane proteins of *Haemonchus contortus* as candidate vaccine antigens in sheep on naturally infected pasture. *Veterinary Parasitology* 98, 285–297.

Sossai, S., Peconick, A.P., Sales-Junior, P.A., Marcelino, F.C., Vargas, M.I. *et al.* (2005) Polymorphism of the *bm*86 gene in south American strains of the cattle tick *Boophilus microplus*. *Experimental & Applied Acarology* 37, 199–214. DOI: 10.1007/s10493-005-3262-7.

Suarez, M., Rubi, J., Pérez, D., Cordova, V., Salazar, Y. *et al.* (2016) Vaccine in the national program for control of bovine ticks *Rhipicephalus microplus* in Venezuela. *Livestock Science* 187, 48–52. DOI: 10.1016/j.livsci.2016.02.005.

Tabor, A.E. (2021) A review of Australian tick vaccine research. *Vaccines* 9, 1030. DOI: 10.3390/vaccines9091030.

Tabor, A., Rodriguez-Valle, M., McGowan, M., Mayer, D., Fowler, E. *et al.* (2017) Cattle vaccination studies using novel anti-cattle tick antigens developed during Beef CRC research. MLA final report B.AHE.0212. Available at: https://www.mla.com.au/contentassets/bb09c2a7f0554bd19b64e3763c46eafe/b.ahe.0212_final_report.pdf (accessed 10 June 2024).

Tan, A.W.L., Francischetti, I.M., Slovak, M., Kini, R.M. and Ribeiro, J.M. (2015) Sexual differences in the sialomes of the zebra tick, *Rhipicephalus pulchellus*. *Journal of Proteomics* 117, 120–144. DOI: 10.1016/j.jprot.2014.12.014.

Trager, W. (1939) Acquired immunity to ticks. *Journal of Parasitology* 25/1, 57–81.

Trentelman, J.J., Teunissen, H., Kleuskens, J.A., Crommert, J., Fuente, J. *et al.* (2019) A combination of antibodies against Bm86 and Subolesin inhibits engorgement of *Rhipicephalus australis* (formerly *Rhipicephalus microplus*) larvae *in vitro*. *Parasites and Vectors* 12/1, 362. DOI: 10.1186/s13071-019-3616-3.

Trimnell, A.R., Davies, G.M., Lissina, O., Hails, R.S. and Nuttall, P.A. (2005) A cross-reactive tick cement antigen is a candidate broad-spectrum tick vaccine. *Vaccine* 23/34, 4329–4341. DOI: 10.1016/j.vaccine.2005.03.041.

Tsuda, A., Mulenga, A., Sugimoto, C., Nakajima, M., Ohashi, K. *et al.* (2001) cDNA cloning, characterisation and vaccine effect analysis of *Haemaphysalis longicornis* tick saliva proteins. *Vaccine* 19, 4287–4296.

Tuboly, T., Yu, W., Bailey, A., Degrandis, S., Du, S. *et al.* (2000) Immunogenicity of porcine transmissible gastroenteritis virus spike protein expressed in plants. *Vaccine* 18, 2023–2028.

van den Berg, J.H., Oosterhuis, K., Schumacher, T.N.M., Haanen, J.B.A.G. and Bins, A.D. (2014) Intradermal vaccination by DNA tattooing. In: Rinaldi, M., Fioretti, D. and Iurescia, S. (eds) *DNA Vaccines. Methods in Molecular Biology*, Vol. 1143. Humana Press, New York.

Van Zee, J.P., Geraci, N.S., Guerrero, F.D., Wikel, S.K., Stuart, J.J. *et al.* (2007) Tick genomics: The *Ixodes* genome project and beyond. *International Journal for Parasitology* 37, 1297–1305. DOI: 10.1016/j.ijpara.2007.05.011.

van Zyl, W.A., Stutzer, C., Olivier, N.A. and Maritz-Olivier, C. (2015) Comparative microarray analyses of adult female midgut tissues from feeding *Rhipicephalus* species. *Ticks & Tick-Borne Diseases* 6/1, 84–90. DOI: 10.1016/j.ttbdis.2014.09.008.

Villar, M., Pacheco, I., Merino, O., Contreras, M., Mateos-Hernández, L. *et al.* (2020) Tick and host derived compounds detected in the cement complex substance. *Biomolecules* 10/4, 555. DOI: 10.3390/biom10040555.

Waldman, J., Xavier, M.A., Vieira, L.R., Logullo, R., Braz, G.R.C. *et al.* (2022) Neuropeptides in *Rhipicephalus microplus* and other hard ticks. *Ticks & Tick-Borne Diseases* 13/3, 101910. DOI: 10.1016/j.ttbdis.2022.101910.

Wang, D., Xiao, Q., Zhang, W., Wang, X., Xue, X. *et al.* (2020) Landscape of ubiquitination events that occur in host skin in response to tick (*Haemaphysalis longicornis*) bitten [sic]. *Developmental and Comparative Immunology* 104, 103572. DOI: 10.1016/j.dci.2019.103572.

Wang, D., Xu, X., Lv, L., Wu, P., Dong, H. *et al.* (2021) Gene cloning, analysis and effect of a new lipocalin homologue from *Haemaphysalis longicornis* as a protective antigen for an anti-tick vaccine. *Veterinary Parasitology* 290, 109358. DOI: 10.1016/j.vetpar.2021.109358.

Wikel, S.K. (1988) Immunological control of hematophagous arthropod vectors: Utilization of novel antigens. *Veterinary Parasitology* 29, 235–264.

Wikel, S.K. (1999) Tick modulation of host immunity: An important factor in pathogen transmission. *International Journal for Parasitology* 29/6, 851–859. DOI: 10.1016/S0020-7519(99)00042-9.

Willadsen, P. (1987) Immunological approaches to the control of ticks. *International Journal for Parasitology* 17/2, 671–677. DOI: 10.1016/0020-7519(87)90145-7.

Willadsen, P. and Kemp, D.H. (1988) Vaccination with “concealed” antigens for tick control. *Parasitology Today* 4/7, 196–198. DOI: 10.1016/0169-4758(88)90084-1.

Willadsen, P. and McKenna, R.V. (1991) Vaccination with ‘concealed’ antigens: Myth or reality? *Parasite Immunology* 13/6, 605–616. DOI: 10.1111/j.1365-3024.1991.tb00556.x.

Willadsen, P. and Jongejan, F. (1999) Immunology of the tick–host interaction and the control of ticks and tick-borne diseases. *Parasitology Today* 15/7, 258–262. DOI: 10.1016/S0169-4758(99)01472-6.

Willadsen, P., McKenna, R.V. and Riding, G.A. (1988) Isolation from the cattle tick, *Boophilus microplus*, of antigenic material capable of eliciting a protective immunological response in the bovine host. *International Journal for Parasitology* 18/2, 183–189. DOI: 10.1016/0020-7519(88)90059-8.

Willadsen, P., Riding, G.A., McKenna, R.V., Kemp, D.H., Tellam, R.L. *et al.* (1989) Immunologic control of a parasitic arthropod. Identification of a protective antigen from *Boophilus microplus*. *Journal of Immunology* 143/4, 1346–1351. DOI: 10.4049/jimmunol.143.4.1346.

Willadsen, P., Kemp, D.H., Cobon, G.S. and Wright, I.G. (1992) Successful vaccination against *Boophilus microplus* and *Babesia bovis* using recombinant antigens. *Memórias Do Instituto Oswaldo Cruz* 87 Suppl III, 289–294.

Willadsen, P., Eisemann, C.H. and Telham, R.L. (1993a) ‘Concealed’ antigens: Expanding the range of immunological targets. *Parasitology Today* 9/4, 132–135. DOI: 10.1016/0169-4758(93)90177-H.

Willadsen, P., Riding, G.A., Jarmey, J. and Atkins, A. (1993b) The nucleotidase of *Boophilus microplus* and its relationship to enzymes from the rat and *Escherichia coli*. *Insect Biochemistry and Molecular Biology* 23/2, 291–295. DOI: 10.1016/0965-1748(93)90010-P.

Willadsen, P., Smith, D., Cobon, G.S. and McKenna, R.V. (1996) Comparative vaccination of cattle against *Boophilus microplus* with recombinant antigen Bm86 alone or in combination with recombinant Bm91. *Parasite Immunology* 18/5, 241–246. DOI: 10.1046/j.1365-3024.1996.d01-90.x.

Wu, Z. and Liu, K. (2021) Overview of vaccine adjuvants. *Medicine in Drug Discovery* 11, 100103. DOI: 10.1016/j.medidd.2021.100103.

Xiong, K., Zabrocki, J., Nachman, R.J. and Pietrantonio, P.V. (2019) Activity of native tick kinins and peptidomimetics on the cognate target G protein-coupled receptor from the cattle fever tick, *Rhipicephalus microplus* (Acari: Ixodidae). *Pest Management Science* 76/10, 3423–3431. DOI: 10.1002/ps.5704.

Wu, P.X., Cui, X.J., Cao, M.X., Lv, L.H., Dong, H.M. *et al.* (2021) Evaluation on two types of paramyosin vaccines for the control of *Haemaphysalis longicornis* infestations in rabbits. *Parasites and Vectors* 14/1, 309. DOI: 10.1186/s13071-021-04812-4.

Wu-Chuang, A., Obregon, D., Mateos-Hernandez, L. and Cabezas-Cruz, A. (2022) Anti-tick microbiota vaccines: How can this actually work? *Biologia* 77/6, 1555–1562. DOI: 10.1007/s11756-021-00818-6.

Wu-Chuang, A., Mateos-Hernandez, L., Maitre, A., Rego, R.O., Šíma, R. *et al.* (2023) Microbiota perturbation by anti-microbiota vaccine reduces the colonization of *Borrelia afzelii* in *Ixodes ricinus*. *Microbiome* 11/1, 151. DOI: 10.1186/s40168-023-01599-7.

Xu, Z., Yan, Y., Zhang, H., Cao, J., Zhou, Y. *et al.* (2020) A serpin from the tick *Rhipicephalus haemaphysaloides*: Involvement in vitellogenesis. *Veterinary Parasitology* 279, 109064. DOI: 10.1016/j.vetpar.2020.109064.

Yuan, C., Yang, Q., Wu, J., Peng, Y., Li, Y. *et al*. (2022) Proteomics reveals the hemolymph components of partially fed *Hyalomma asiaticum* ticks. *Ticks & Tick-Borne Diseases* 13/6, 102032. DOI: 10.1016/j.ttbdis.2022.102032.

Zheng, W., Hu, H., Jiang, J., Sun, X., Fu, R. *et al*. (2022) *Haemaphysalis longicornis* calreticulin is not an effective molecular tool for tick bite diagnosis and disruption of tick infestations. *Veterinary Parasitology* 309, 109775. DOI: 10.1016/j.vetpar.2022.109775.

Zhou, J., Gong, H., Zhou, Y., Xuan, X. and Fujisaki, K. (2006) Identification of a glycine-rich protein from the tick *Rhipicephalus haemaphysaloides* and evaluation of its vaccine potential against tick feeding. *Parasitology Research* 100/1, 77–84. DOI: 10.1007/s00436-006-0243-7.

Zivkovic, Z., Esteves, E., Almazán, C., Daffre, S., Nijhof, A.M. *et al*. (2010a) Differential expression of genes in salivary glands of male *Rhipicephalus* (*Boophilus*) *microplus* in response to infection with *Anaplasma marginale*. *BMC Genomics* 11, 186. Available at: http://www.biomedcentral.com/1471-2164/11/186 (accessed 4 January 2025).

Zivkovic, Z., Torina, A., Mitra, R., Alongi, A., Scimeca, S. *et al*. (2010b) Subolesin expression in response to pathogen infection in ticks. *BMC Immunology* 11, 7. Available at: http://www.biomedcentral.com/1471-2172/11/7 (accessed 4 January 2025).

6 Barriers to Commercial Success

Abstract
Only one antigen, discovered more than 30 years ago, has thus far been commercialized as a tick vaccine. Many other potential antigens have since been described and tested. The threat posed by ticks to human and animal health has not abated. It seems logical to assume that nor has the need for greater immunological engagement in the management of ticks. The reasons for failure to meet this need are many-fold and are seldom discussed openly. Their roots seem to lie variously in science, economics and human psychology, adding up to an apparently lacklustre market potential.

The notion of immunity to ticks and their toxins is not new, nor is the technology to manufacture vaccines containing recombinant subunit antigens that could offer protection. The fact that immunity to ticks is a more sustainable approach to tick management than reliance on chemical acaricides is self-evident.

Figure 6.1 provides graphic evidence of ongoing interest in the subject in the form of a number of recent scientific publications (de la Fuente and Estrada-Peña, 2019). de la Fuente (2021) lists a catalogue of translational biotechnology developments in the more than 25 years since the first and only vaccines were registered for the control of ticks.

At the time of writing, the absence of more commercial vaccines against ticks than just Gavac® can thus not be ascribed to a knowledge deficit, nor a lack of technological know-how. But the enormity of the combined challenges of reducing tick burdens and tick-borne pathogen infection, multiplication and transmission has led to an underestimation of the potential of vaccines as a safe, effective and sustainable intervention against ticks and tick-borne diseases, and probably contributes to the continued reliance on chemical tick control (de la Fuente *et al.*, 2017; de la Fuente and Estrada-Peña, 2019). Efforts to address the diagnosis, prevention and treatment of tick-borne diseases in animals and humans seems to have overshadowed consideration of vaccines against the vector as an early intervention step in tick-borne disease management.

Possible reasons for the fact that ticks on livestock are not more widely managed by vaccination have been propounded before (de la Fuente *et al.*, 2007; de la Fuente and Estrada-Peña, 2019) and are explored further in this chapter. It is highly likely that immunization on its own will be inadequate for satisfactory tick management, and that there will be the need for integration with other control modalities.

6.1 Market Failure

In simplistic terms, if there is a market need for a good or a service, sooner or later an entrepreneur will offer a solution to satisfy this need. The customer may see sufficient benefit accruing from the good or service to be prepared to pay for it. The entrepreneur will perceive there to be sufficient profitability and will embark upon the enterprise.

Livestock parasites posed a sufficient threat to profitable livestock production at the beginning of the 20th century for a vast global chemical veterinary pharmaceutical industry to develop, albeit mostly as an adjunct to the much larger agricultural chemicals market. Marketing campaigns were largely based on claims that demonstrable productivity, health and welfare gains in treated animals outweighed the direct and ancillary costs of using these products.

DOI: 10.1079/9781800625761.0006

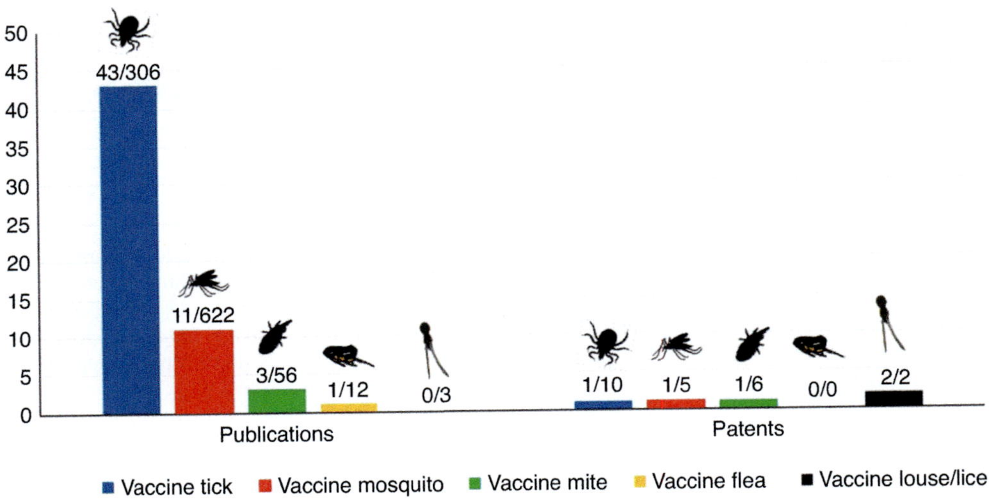

Fig. 6.1. Publications and patents relating to ectoparasite vaccines from 2017 to 29 May 2019. From de la Fuente and Estrada-Peña (2019) under the terms and conditions of the Creative Commons Attribution (CC BY) License.

Tactful reference to 'company restructuring' as an obstacle to the widespread success of Bm86 (de la Fuente *et al.*, 2007) obscures the fact that commercialization of this antigen in vaccine form is unlikely to have happened without substantial initial financial investment from government sources, filling the gap left by commercial lack of interest. There are strong indications that ongoing market failure is a stumbling block to entry of new vaccines to the market (Schröder, 2023).

6.1.1 Market potential

In strictly commercial terms, it is important to distinguish between the concepts of a 'market need' and 'market potential'. As dire as the need for a health management solution might be, this does not translate into market potential unless someone is prepared to pay for the solution. In such instances of market failure, the need might have to be met by charitable donations or by concerted government subvention, which further weakens consumer demand.

A good example of a solution for which a sufficient market potential is unlikely to exist is a vaccine against a tick toxin, despite numerous attempts (Crause *et al.*, 1994; Masina, 1999; Masina and Broady, 1999; Rodriguez-Valle *et al.*, 2021). There is no argument about the gravity of tick intoxication, which invariably has fatal consequences unless treated assertively, but the market potential for a vaccine is doubtful. Three possible market segments for such a vaccine can be envisaged.

The annual number of human cases of tick intoxication, as a percentage of the whole population, is unlikely to warrant the expense of manufacturing even one batch of human vaccine. This is likely to be true even where human exposure to ticks is considered to be common, but the main concern seems to be borreliosis rather than tick toxicity (Hook *et al.*, 2015). Adults who have not yet suffered from tick envenomation either do not venture into bushland often enough for it to be a problem or, if they do, take other anti-tick bite precautions to limit their risk.

The same argument almost certainly holds true for the majority of urbanized companion animals. Veterinary antivenene sales are probably the best indicator of the low percentage of cat and dog tick paralysis cases when measured against the entire population. Cared-for pets are, in addition to a vigorously commercially promoted vaccination regime against various infectious diseases, also mostly subject to stringent prophylactic ectoparasite control with convenient systemic or topical formulations.

Livestock can, and in some areas do, suffer from tick toxicity. For none of the cited examples (see section 1.3.2, this volume) does an antitoxin vaccine offer a commercially attractive solution, either because the risk of intoxication is deemed too low or because cost-effective alternative solutions already exist.

The market seems to be failing in the case of antiparasitic vaccines for livestock, with very few exceptions. This might be attributable to a much smaller potential market volume when compared to chemicals (de la Fuente and Estrada-Peña, 2019). Whereas chemicals have to be applied regularly to remain effective (an incentive for developing formulations with extended durations of efficacy), a vaccine is likely to be applied only a limited number of times in each animal's lifetime. The expected profit margin on a vaccine is probably also much smaller than on a dose of chemical. This might be because vaccines are perceived as inexpensive 'natural' products.

The Caribbean niche market for Gavac® is unique in that the vaccine protects cattle against the most important tick and the diseases it transmits in the region, and the husbandry system allows for regular mustering of cattle for booster vaccinations. The fact that the vaccine production facility is government owned might also protect the product from market turbulence.

6.1.2 The perceived cost of the solution

Synthetic chemicals

Especially in the case of remedies for animals destined for human consumption, generating the requisite data to demonstrate the safety of the chemical, its metabolites and their possible residues to consumers requires considerable investment that has to be weighed against the potential revenue and profit, once the product reaches the market, which seldom occurs in under 7 years and might take longer. Economies of scale have resulted in a diminishing number of chemical manufacturers dominating the world market for parasiticides, and shrinkage in the palette of chemicals available for treating livestock.

The reliance on chemicals by livestock producers is precarious, and unlikely to be sustainable for a variety of reasons. Although the volume of chemicals needed for treating livestock is vast, the quicker path to market and attractive profit margins on small pack sizes for companion animals make this the preferred market segment for most manufacturers. This is evidenced by a history of mergers and acquisitions, often leading to the closing down of the animal health divisions of multinational companies during the decades spanning the turn of the 20th century. See 'company restructuring' (de la Fuente *et al.*, 2007).

Exposing a parasite population to a chemical which leaves behind some survivors invariably leads to selection for resistance against that chemical. Other than possibly the newest of chemical groups, it is difficult to conjure up a synthetic antiparasitic molecule that is not affected by some form of resistance (see section 2.2.1, this volume). Environmental pollution and human exposure resulting from accumulating spillage or excretion of chemicals and/or their metabolites are often cited as cause for concern in support of movements to reduce reliance on these substances. Possibly less obvious as a non-sustainable factor is the fact that most synthetic parasiticides rely for their feedstock on refined crude oil, which has to be regarded as a finite resource.

Vaccines

Few of these arguments against the sustainability of chemical acaricides apply to vaccines. An attractive benefit offered by vaccines over chemicals is a much quicker path to market, without the need for voluminous human, target animal and environmental safety data requiring several years to generate. Intellectual property ownership might be seen as vulnerable (see section 6.2), but the considerable volume of information in the public domain on potential vaccines against ticks could mean that much of the initial product development investigative work (antigen selection and screening, formulation development, route of administration) has already been done and need not be repeated.

Some of the published Australian research has been cofunded by taxpayers and producer organizations, such as the Australian Meat Research Committee (Willadsen, 1976; Willadsen *et al.*, 1978; Agbede and Kemp, 1986; Johnston *et al.*, 1986; Kemp *et al.*, 1986), Beef CRC3 (both now defunct) and Meat and Livestock Australia (Playford, 2005; Tabor, 2011; Meeusen *et al.*, 2013; Lew-Tabor *et al.*, 2014; Lew-Tabor and Rodriguez-Valle, 2016; Tabor *et al.*, 2017; Mahony *et al.*, 2019), one of the current 15 rural research and development corporations (www.ruralrdc.com.au).

6.1.3 Technical obstacles

Global pharmaceutical manufacturers relying on their expertise in synthetic chemistry might find the paradigm shift to the more biological approach of antigen production difficult. Once the appropriate antigen(s) has/have been selected, they must be produced in commercial quantities. Knowledge of the immunological basis for resistance to ticks will contribute to the selection of adjuvants and delivery systems for vaccines that are practically useful (Willadsen, 1987).

Translating laboratory research results into practical parasite biocontrol methods is difficult. In the case of a vaccine against ticks, the rate-limiting step in making scientific progress has been said to be the resource constraint on evaluating laboratory research results appropriately in large animals (Willadsen, 2006) (see section 5.6, this volume).

Vaccine technology has advanced to the point where attenuated or inactivated organisms are no longer seen as desirable vaccine candidates. Recombinant exogenous or endogenous expression of antigenic proteins or precursors, or synthetic antigenic epitopes, are likely to gain preference. Scaling of production could improve efficiency to the point of product profitability. Technological advances may potentially open the way for small, boutique and niche market entrepreneurs.

6.2 Intellectual Property (IP) Vulnerability

Protection of IP in the form of patents on newly discovered molecules has been an important safety net in the chemical industry's continued investment in the search for novel advantage. The period of patent protection of approximately 18 years has to be exploited efficiently for product development and the generation of registration data, followed by a period of profitable marketing to recoup the investment, invest in ongoing research and satisfy the demands of company shareholders. But patents for parasiticides have had a chequered history.

New molecules are invariably based on a newly discovered mode of action, aimed at a physiological process essential for the parasite's survival. The patent description must be very precise to prevent the exploitation of alternative chemical paths to the same objective. The benzimidazoles (BZs) are a good example. They entered the anthelmintic market with the publication of the thiabendazole (TBZ) patent in 1961 and revolutionized internal parasite control in livestock in terms of safety and efficacy. During the ensuing 7–20 years, during which TBZ enjoyed patent protection, a plethora of BZ molecules appeared, some with unwanted side-effects but mostly with improved potency and wider efficacy spectra, e.g. oxibendazole (1968), parbendazole (1968), cambendazole (1969), flubendazole (1971), mebendazole (1971), fenbendazole (1973) and albendazole (1975), as well as the prodrugs oxfendazole (1974), febantel (1975) and netobimin (1982) (Lanusse *et al.*, 1990; O'Neil *et al.*, 2013).

Recognition of IP rights and enforcement of patent protection are not globally consistent. This places a geographic restriction on the market potential of a new discovery and the ongoing threat of so-called 'pirate' products while the patent is valid, and the invariable flood of generic copies once the patent lapses. Regulatory authorities do not demand the same amount of information for generic remedies as is required for the pioneer products. Evidence of bioequivalence of the generic formulation with the pioneer is often all that is needed for the same label claims to be granted.

Protection of the IP of a discovery of a natural phenomenon, for example the nucleotide sequence of a gene encoding a specific protein, is likely to be more precarious than that of an invention (creating something that did not exist before). In the case of a vaccine, IP might lie in the process of producing or expressing the antigen, or in the formulation and adjuvant content, and might be better protected by confidentiality rather than by patent.

Using knowledge about an antigenic epitope to design a synthetic polypeptide or protein construct might be one solution to this problem. A series of investigations of a number of candidates led to a patent being taken out on SBm7462® (Patarroyo *et al.*, 2002, 2009, 2020), aimed at [*B.*] *R. microplus*. Synthetic polypeptide chimeras of combined subolesin and other proteins have also been used as antigens for immunization against ticks (Moreno-Cid *et al.*, 2013; Contreras and de la Fuente, 2016; Contreras *et al.*, 2020; Hassan *et al.*, 2020).

6.3 Unrealistic or Unattainable Expectations

Tick vaccines cannot prevent tick infestation, nor do they result in high tick mortality. They can reduce tick burdens and transmission of tick-borne pathogens by reducing the fecundity of adult ticks through interfering with tick feeding, development and reproduction (Floyd *et al.*, 1995). A consistent vaccination regime can be expected to result in the free-living tick population diminishing to tolerable or insignificant levels over time (Schröder, 2023).

Most of the information on field efficacy of vaccination against tick infestation pertains to cattle, but results have also been published for other livestock, companion animals and wild animals (de la Fuente *et al.*, 2017). Vaccine efficacy can be enhanced by combining immunogenically protective epitopes from different proteins and by appropriate adjuvants and presentation methods (de la Fuente and Estrada-Peña, 2019).

6.3.1 Percentage efficacy

Acaricidal efficacy, expressed as a percentage, is calculated on the composite reduction in numbers of adult female ticks successfully completing a bloodmeal, mass of eggs laid by successful ticks and the hatchability of such eggs. It is the first of these three criteria which is most visibly and dramatically demonstrable for chemicals, with the latter two added in the event that some ticks do engorge and detach. The same criteria have been used for the assessment of vaccines. The degree of protection against tick infestation from immunization with a variety of antigens has been underwhelming thus far, when compared with commercial chemical acaricides (Graf *et al.*, 2004; Playford, 2005; Tabor, 2021).

Switching the mindset from chemical acaricide to immunological tick control requires a number of basic but obvious premises.

- The immune response is not an acaricide. It does not cause an immediate and dramatic drop in parasitic tick numbers, as is usually seen when a novel chemical mode of action is employed before resistance selection has occurred.
- The immune response is not repellent – the tick needs to infest the host in order to be confronted with immunity.
- Depending on where in the tick's physiology, anatomy and life history the target antigen is situated or expressed, the tick's surrender to the immune response might vary in the form and timing of its onset.
- The visible effects of a successful vaccination campaign against ticks are unlikely to become evident other than after a few seasons, allowing the residual free-living tick population to diminish with minimal replenishment from the immunized hosts.
- The requisite paradigm shift to acceptance of these realities will no doubt require substantial commercial promotional effort.

The relatively crude *H. contortus* gut antigen reduced worm burdens by 'up to 72%' (Smith *et al.*, 1994), which did not preclude the Barbervax® vaccine from commercialization. Examples abound of diligent but persistent immunization with imperfect vaccines making significant inroads into disease prevalence (Dhand *et al.*, 2013, 2016; Green *et al.*, 2021), meaning that unrealistic expectations of a tick vaccine ought to be reconsidered.

Several factors can potentially mitigate against a vaccine achieving 90–95% efficacy, a threshold below which a chemical runs the risk of being deemed ineffective (Graf *et al.*, 2004; Holdsworth *et al.*, 2006; Trentelman *et al.*, 2019), or up against tick resistance (Holdsworth *et al.*, 2006). Individual host variations in immune competence, either genetic or due to physiological status, antigenic diversity among tick strains and a natural waning of antibody titre in the absence of a 'boosting' stimulus by a concealed antigen are but three that come to mind.

A tick vaccine will probably provide most benefit when it is used in an integrated control programme that includes other modes of intervention (Mendoza-Martínez *et al.*, 2021).

6.3.2 Efficacy spectrum

Although much of the sequence of the Bm86 gene is conserved in other tick genera and species (see section 5.2.5, this volume), the antigen does not elicit sufficiently effective protection against them. Amino acid and nucleotide sequence variability between *R. microplus* and *R. australis* isolates also limit the wider utility of the vaccine for these species.

Vaccination against just one tick species is not commercially feasible. The ideal would be a vaccine containing antigens of multiple tick species, or both ticks and tick-borne pathogens (Parthasarathi *et al.*, 2021).

Judging by the considerable number of promising conserved antigens and the feasibility of an mRNA cocktail encoding a number of antigenic proteins (see Chapter 5, this volume), the possibility of a single vaccine against ticks on livestock on a global scale no longer seems far-fetched. Should customization of the vaccine be necessary to cater for geographic and host differences or variations, the recombinant technology is by now nimble enough for that not to be an insurmountable problem.

6.3.3 Duration of immunity

Any immune response wanes over time, unless it is boosted. The Achilles heel of a tick vaccine using a concealed antigen is that natural exposure to tick infestation does not serve any boosting purpose – animals need to be revaccinated. Under extensive husbandry conditions, such as prevail in most of northern Australia, the cost of mustering cattle at regular intervals rules out the possibility of handling animals more often than once per year. Although somewhat whimsical, the thought of a rapid titre test as an indicator of the need for revaccination might be a welcome adjunct to a commercial vaccine.

Under these conditions, a commercially successful vaccine will be the one that provides immune protection, if not for the full 12 months between cattle musters then at least for the majority of the active tick season (6–7 months). One can but look wistfully at an oil-based vaccine against botulism in cattle that only needs to be given once in 3 years and wish that this were possible for ticks (Brown *et al.*, 1999; Fordyce and Emery, 2009).

An attractive alternative might be an orally administered booster which could be formulated in, for example, pelleted feed supplement. But mRNA vaccines formulated as replicons might offer a way past this obstacle.

6.4 Sylvatic Hosts

The presence of an unimmunized sympatric or synanthropic population of hosts can sustain a tick population and pose a threat to the success of a livestock vaccination campaign (de la Fuente and Estrada-Peña, 2019). This problem is, however, not unique to vaccines. In some instances, innovation has enabled the application of chemicals to some of the wild host population (Duncan and Monks, 1992; Burridge *et al.*, 2004), while in others, chemical treatment of livestock caused a displacement of ticks to less favourable environments (Norval *et al.*, 1994). Vaccine delivery using viral vectors might offer a solution (de la Fuente and Estrada-Peña, 2019).

References

Agbede, R.I.S. and Kemp, D.H. (1986) Immunization of cattle against *Boophilus microplus* using extracts derived from adult female ticks: Histopathology of ticks feeding on vaccinated cattle. *International Journal for Parasitology* 16/1, 35–41.

Brown, A.T., Gregory, A.R., Ellis, T.M. and Hearnden, M.N. (1999) Comparative immunogenicity of two bivalent botulinum vaccines. *Australian Veterinary Journal* 77/6, 388–391. DOI: 10.1111/j.1751-0813.1999.tb10314.x.

Burridge, M.J., Simmons, L.A., Ahrens, E.H., Naudé, S.A.J. and Malan, F.S. (2004) Development of a novel self-medicating applicator for control of internal and external parasites of wild and domestic animals. *Onderstepoort Journal of Veterinary Research* 71, 41–51.

Contreras, M. and de la Fuente, J. (2016) Control of *Ixodes ricinus* and *Dermacentor reticulatus* tick infestations in rabbits vaccinated with the Q38 Subolesin/Akirin chimera. *Vaccine* 34/27, 3010–3013. DOI: 10.1016/j.vaccine.2016.04.092.

Contreras, M., San José, C., Estrada-Peña, A., Talavera, V., Rayas, E. *et al.* (2020) Control of tick infestations in wild roe deer (*Capreolus capreolus*) vaccinated with the Q38 Subolesin/Akirin chimera. *Vaccine* 38/41, 6450–6454. DOI: 10.1016/j.vaccine.2020.07.062.

Crause, J.C., Wyngaardt, S. and Neitz, A.W.H. (1994) A shared epitope found in the major paralysis inducing tick species of Africa. *Experimental & Applied Acarology* 18, 51–59.

de la Fuente, J. (2021) Translational biotechnology for the control of ticks and tick-borne diseases. *Ticks and Tick-Borne Diseases* 12, 101738. DOI: 10.1016/j.ttbdis.2021.101738.

de la Fuente, J. and Estrada-Peña, A. (2019) Why new vaccines for the control of ectoparasite vectors have not been registered and commercialized? *Vaccines* 7/3, 75. DOI: 10.3390/vaccines7030075.

de la Fuente, J., Almazán, C., Canales, M., Lastra, J.M.P., Kocan, K.M. *et al.* (2007) A ten-year review of commercial vaccine performance for control of tick infestations on cattle. *Animal Health Research Reviews* 8/1, 23–28. DOI: 10.1017/S1466252307001193.

de la Fuente, J., Contreras, M., Estrada-Peña, A. and Cabezas-Cruz, A. (2017) Targeting a global health problem: Vaccine design and challenges for the control of tick-borne diseases. *Vaccine* 35/38, 5089–5094. DOI: 10.1016/j.vaccine.2017.07.097.

Dhand, N.K., Johnson, W.O., Eppleston, J., Whittington, R.J. and Windsor, P.A. (2013) Comparison of pre- and post-vaccination ovine Johne's disease prevalence using a Bayesian approach. *Preventive Veterinary Medicine* 111/1-2, 81–91. DOI: 10.1016/j.prevetmed.2013.03.003.

Dhand, N.K., Eppleston, J., Whittington, R.J. and Windsor, P.A. (2016) Changes in prevalence of ovine paratuberculosis following vaccination with Gudair®: Results of a longitudinal study conducted over a decade. *Vaccine* 34/42, 5107–5113. DOI: 10.1016/j.vaccine.2016.08.064.

Duncan, I.M. and Monks, N. (1992) Tick control on eland (*Taurotragus oryx*) and buffalo (*Syncerus caffer*) with flumethrin 1% pour-on through a Duncan applicator. *Journal of the South African Veterinary Association* 63/1, 7–10.

Floyd, R.B., Sutherst, R.W. and Hungerford, J. (1995) Modelling the field efficacy of a genetically engineered vaccine against the cattle tick, *Boophilus microplus*. *International Journal for Parasitology* 25/3, 285–291. DOI: 10.1016/0020-7519(94)00084-2.

Fordyce, G. and Emery, T. (2009) Investigation of effectiveness of practical vaccination protocols for reproductive wastage in north Australian breeder herds. MLA final report B.NBP.0510. Available at: https://www.mla.com.au/research-and-development/search-rd-reports/?q=b.nbp.0510&sort=1 (accessed 4 August 2024).

Graf, J.F., Gogolewski, R., Leach-Bing, N., Sabatini, G.A., Molento, M.B. *et al.* (2004) Tick control: An industry point of view. *Parasitology* 129, S427–S442. DOI: 10.1017/S0031182004006079.

Green, A.C., Plain, K.M., Eppleston, J., Martinez, E., Emery, D. *et al.* (2021) Continuity in ovine Johne's disease vaccination practices despite a decline in clinical disease. *Australian Veterinary Journal* 99/9, 392–394. DOI: 10.1111/avj.13092.

Hassan, I.A., Wang, Y., Zhou, Y., Cao, J., Zhang, H. *et al.* (2020) Cross protection induced by combined Subolesin-based DNA and protein immunizations against adult *Haemaphysalis longicornis*. *Vaccine* 38/4, 907–915. DOI: 10.1016/j.vaccine.2019.10.076.

Holdsworth, P.A., Kemp, D., Green, P., Peter, R.J., de Bruin, C. *et al.* (2006) World Association for the Advancement of Veterinary Parasitology (W.A.A.V.P.) guidelines for evaluating the efficacy of acaricides against ticks (Ixodidae) on ruminants. *Veterinary Parasitology* 136/1, 29–43. DOI: 10.1016/j.vetpar.2005.11.011.

Hook, S.A., Nelson, C.A. and Mead, P.S. (2015) U.S. public's experience with ticks and tick-borne diseases: Results from national HealthStyles surveys. *Ticks & Tick-Borne Diseases* 6, 483–488. DOI: 10.1016/j.ttbdis.2015.03.017.

Johnston, L.A.Y., Kemp, D.H. and Pearson, R.D. (1986) Immunization of cattle against *Boophilus microplus* using extracts derived from adult female ticks: Effects of induced immunity on tick populations. *International Journal for Parasitology* 16/1, 27–34.

Kemp, D.H., Agbede, R.I.S., Johnston, L.A.Y. and Gough, J.M. (1986) Immunization of cattle against *Boophilus microplus* using extracts derived from adult female ticks: Feeding and survival of the parasite on vaccinated cattle. *International Journal for Parasitology* 16/2, 115–120.

Lanusse, C.E., Ranjan, S. and Prichard, R.K. (1990) Comparison of pharmacokinetic variables for two injectable formulations of netobimin administered to calves. *American Journal of Veterinary Research* 51/9, 1459–1463.

Lew-Tabor, A.E. and Rodriguez-Valle, M. (2016) A review of reverse vaccinology approaches for the development of vaccines against ticks and tick-borne diseases. *Ticks and Tick-Borne Diseases* 7, 573–585. DOI: 10.1016/j.ttbdis.2015.12.012.

Lew-Tabor, A.E., Bruyeres, A.G., Zhang, B. and Rodriguez-Valle, M. (2014) *Rhipicephalus (Boophilus) microplus* tick in vitro feeding methods for functional (dsRNA) and vaccine candidate (antibody) screening. *Ticks & Tick-Borne Diseases* 5/5, 500–510. DOI: 10.1016/j.ttbdis.2014.03.005.

Mahony, T.J., Kobaisi, M.A. and Mainwaring, D.E. (2019) Testing and verification of a single-dose cattletick vaccine. MLA final report B.AHE.0316. Available at: https://www.mla.com.au/research-and-development/search-rd-reports/?q=b.ahe.0316&sort=1 (accessed 25 April 2024).

Masina, S. (1999) The sequence, expression and immunological characterisation of the HT-1 neurotoxin from the Australian paralysis tick *Ixodes holocyclus*. PhD thesis, University of Technology, Sydney, Australia.

Masina, S. and Broady, K.W. (1999) Tick paralysis: Development of a vaccine. *International Journal for Parasitology* 29, 535–541.

Meeusen, E.N., de Veer, M., Hertzog, P.J., Stear, M.J., Mallard, B.A. *et al.* (2013) New approaches to innate immunity in livestock and the potential formanipulation – review. MLA final report B.BSC.0321. Available at: https://www.mla.com.au/research-and-development/search-rd-reports/?q=b.bsc.0321&sort=1 (accessed 15 October 2023).

Mendoza-Martínez, N., Alonso-Diaz, M.A., Merino, O., Fernandez-Salas, A. and Lagunes-Quintanilla, R. (2021) Protective efficacy of the peptide Subolesin antigen against the cattle tick *Rhipicephalus microplus* under natural infestation. *Veterinary Parasitology* 299, 109577. DOI: 10.1016/j.vetpar.2021.109577.

Moreno-Cid, J.A., Pérez de la Lastra, J.M., Villar, M., Jiménez, M., Pinal, R. *et al.* (2013) Control of multiple arthropod vector infestations with subolesin/akirin vaccines. *Vaccine* 31/8, 1187–1196. DOI: 10.1016/j.vaccine.2012.12.073.

Norval, R.A.I., Perry, B.D., Meltzer, M.I., Kruska, R.L. and Booth, T.H. (1994) Factors affecting the distributions of the ticks *Amblyomma hebraeum* and *A. variegatum* in Zimbabwe: Implications of reduced acaricide usage. *Experimental & Applied Acarology* 18, 383–407.

O'Neil, M.J., Heckelman, P.E., Dobbelaar, P.H. and Roman, K.J. (eds) (2013) *The Merck Index*, 15th edn. Royal Society of Chemistry, Cambridge.

Parthasarathi, B.C., Kumar, B. and Ghosh, S. (2021) Current status and future prospects of multi-antigen tick vaccine. *Journal of Vector-Borne Diseases* 58, 183–192.

Patarroyo, J.H., Portela, R.W., Castro, R.O., Pimentel, J.C., Guzman, F. *et al.* (2002) Immunization of cattle with synthetic peptides derived from the *Boophilus microplus* gut protein (Bm86). *Veterinary Immunology and Immunopathology* 88, 163–172.

Patarroyo, J.H., Vargas, M.I., González, C.Z., Guzmán, F., Martins-Filho, O.A. *et al.* (2009) Immune response of bovines stimulated by synthetic vaccine SBm7462 against *Rhipicephalus (Boophilus) microplus*. *Veterinary Parasitology* 166/3-4, 333–339. DOI: 10.1016/j.vetpar.2009.09.036.

Patarroyo, J.H., Sousa Neves, E., Fidelis, C.F., Tafur-Gómez, G.A., Araujo, L. *et al.* (2020) Bovine immunisation with a recombinant peptide derived from synthetic SBm7462(R) (Bm86 epitope construct) immunogen for *Rhipicephalus microplus* control. *Ticks & Tick-Borne Diseases* 11/5, 101461. DOI: 10.1016/j.ttbdis.2020.101461.

Playford, M. (2005) Review of research needs for cattle tick control. MLA final report AHW.054A. Available at: https://www.mla.com.au/research-and-development/search-rd-reports/?q=ahw.054a&sort=1 (accessed 25 April 2024).

Rodriguez-Valle, M., McAlister, S., Moolhuijzen, P.M., Booth, M., Agnew, K. *et al.* (2021) Immunomic investigation of holocyclotoxins to produce the first protective anti-venom vaccine against the australian paralysis tick, *Ixodes holocyclus*. *Frontiers in Immunology* 12, 744795. DOI: 10.3389/fimmu.2021.744795.

Schröder, J. (2023) Continuing the search for a tick vaccine. In: *Proceedings of the Northern Beef Research Update Conference*, North Australia Beef Research Council, Darwin, Australia, August 22–25, 2023, pp. 90–94.

Smith, W.D., Smith, S.K. and Murray, J.M. (1994) Protection studies with integral membrane fractions of *Haemonchus contortus*. *Parasite Immunology* 16/5, 231–241.

Tabor, A. (2011) Selection of novel tick antigens using vaccination-challenge studies in cattle. MLA Final Report B.AHE.0024. Available at: https://www.mla.com.au/research-and-development/search-rd-reports/?q=%22b.ahe.0024%22&sort=1 (accessed 25 April 2024).

Tabor, A.E. (2021) A review of Australian tick vaccine research. *Vaccines* 9, 1030. DOI: 10.3390/vaccines9091030.

Tabor, A., Rodriguez-Valle, M., McGowan, M., Mayer, D., Fowler, E. *et al.* (2017) Cattle vaccination studies using novel anti-cattle tick antigens developed during Beef CRC research. MLA Final Report B.AHE.0212. Available at: https://www.mla.com.au/research-and-development/search-rd-reports/?q=b.ahe.0212&sort=1 (accessed 25 April 2024).

Trentelman, J.J., Teunissen, H., Kleuskens, J.A., Crommert, J., Fuente, J. *et al.* (2019) A combination of antibodies against Bm86 and Subolesin inhibits engorgement of *Rhipicephalus australis* (formerly *Rhipicephalus microplus*) larvae *in vitro*. *Parasites and Vectors* 12/1, 362. DOI: 10.1186/s13071-019-3616-3.

Willadsen, P. (1976) Allergenic activity of an esterase from *Boophilus microplus*. *FEBS Letters* 72/2, 346–349.

Willadsen, P. (1987) Immunological approaches to the control of ticks. *International Journal for Parasitology* 17/2, 671–677. DOI: 10.1016/0020-7519(87)90145-7.

Willadsen, P. (2006) Tick control: Thoughts on a research agenda. *Veterinary Parasitology* 138/1-2, 161–168. DOI: 10.1016/j.vetpar.2006.01.050.

Willadsen, P., Williams, P.G., Roberts, J.A. and Kerr, J.D. (1978) Responses of cattle to allergens from *Boophilus microplus*. *International Journal for Parasitology* 8, 89–95.

7 Discussion and Conclusions

The direct and indirect impacts of tick infestation on successful livestock production are impossible to measure and difficult to estimate. Ticks are adaptable and can survive under diverse environmental and meteorological conditions. They are obligate parasites, requiring more than one bloodmeal, on a diverse range of vertebrate hosts, to complete their life cycles. In the course of their feeding, they cause harm and can transmit disease, often with fatal consequences for animals and humans. Tick saliva contains a range of chemicals with harmful effects either locally at the bite wound and/or systemically in the form of allergies and toxicoses, of which paralysis is most prevalent (see Chapter 1, this volume). In balanced ecosystems, hosts and ticks coexist, and ticks can be regarded as one of the fitness selection factors in a healthy host population. But increasing human food demand leads to greater host stocking densities, invariably disturbing this equilibrium, making the impost of tick infestation on profitable livestock production intolerable and prompting anthropogenic intervention.

A number of obstacles potentially limit the success of tick infestation of a suitable host. Free-living ticks are subject to predation, acaripathogenic fungi, nematodes and parasitoid wasps and harsh environmental conditions such as bushfires, sunlight exposure and starvation. The role of viruses pathogenic to ticks and their potential exploitation for biological control need further investigation. Parasitic ticks can be reduced in number by host grooming and insectivorous birds.

There are numerous anthropogenic impacts on their survival, of which the application of chemical acaricides has had the biggest effect (see Chapter 2, this volume). None of the non-chemical factors that might sustainably be useful for keeping tick populations to acceptable levels have thus far lent themselves to commercial application or universal adoption. Reliance on chemicals, regardless of their origin, the mainstay of managing the threat posed by ticks to human and animal health for more than a century, is not sustainable for various reasons. Tick resistance to most acaricidal chemicals has proven to be the inevitable consequence of every discovery of a novel mode of action. Vastly improved potency of modern chemicals has allowed the use of smaller quantities but the environmental impact of chemical pesticides on beneficial arthropod populations is cause for increasing alarm. The threat to human health of chemical residues in food is the reason for increased regulatory scrutiny and greater demand for safety data. The fact that fossil fuel constitutes the feed stock for most of the chemical industry is probably the least considered aspect of general unease about continued exploitation of this dwindling resource.

Parasitic ticks also have to overcome a staged host defence, commencing with innate resistance and host behaviour. Tick infestation, even of a naïve host, sets in train a cascade of chain reactions in what is initially an allergic type of inflammatory response. Ticks have evolved in dealing with these defence mechanisms with anticoagulant, anti-inflammatory and immunomodulatory components in their saliva, rendering innate resistance and immunity only partially effective, even in fit hosts. The Zebu breeds of cattle are innately more resistant to ticks than European breeds, as evidenced by the fewer ticks they carry when exposed to the same infestation challenge. Especially in extensive enterprises, where regular cattle mustering for acaricidal treatment is prohibitively expensive, reliance on the genotypic innate resistance is the mainstay of tick management (see Chapter 3, this volume). But beef from Zebu cattle is

DOI: 10.1079/9781800625761.0007

perceived by fastidious consumers to be of a lower eating quality than that from European breeds. This market signal therefore militates against continued reliance on this heritable tick defence.

Repeated tick infestations stimulate the host's immune system to mount cellular and humoral immune responses to thwart the tick's successful completion of a bloodmeal. Antibodies to a variety of tick antigens have been demonstrated in immune hosts. The visible outcome of this adaptive immunity in response to natural infestation is the smaller numbers of ticks carried when compared with the tick burdens on naïve hosts and, on closer inspection, the smaller size of replete female ticks and their reduced fertility and fecundity. But ticks have also evolved modulatory mechanisms for adaptive immunity, so this protection is not absolute, does not prevent transmission of tick-borne disease and is insufficient to satisfy commercial livestock production demands (see Chapter 4, this volume). Hyperimmune serum can be used for treating cases of tick paralysis, with due consideration of the attendant risks.

The use of tick antigens not encountered by the host's immune system in the usual course of tick infestation, so-called 'hidden' or 'concealed' antigens, has thus far proven to be the most effective method for eliciting a protective immune response. It avoids the evolutionary evasive mechanisms that ticks have acquired to deal with the host's adaptive immunity. It also avoids the redundancy in tick salivary proteins, both in function and in life-stage synchrony. The Bm86 gut antigen, isolated from [*B. microplus*] *R. australis* late in the 20th century was the first, and is thus far the only, such antigen to be successfully commercialized. Genomic diversity in the Bm86 gene between different isolates of *R. microplus* and *R. australis*, and proteomic diversity in the amino acid sequences of the antigens encoded by these genes, coupled with the relatively narrow spectrum of anti-tick efficacy, limits the geographic application of Bm86-containing vaccine beyond the Caribbean countries, where it has successfully reduced reliance on chemical acaricides by ca. 70%.

Numerous alternative concealed antigens have since been discovered and tested (see Chapter 5, this volume). This promises the possibility of a vaccine containing a combination of antigens, some of them sufficiently conserved to allow an efficacy spectrum wide enough to have global commercial appeal for use in cattle, and possibly sheep and goats. Technological developments offer the ability for expression of these recombinant proteins in commercial quantities. Formulating these vaccines to enable sustained release of the antigen such that only one administration is required for season-long protection would vastly improve their market suitability.

The market share of vaccines in animal health management is smaller by several degrees of magnitude than that of chemicals such as antimicrobials, anthelmintics, acaricides and insecticides (see Chapter 6, this volume). Vaccines are used in smaller volumes, partly because they need to be administered less frequently. The degree of efficacy expected from successful chemical acaricides has not yet been attained by immunization with any tick antigen. This perceived 'poor efficacy' will remain one of the barriers to adoption of vaccines against ticks until producer expectations can be scaled back to realistic levels, and until the benefits of a more sustainable approach are recognized and accepted. The most benefit from a tick vaccine will probably be derived when it is used in a multimodal integrated management programme.

The antigens in vaccines are mostly discoveries of naturally occurring phenomena, rather than inventions, which makes Intellectual Property protection in the form of patents problematic. The invention of a novel chemical molecule is invariably patentable, which allows roughly 18 years' 'protection' from direct commercial competition, during which the patent holder can reap profits to recoup prior investments in product development and invest in the search for new inventions. In vaccine production, keeping innovative production methods secret is one competitive advantage on which an entrepreneur can rely. But protectable Intellectual Property is likely also to lie in the composition of synthetic antigens designed *in silico* and expressed by modern molecular techniques.

Index

Note:- Page numbers in **bold** type refer to **figures.** Page numbers in *italic* type refer to *tables.*

Printed and bound by CPI Group (UK) Ltd, Croydon, CR0 4YY

13/09/2026

14961113-0008